LIMITED RADIOGRAPHY

THIRD EDITION

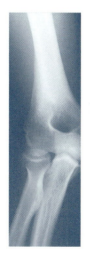
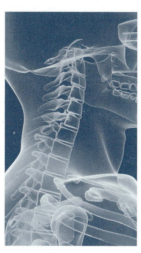
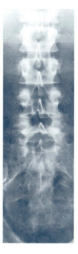

Frances E. Campeau, MA, RT(R)(M), FAEIRS

*Professor Emerita of the former University of Louisville,
Radiologic Technology Program*

Jeana Fleitz, MEd., RT(R)(M)

*Program Administrator and Consultant to the Kentucky
Department of Education*

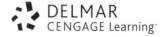

DELMAR
CENGAGE Learning

Australia • Brazil • Japan • Korea • Mexico • Singapore • Spain • United Kingdom • United States

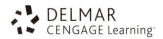

Limited Radiography, Third Edition
Frances E. Campeau, Jeana Fleitz

Vice President, Career and Professional Editorial: Dave Garza

Director of Learning Solutions: Matthew Kane

Senior Acquisitions Editor: Sherry Dickinson

Managing Editor: Marah Bellegarde

Product Manager: Natalie Pashoukos

Editorial Assistant: Anthony Souza

Vice President, Career and Professional Marketing: Jennifer Ann Baker

Marketing Director: Wendy Mapstone

Senior Marketing Manager: Michelle McTighe

Marketing Coordinator: Erica Ropitzky

Production Director: Carolyn Miller

Production Manager: Andrew Crouth

Senior Content Project Manager: James Zayicek

Senior Art Director: David Arsenault

For product information and technology assistance, contact us at
Professional & Career Group Customer Support, 1-800-648-7450

For permission to use material from this text or product, submit all requests online at **cengage.com/permissions**
Further permissions questions can be e-mailed to
permissionrequest@cengage.com

Library of Congress Control Number: 2009927658

ISBN-13: 978-1-435-48112-1

ISBN-10: 1-435-48112-7

Delmar
5 Maxwell Drive
Clifton Park, NY 12065–2919
USA

Cengage Learning products are represented in Canada by Nelson Education, Ltd.

For your lifelong learning solutions, visit **delmar.cengage.com**

Visit our corporate website at **cengage.com**

Printed in the United States of America
3 4 5 6 7 17 16 15 14 13

DEDICATION

To my wonderful mother and father, Faye and Dewey, whose loving care and sustained support always gave me the courage and the drive to meet my goals. Also, to my loving sister, Helen and Ann, and to my brother David.

Frances E. Campeau

To my family and loved ones: my husband Don Moore, Deanna Hansen, Jennifer Love, and to the "little ones," Piper and Teague, for allowing me time to pursue my dreams.

Jeana Fleitz

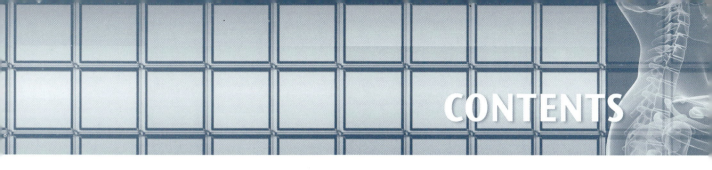

CONTENTS

INDEX OF TABLES

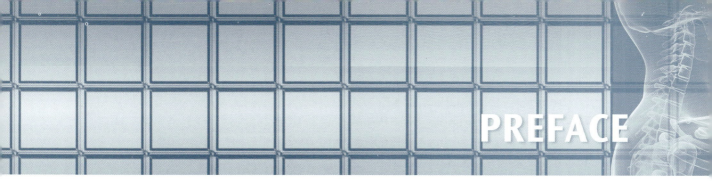

The goal of this third edition is twofold: (1) to meet the needs of the radiographer in limited practice, including upgrading the performance standards in these areas of practice, and (2) to provide students with a fundamental imaging foundation so that they are competent clinical practitioners capable of producing diagnostic images while subjecting patient and health care personnel to minimum radiation exposure. The terms *radiography, radiographic, imaging*, and *images* are used interchangeably in keeping with past, current, and rapidly evolving medical imaging technology. This is necessary in order to meet the needs of limited radiography operators who work in different environments, that is, offices and clinics in urban and rural areas.

The authors recognize that currently the scope of practice, educational requirements, and licensure requirements for limited radiography practice vary from state to state with no overarching federal regulations. Therefore, practitioners will need to become acquainted with their respective state requirements.

This book is not meant to be a comprehensive text on the radiologic sciences. It is, more importantly, written to present basic concepts with the intent that students will be able to apply the information appropriately in clinical applications.

Features

The updated book has sixteen chapters. Each chapter includes the following:

- Outline
- Objectives
- Key terms
- Review questions

New to the Third Edition

We have written four new chapters: Chapter 8, Basic Positioning and Patients with Special Needs; Chapter 10, Digital Radiography and PACS; Chapter 11, Radiographic Pathology; and Chapter 14, Imaging Specialties. The remaining twelve chapters have been revised with updates but retain their basic concepts. Some chapter numbers have changed in order to build a logical sequence of content. However, instruction of content may be utilized according to program curriculum design.

It is necessary to mention that Chapter 8 is intended to address basic concepts of positioning and body structure relative to producing images of patients with special needs (i.e., pediatrics and geriatrics in this text). There are several excellent positioning and anatomy books; thus, this book focuses on imaging concepts, radiation protection, and evolving technologies as they relate to limited radiography. The chapter on radiographic pathology is included in the book as an enhancement to the scope of knowledge for limited radiography. The chapters on digital radiography and PACS and imaging specialties are clearly needed at any level of program study; thus, they are included in this revised edition.

Instructor's Resources

Other changes are reflected in the Instructors Manual. All of the tasks in the previous editions of the textbook have been moved to the Instructors Manual. This will give the instructor a more flexible use of the tasks. Also, answers for chapter reviews, along with competency checklists for procedural tasks listed in the appendices, are now included in the Instructors Manual. New to the Instructors Manual are the identification of critical thinking skills needed for student development and tips for instructors to assist in student application of radiographic procedures.

Acknowledgements

The authors believe that the role of the limited radiographer continues to progress with the rapid growth in imaging technology. As the first to support the limited radiographer with a textbook, our commitment is stronger today by providing an updated edition to meet the current state of the occupation. We have made every effort to utilize many resources and content experts to update and expand this third edition of *Limited Radiography*.

We are again indebted to Ms. Nancy C. Roubieu for her input to the manuscript and editing of some chapters. Also, to Dr. Don Pack for his contribution in current technology. We are grateful to the book reviewers who are always very helpful in evaluating the content. Because no one operates in a vacuum, we appreciate everyone who has been willing to look at this revised edition in any way.

Frances E. Campeau, *MA, RT(R)(M), FAEIRS*
Jeana Fleitz, *MEd, RT(R)(M)*

Reviewers

James J. Byrne, MEd, RT(R)
Radiography Program Coordinator
Columbus State Community College
Columbus, Ohio

Donna Collentine, RT(R), MA
Radiography Program Director
Cape Fear Community College
Wilmington, NC

Dr. Pawen Dhokal, DC
Owner, ELITE Health Clinics
Owner, EXCEL Clinics (Excellence in Clinical Education & Learning)
Co-Founder of Image Radiology Seminars
Dean of Medical Specialties and Health Care Administration Program, CCSD
Radiology Instructor
California College, San Diego
San Diego, CA

Shanna Gallaher
PTR Instructor/Program Manager
The Bryman School of Phoenix
Phoenix, AZ

Eva Oltman, MEd, CPC, CMA, LMR, EMT
Divison Chair of Allied Health
Jefferson Community and Technical College
Louisville, KY

Michele R. Wells, BS, RT(R)(M), RDMS
Radiography Program Director
York Technical College
Rock Hill, SC

Lisa Wood, MS, RT
Professor
Salt Lake Community College
Salt Lake City, UT

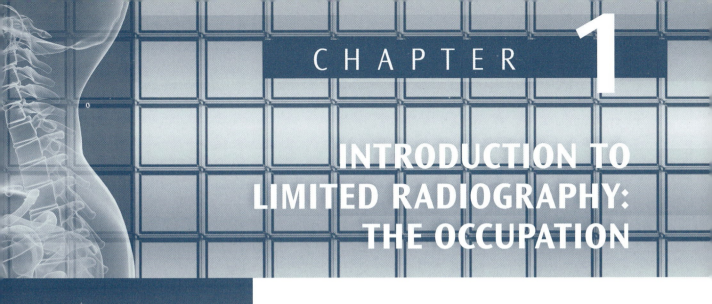

CHAPTER 1

INTRODUCTION TO LIMITED RADIOGRAPHY: THE OCCUPATION

Key Terms

American Registry of Radiologic Technologists (ARRT)

American Society of Radiologic Technologists (ASRT)

Bone Densitometry Equipment Operators

Certification

Consumer-Assurance of Radiologic Excellence (RadCARE) Bill

Consumer-Patient Radiation Health and Safety Act

Continuing Education

Joint Review Committee on Education in Radiologic Technology (JRCERT)

Limited Radiographer

Limited Scope of Practice in Radiography

Limited X-ray Machine Operator Standards (ASRT)

Radiologic Technologist

Registration

Chapter Outline

Introduction
History, Purpose, and Functions
Philosophy Statement
Occupational Scope of Practice
General Requirements
Scope of Practice
Education
Continuing Education and Professional Organizations
Occupational Progress and Professionalization
The Future

Objectives

Upon completion of the chapter, the student will meet the following objectives by verifying knowledge of the facts and principles presented through oral and written communication at a level deemed competent.

○ Select the correct definition of the chapter key terms.
○ Differentiate between the role and function of the American Society of Radiologic Technologists (ASRT), Joint Review Committee on Education in Radiologic Technology (JRCERT), and the American Society of Radiologic Technologists (ASRT).

1

⊃ Recall the five primary and twelve post-primary certification examinations offered by the ARRT.

⊃ Recall the ASRT definition of a radiologic technologist and a limited x-ray machine operator.

⊃ Discuss the differences between basic noncontrast x-ray examinations and those requiring the use of contrast media.

⊃ Research and list potential employment opportunities (in your community/ state) for limited radiographers.

⊃ Identify where to obtain information about particular states' limited radiography certification.

⊃ Describe the impact of the Consumer-Patient Radiation Health and Safety Act on the development of the limited radiography occupation.

⊃ Research and summarize in a paragraph, the status of the CARE bill.

⊃ Write a paragraph about the intent of continuing education (CE) after attaining initial certification in limited radiography. (Include a particular states' CE requirements for renewal of the initial certification or license.)

Introduction

Does the term limited radiography designate a new occupation emerging within the radiological sciences, or does it designate a skill level within the radiological sciences consisting of limited radiography tasks performed by a myriad of workers in medical offices, clinics, and ambulatory care centers?

Why are individuals who operate radiation-producing equipment coming under state and federal guidelines and regulations that address the establishment of minimum educational standards, competency testing, and continuing education? Who are limited radiographers, how are they educated, and where are they employed? Do limited radiographers and radiologic technologists share a common professional role but differ in their level of responsibility and scope of practice? These are just a few of the many questions being asked today about limited radiography and individuals called limited radiographers. This chapter will focus on the essential characteristics of limited radiography as an occupation.

In 2007, the American Society of Radiologic Technologists (ASRT) published standards for limited x-ray machine operators. "The practice standards define the practice and establish general criteria to determine compliance. Practice standards are authoritative statements established by the radiologic technology profession for judging the quality of practice, service, and education" (American Society of Radiologic Technologists, 2007).

The practice of radiography constantly changes as a result of a number of factors including technological advances, market and economic forces, and statutory and regulatory mandates. "While a minimum standard of acceptable performance is appropriate and should be followed by all limited x-ray machine operators, it is appropriate to assume that the practice is the same in all regions of the United States. Community custom, state statute, or regulation may dictate practice parameters. Wherever there is a conflict between these standards and state or local statutes and regulations, the state or local statutes and regulations supersede these standards" (ASRT, 2007).

"The standards are divided into five sections: scope of practice, clinical performance, quality performance, professional performance, and advisory opinion" (ASRT, 2007). A complete copy of *The Practice Standards for Medical Imaging and Radiation Therapy Limited X-ray Machine Operator Standards* is included in the appendix.

The following statement is from *The Limited X-ray Machine Operator Standards* and helps to distinguish the occupation within the radiological sciences.

> The operation of x-ray equipment in a limited scope is performed by a segment of health care employees responsible for the administration of ionizing radiation to humans and animals for diagnostic, therapeutic, or research purposes. A limited x-ray machine operator performs radiographic procedures and related techniques within the scope of practice, producing images for the interpretation by a licensed independent practitioner. A limited x-ray machine operator acquires additional images at the request of a licensed independent practitioner or radiologic technologist.
>
> An interdisciplinary team of radiologists, radiologic technologists, and support staff plays a critical role in the delivery of health services: the limited x-ray machine operator plays a supporting role through the performance of radiographic examinations within the scope of practice.

General requirements, education, and certification included in the practice standards will be discussed later in this chapter.

History, Purpose, and Functions

In November 1895, Wilhelm Conrad Roentgen announced his discovery of a new kind of radiant energy. Investigating conduction of electrons through a partially evacuated glass tube, he found that a plate coated with a fluorescent material emitted light when struck by rays from the glass tube. Using the nomenclature for the algebraic unknown ("X"), Roentgen called the mysterious new light "X ray." In the early years, Roentgen and others used X rays to diagnose bone fractures, examine internal organs, and locate foreign objects in tissues.

In the late 1800s and early 1900s, as medical applications of x-rays expanded, there was a need for people to operate x-ray equipment. In one historical account of the radiography profession on its 100th year (1995) of existence, the authors refer to those early radiographers as "the shadow-makers" (ASRT, 1995).

As the number of those early "shadow-makers" increased, a sense of community among scientists, doctors, photographers, and workers was formed. From humble beginnings, three major organizations exist today that have a major influence on the radiography profession: these being the American Registry of Radiologic Technologists (ARRT), the Joint Review Committee on Education in Radiologic Technology (JRCERT), and the American Society of Radiologic Technologists (ASRT).

The ARRT is the largest certifying body in the radiological profession with more than 275,000 registered technologists as of April 2008 (American Registry of Radiologic Technologists, 2008a). The ARRT's mission is to promote high standards of patient care by recognizing qualified individuals in medical imaging, interventional procedures, and radiation therapy (ARRT, 2008a). The ARRT's primary role is to test and certify technologists and administer continuing education (CE) and ethics requirements for their annual registration (Kollmer, 2005).

The Joint Review Committee on Education in Radiologic Technology (JRCERT) is the profession's largest programmatic accrediting agency. The JRCERT reviews a program's admissions policy, curriculum, academic practices, and faculty qualifications. The intent of such reviews is to ensure that minimum educational standards are met and that students are appropriately qualified to practice (Kollmer, 2005; Joint Review Committee on Education in Radiologic Technology, 2008).

The American Society of Radiologic Technologists (ASRT) is the world's largest and oldest membership association for medical imaging technologists and radiation therapists (ASRT, 2009). The ASRT provides members with educational opportunities, promotes radiologic technology as a career, and monitors state and federal legislation that affects the profession (ASRT, 2009). The ASRT is also responsible for establishing standards of practice for the radiological science profession and developing educational curriculum (ASRT, 2009).

Today, because of scientific advancements in equipment design, medical imaging, a branch of medical science that uses radiant energies, has a far wider scope of application. As such, skilled professionals are needed to assist in these imaging procedures, and the ARRT offers certification in five primary pathways

---

Certifications Offered

Primary Pathways and Certifications

- Radiography
- Nuclear Medicine Technology
- Radiation Therapy
- Sonography
- Magnetic Resonance Imaging

Post-Primary Pathways and Certifications

- Mammography
- Computed Tomography
- Magnetic Resonance Imaging (Note: Both a primary and post-primary track)
- Quality Management
- Bone Densitometry
- Cardiac-Interventional Radiography
- Vascular-Interventional Radiography
- Cardiovascular-Interventional Radiography (Note: No longer available for new candidates)
- Sonography (Note: Both a primary and post-primary track)
- Vascular Sonography
- Breast Sonography

FIGURE 1-1 Overview of the ARRT primary and post-primary pathways and certifications

Adapted from information listed on the ARRT website available at http://www.arrt.org.
Accessed November 12, 2008.

and twelve post-primary certifications (ARRT, 2008c). Figure 1-1 is an overview of these areas of practice and Figure 1-2 provides information about the supporting primary categories for post-primary tracks. (ARRT, 2008c; ARRT, 2008h). The ARRT website (www.arrt.org) provides extensive information about eligibility requirements and content specifications for each primary and post-primary examination.

Although diversity and specialization exist within the radiological sciences, a core of knowledge and skills is common to all radiographers. Beyond this basic core, there are distinct differences between the scope of practice of a limited radiographer and a radiologic technologist. The differences (educational and scope of practice) between a radiologic technologist and a limited radiographer are readily apparent in the following description.

In 2003, the American Society of Radiologic Technologists (ASRT) Commission on Education offered resolution 03-2.02B, which provides definitions to distinguish important differences between the professional and educational qualifications of personnel in diagnostic medical imaging (McElveny & Olmstead,

FIGURE 1-2 ARRT primary pathways supporting categories for post-primary tracks and certifications

	Radiography is a supporting category for	Nuclear Medicine Technology* is a supporting category for	Radiation Therapy is a supporting category for	Sonography** is a supporting category for	Magnetic Resonance Imaging is not a supporting category for other certifications
Mammography	x				
Computed Tomography	x	x	x		
Magnetic Resonance Imaging	x	x	x	x	
Quality Management	x	x	x		
Bone Densitometry	x	x	x		
Cardiac-Interventional Radiography	x				
Vascular-Interventional Radiography	x				
Sonography	x	x	x	x	
Vascular Sonography	x	x	x	x	
Breast Sonography***				x	
Radiologist Assistant	x				

*Supporting category of NMT may be through ARRT or NMTCB
**Supporting category of Sonography may be through ARRT or ARDMS
***Mammography also serves as a supporting category for Breast Sonography
Adapted from information listed on the ARRT Website available at http://www.arrt.org. Accessed September 8, 2008.

2003; Clements, 2003). A radiologic technologist is defined as an individual who has graduated from a nationally accredited education program in the radiologic sciences and is registered with the ARRT or an equivalent national organization or holds a full state license (McElveny & Olmstead, 2003; Clements, 2003). Radiologic technologists perform both basic and contrast radiographic procedures as supervised by a licensed independent practitioner. These procedures may be performed in hospitals or other medical care settings.

A limited x-ray machine operator (i.e., limited radiographer) is defined as an individual other than a radiologic technologist who performs diagnostic x-ray procedures on selected anatomical sites. The ASRT resolution also recommends that the term limited x-ray machine operator replace other titles used by states and employers such as "radiologic technician," "x-ray technician," or "limited permitee" (McElveny & Olmstead, 2003; Clements, 2003; Chang, 2006; Tuggle, 2002). The use of the title limited x-ray machine operator was selected because it is used by the ARRT and also the title used in the proposed Consumer Assurance of Radiologic Excellence (RadCARE) bill, which will be discussed later in this chapter.

For purposes of brevity, the authors will use the term limited radiographer when referring to limited x-ray machine operators.

A limited radiographer may have completed formal allied health education in a program such as nursing, medical assisting, medical technology, respiratory therapy, or physical therapy. Such programs generally do not provide radiography education; however, cross training, or a multiskilled approach, is common in medical assisting programs. Individuals from allied health educational programs who have not received formal limited radiography education may acquire radiography skills by less traditional methods, such as on-the-job training, correspondence courses, or independent study programs.

A limited radiographer performs basic noncontrast media x-ray examinations under the supervision of a licensed practitioner of the healing arts. Limited radiographers generally do not perform specialized x-ray or fluoroscopic procedures. These procedures often include the use of contrast media and require specific education and training beyond the scope of the duties of a limited radiographer.

Limited radiographers usually are employed in medical offices and outpatient and ambulatory care clinics; in some states, they are also employed in hospitals. A variety of occupational titles exists for workers/staff who perform limited radiography tasks; such titles vary from one area of the United States to another. Thus, the limited radiographer may be called a limited license radiographer, radiographic assistant, limited medical radiographer, practical technologist, limited permittee, limited x-ray technician, or basic x-ray machine operator.

Radiographers may be further classified by state laws that regulate the scope of practice. A number of states recognize multiple Limited Permittee categories for radiographers: chest, extremities, gastrointestinal, skull, torso-skeletal, dermatology, genito-urinary, leg and podiatric, dental laboratory, and photofluorographic chest. If the reader should desire additional information about classification of radiographers and radiographic tasks in a particular state, contact that state's Radiation Control Office. A list of individual state radiation control offices is available on the ARRT website: www.arrt.org.

In 1981, Public Law 97-35 (the Consumer-Patient Radiation Health and Safety Act) was enacted in response to growing concern and awareness about potential long-term effects from radiation exposure (Chang, 2006). The act gave Congress the power to protect consumers and patients from unnecessary or excessive radiation exposure. To do so, Congress established the following objectives (Chang, 2006).

1. Provide for the establishment of minimum standards by the federal government for the accreditation of education programs for persons who administer radiologic procedures and for certification of such persons.
2. Ensure that medical and dental radiologic procedures are consistent with rigorous safety precautions and standards.

On December 11, 1985 in the *Federal Register*, the Secretary of Health and Human Services issued 42 CFR Part 75—minimum Standards for Accreditation of Educational Programs For, and the Credentialing of Radiologic Personnel; Final Rule (ASRT, 1995). These standards are intended for use by states in implementing Public Law 97-35.

On June 5, 2003, Senators Michael Enzi, R-Wyoming, and Edward M. Kennedy, D-Massachusetts, introduced a bill in the U.S. Senate, The Consumer-Assurance of Radiologic Excellence, or RadCARE bill (McElveny, 2005). The RadCARE bill directs the U.S. Secretary of Health and Human Services to establish minimum educational and credentialing standards for personnel who plan and deliver radiation therapy and perform all types of diagnostic imaging procedures except medical ultrasound. The bill would amend the Consumer-Patient Radiation Health and Safety Act, a 1981 law that established federal minimum standards for the education and credentialing of radiologic technologists. When President Ronald Reagan signed the 1981 act into law, compliance by the states was made voluntary rather than mandatory. As a result of this federal initiative, only 37 states have enacted full licensure laws or regulations for radiographers, 29 for radiation therapists, and 23 for nuclear medicine technologists. In states without regulations, individuals are permitted to perform radiologic procedures without any formal education (McElveny, 2005; Chang, 2005).

The RadCARE bill would improve the quality of patient care by ensuring that personnel who perform radiologic examinations and procedures are well trained, and the legislation also would protect taxpayer money by limiting Medicare and Medicaid reimbursement only to facilities whose personnel are properly qualified. The measure also would allow for alternative standards if the minimum federal standard were not accommodating for rural areas.

In 2008, the U.S. House of Representatives and U.S. Senate approved a Medicare bill (H.R. 6331) which included a section directing the Secretary of Health and Human Services to establish standards for personnel who perform computed tomography (CT), magnetic resonance imaging (MRI), and positron emission tomography (PET) procedures (ASRT, 2008). The bill excludes x-ray, fluoroscopy, and ultrasonography, as well as radiation therapy (ASRT, 2008).

The ASRT supports calling Senators and Representatives immediately to ask that they move the CARE bill (H.R. 583 and S. 1042) to the floor and ensure all medical imaging and radiation therapy patients have procedures performed by qualified personnel (ASRT, 2008). Updated information on the status of these bills may be found on the ASRT's website www.asrt.org.

Philosophy Statement

In its relation to a health care profession, a philosophy statement speaks to the motivating concepts or principles guiding the practice of that profession. Thus, the authors offer the following philosophy statement to express the scope of practice for limited radiography. This statement attempts to capture the intent of the Consumer-Patient Radiation Health and Safety Act and the RadCARE/CARE bill, which will be discussed later in this chapter.

A limited radiographer is a multiskilled person dedicated to assisting in many aspects of medical care. These duties are at the request of and under the supervision of a licensed practitioner of the healing arts. The limited radiographer's scope of practice is confined to radiography of anatomic parts and body regions as regulated by applicable state laws. Although their scope of practice may be confined by law, limited radiographers must have the depth of knowledge and understanding necessary for each radiographic task to ensure skill competency and safety as a practitioner. Competence in the occupation also requires that a limited radiographer demonstrate professional characteristics, adhere to ethical and legal standards of medical practice, communicate effectively, and recognize and respond to emergencies to provide maximum protection to the patient.

Occupational Scope of Practice

Job requirements and responsibilities of a limited radiographer vary from office to office or other practice site; particular qualifications and responsibilities depend upon the medical specialty or geographic area of employment. The scope of duties limited radiographers perform also depends upon applicable state laws. Regardless of these differences, limited radiographers must possess a basic core of knowledge and skills.

General Requirements

The following general requirements are from the ASRT *Limited X-ray Machine Operator Standards*.

> Limited x-ray machine operators must demonstrate an understanding of human anatomy, physiology, pathology, and medical terminology. Limited x-ray machine operators must maintain a high degree of accuracy in radiographic positioning and exposure technique. They must maintain knowledge of radiation protection and safety. Limited x-ray machine operators perform radiographic procedures within their scope or assist the licensed independent practitioner or radiologic technologist in the completion of radiographic procedures.
>
> Limited x-ray machine operators must remain sensitive to the physical and emotional needs of the patient through good communication, patient monitoring, and patient care skills. Limited x-ray machine operators use ethical judgment and critical thinking. Quality improvement and customer service allows the limited x-ray machine operator to be a responsible member of the health care team by continually assessing performance. Limited x-ray machine operators engage in ongoing education to enhance patient care, public education, knowledge, and technical competence while embracing lifelong learning (ASRT, 2007).

Scope of Practice

The ASRT practice standards for limited x-ray machine operators serve as a guide for appropriate practice. "Standards provide role definition that can be used by individual facilities to develop job descriptions and practice parameters. Those outside the imaging, therapeutic, and radiation science community can use the standards as an overview of the role and responsibilities" (ASRT, 2007).

The following scope of practice statement is from the ASRT *Limited X-ray Machine Operator Standards*.

1. Performing radiographic procedures limited to education or the specific area of anatomical interest based on training and licensure/certification.
2. Corroborating patient's clinical history with procedure, ensuring information is documented and available for use by a licensed independent practitioner.

3. Maintaining confidentiality of the patient's protected health information in accordance with the Health Insurance Portability and Accountability Act.
4. Preparing the patient for procedures, including providing instructions to obtain desired results, gain cooperation, and minimize anxiety.
5. Operating radiography equipment to obtain static image.
6. Upon completion of proven competency level, positioning patient to best demonstrate anatomic area of interest, respecting patient ability and comfort.
7. Assisting a licensed independent practitioner or radiologic technologist during radiographic procedures.
8. Immobilizing patients as required for appropriate examination.
9. Determining radiographic technique exposure factors.
10. Applying principles of radiation protection to minimize exposure to patient, self, and others.
11. Evaluating images for positioning, centering, appropriate anatomy, and overall image quality.
12. Evaluating radiographs or images for technical quality, ensuring proper identification is recorded.
13. Assuming responsibility for provision of physical and psychological needs of patients during procedures.
14. Initiating first-aid and assisting with basic life support action when necessary.
15. Assisting the licensed independent practitioner or radiologic technologist in providing patient education.
16. Observing universal precautions.
17. Applying the principles of patient safety during all aspects of radiographic procedures including assisting and transporting patients.

The more experienced limited radiographer may become an office or clinic manager, supervising other personnel and coordinating the overall operations of a medical practice.

Basic to the occupation is the ability and desire to perform as a cooperative member of a medical team. A good perspective from which to view the occupation is to think of it as being "service oriented" rather than "task oriented." The purpose is to function as a medical team member and to help provide quality care for the person undergoing x-ray examinations.

Education

During the years when limited radiography was beginning to develop as a distinguishable job category, it was a common practice for allied health workers to learn radiography on the job. Of course, some of these individuals had completed formal educational programs in related fields, such as in nursing, medical technology, or medical assisting; however, most of these workers trained in other fields did not have prior education in radiography per se and learned radiographic procedures on the job.

A number of factors, such as consumer awareness of the dangers of radiation and state compliance with the Consumer-Patient Radiation Health and Safety Act, have resulted in the limited radiographer's occupation becoming more than just a series of tasks that can be taught in an on-the-job learning situation. Rather, a structured competency-based educational system is needed to assure that the limited radiographer is a skilled and safe practitioner. A minimum task list is provided in the publication *Task Inventory for Radiography*, available from The American Registry of Radiologic Technologists, 1255 Northland Drive, Mendota Heights, MN 55120.

Many states have adopted the Standards for the Accreditation of Educational Programs for, and the Credentialing of Radiologic Personnel provided by the Department of Health and Human Services, 42 CFR Part 75; December 1985. The *Limited X-ray Machine Operator Standards* published (2007) by the ASRT also provides guidance for the development of limited radiography training programs.

Implementation of limited radiography training programs varies from state to state. Some states have developed essentials and guidelines for formal limited radiography educational programs and alternatives—for example, correspondence or independent study programs combined with a supervised on-the-job clinical experience. The scope of limited radiography training programs generally is based on the ARRT content specifications for the examination for the limited scope of practice in radiography (ARRT, 2008g). The full content of the specifications is available on the ARRT website www.arrt.org.

Limited radiography education may be included with other health occupational programs, such as medical assistant or laboratory technician. Some states have limited radiography education programs designed to admit such individuals as registered nurses or licensed practical or vocational nurses, laboratory technologists, chiropractic or medical assistants, physician assistants, or paramedics.

The American Registry of Radiologic Technologists (ARRT), founded in 1922, has as its purpose the study and elevation of standards of radiologic technology as well as the examining and certifying of eligible candidates. By 2008, the ARRT had five primary and eleven post-primary certification examinations plus several examination programs used solely for state licensing. Refer to Figures 1-1 and 1-2 for a list of the primary and post-primary examinations. There are several terms associated with attaining recognized competency in radiography. These include certification, registration, and licensing. The ARRT uses the following definitions to differentiate between the terms; however, states adopting regulations concerning those who operate medical imaging equipment may use different definitions (ARRT, 2008b; 2008f). Additional information regarding state regulations may be obtained from the ARRT website www.arrt.org.

- "Certification is a one-time process of initially recognizing individuals who have satisfied certain standards within a profession." A person is certified by ARRT or a state agency after meeting educational preparation standards, complying with ethics standards, and passing a certification examination (ARRT, 2008b).
- Registration is a procedure required to maintain an active status of the certification. Registration refers to individuals who have already fulfilled the requirements for initial certification, and continue to meet the requirements for registration. The time frame for the registration cycle may be different for each state but the ARRT registration is an annual procedure (ARRT, 2008f).
- Licensing most commonly is used in referring to state laws. "The State not ARRT is the authority that administers the license and grants an individual permission to practice radiography within that state. Application for and renewal of a state license are separate from ARRT processes" (ARRT, 2008b; 2008f).

ARRT examinations available to states for licensing purposes include the *Limited Scope of Practice in Radiography* and the Bone Densitometry Equipment Operators examinations. As of 2008, 35 states utilize ARRT administered examinations for state licensing (ARRT, 2008a). ARRT examination handbooks are available for both examinations from the ARRT website www.arrt.org (ARRT, 2008e; 2008f).

In order to attain initial registration and certification, the candidate must attest that certain requirements have been met. The ARRT cites the basic requirements in their "Equation for Excellence" to be three components: ethics, education, and examination; however, individual states may impose additional requirements as stated in their regulations (ASRT, 1995).

The ARRT's ethics standards require that the person be of good moral character and must not have engaged in conduct inconsistent with the ARRT Rules of Ethics (ASRT, 1995). Figure 1-3 provides examples of the questions an applicant for certification in limited radiography may expect to answer (ARRT, 2008d). Note that the states may ask very specific questions, which the candidates are required to answer, such as have you:

- Any medical condition(s) which in any way impair or limit your ability to perform as a radiologic technologist?;
- Been engaged in the illegal or improper use of drugs or other chemical substance?;

STATE DEPARTMENT OF PUBLIC HEALTH
BUREAU OF RADIOLOGICAL HEALTH

DIAGNOSTIC RADIOGRAPHY "PERMIT TO PRACTICE" APPLICATION

Instructions for completing this form:
1. Print or type the required information. Provide the appropriate document(s).
2. Send the completed form and a $60 initial fee in a check or money order made payable to:
   State Department of Public Health, Bureau of Radiological Health
   Main State Office Building, 4th Floor, 123 East 9th Street, Anywhere, US 01234
If you have any questions, please contact: Joe Smith 555/123-4567; jsmith@sdph.state.us

----

Applicant's Name: _____ Home Phone Number _____

Home Mailing Address: _____ email address _____

City: _____ State: _____ Zip: _____

Date of Birth: _____ Social Security #: _____
          [ ] High School Graduate   [ ] GED Certification

This application is for a:

[ ] General Permit   [ ] Limited Permit in: [ ] Chest   [ ] Extremities   [ ] Spines   [ ] Sinus

1. General permit. Provide a copy of the ARRT card or proof that you have passed the ARRT certification test or provide your ARRT
   Reg. #_____. Current membership in the ARRT is not required. If you have not passed the ARRT test,
   you must pass it before this permit can be issued.
2. Limited permit. Include a copy of proof that you have passed the limited test and a copy of proof of completion of your limited training course.
   A letter from your instructor stating you have completed the limited competencies meets the training requirement. If you have not passed the
   ARRT limited test, you must pass it before this permit can be issued. To take the limited test, submit a testing application to the SDPH.

Name of training school graduating from: _____

If you have a current, expired, or inactive permit or license in another state, please provide the state and type of

license:_____
Have you ever had a permit or license suspended or revoked? [ ] no [ ] yes. If yes, please state the circumstances.

_____

Current Employer in radiography: _____ Phone number _____

Employer's Address: _____

City: _____ State: _____ Zip: _____
If you are not currently working in radiography, please provide the name and address of your last radiography employer and the dates of your
employment:
Date: _____ Employer: _____

Employer address: _____

Have you:
1. Any medical condition(s) which in any way impair or limit your ability to perform as a radiologic technologist? [ ] yes [ ] no   Please specify

_____

2. Been engaged in the illegal or improper use of drugs or other chemical substance? [ ] yes [ ] no

3. Been convicted of a misdemeanor or felony that may impair or limit your ability to perform diagnostic radiography? Please explain. You
   must answer "yes" even if the matter has been expunged from the record. [ ] yes [ ] no

4. Had any disciplinary action brought against you in connection with a certificate or license issued from a certifying or licensing entity?
   [ ] yes [ ] no   Please explain.

5. Been found guilty of incompetence or negligence during your performance as a diagnostic radiographer? [ ] yes [ ] no   Please explain.

Privacy Act Notice: Disclosure of your social security number on this application is required by 42 U.S.C. § 666(a)(13) and State Code
§ 252J.8(1). The number will be used in connection with the collection of child support obligations and as an internal means to accurately
identify licensees, and may be shared with taxing authorities as allowed by law including State Code § 421.18.

1. I will allow a representative of the State Department of Public Health to comprehensively evaluate whether or not I meet the training
   standard.

2. The information provided on this form and enclosure(s) is truthful and accurate.

3. My name and address may be sent to companies requesting it for continuing education promotions or employment opportunities.

_____   _____
Signature of Applicant   Date
Revised 4/1/2008

Guidelines to continuing education can be found on our website.

FIGURE 1-3 Diagnostic radiography "permit to practice" application
Source: Delmar, Cengage Learning.

- Been convicted of a misdemeanor or felony that may impair or limit your ability to perform diagnostic radiography? Please explain. You must answer "yes" even if the matter has been expunged from the record;
- Had any disciplinary action brought against you in connection with a certificate or license issued from a certifying or licensing entity?; and
- Been found guilty of incompetence or negligence during your performance as a diagnostic radiographer? (ARRT, 2008d)

In many, but not all, of the states that credential limited radiographers, after attaining the initial credential, continuing education (CE) is required for ongoing renewal. The purpose and scope of continuing education will be discussed later in this chapter.

The ARRT provides examinations covering limited scope of practice in radiography and bone densitometry equipment operator, by agreement, to states requiring licensing of radiographers (ARRT, 2008d; 2008e). The limited scope of practice in radiography examination content specifications (see Table 1-1) provides for a 100-question core module that includes four major sections and five separate selected radiographic procedure modules (chest, extremities, skull/sinuses, spine, and podiatric radiography) (ARRT, 2008e). The 100-question core module of the examination covers information appropriate for all candidates. The bone densitometry equipment operators examination content specifications provides a total of 60 test questions that include eight major sections, shown in Table 1-2 (ARRT, 2008d).

All test questions on the ARRT limited scope of practice in radiography examination and the bone densitometry equipment operators examination are in a multiple-choice format. The ARRT provides a recommended pass-fail rate; however, each state is responsible for setting a passing score. The ARRT provides examination scores directly to states who maintain the responsibility of notifying candidates.

Licensing states, through legislation, set forth the particular requirements that candidates must meet to be eligible to take one of the examinations. These requirements address which specific sections of the ARRT examination that candidates must satisfactorily complete. Refer to Figure 1-4, which is an example of an application for the Limited Scope of Practice in Radiography and lists the various sections of the examination that may be required.

Individuals are limited to three attempts to pass an examination and must complete the attempts within a three-year period. Individuals failing three times within the timeframe may retake the examination within one year of the third attempt after completing remedial activities acceptable to the state agency utilizing the examination.

TABLE 1-1   Content Specifications for the Examination for the Limited Scope of Practice in Radiography (ARRT, 2008f)

Core Module	Number of Questions	Testing Time
Radiation protection	35	
Equipment operation and quality control	12	
Image production and evaluation	38	
Patient care and education	15	
Total questions	100	1 hour and 40 minutes

Radiographic Procedures	Modules Number of Questions	Testing Time
Chest	20	20 minutes
Extremities	25	25 minutes
Skull/sinuses	20	20 minutes
Spine	25	25 minutes
Podiatric radiography	20	20 minutes

TABLE 1-2   Content Specifications for the Bone Densitometry Equipment Operators Examination (ARRT, 2008d)

Major Sections	Number of Questions
Basic concepts	12
Equipment operation & quality control	9
Radiation safety	9
DXA Scanning of the finger	4
DXA Scanning of heel	4
DXA Scanning of forearm	6
DXA Scanning of lumbar spine	8
DXA Scanning of proximal femur	8
	60 questions*

*An additional 20% of the test may be pilot questions.

For further information, contact the American Registry of Radiologic Technologists at 1255 Northland Drive, St. Paul, Minnesota 55120-1155.

Application for the Limited Scope
of Practice in Radiography Examination

IF THIS FORM IS NOT COMPLETED IN ITS ENTIRETY AND/OR TESTING FEE IS NOT INCLUDED, IT WILL BE RETURNED TO YOU.

Name: _____
    (Last Name)   (First Name)   (Middle Name)

Address: _____
    (Street Address - NOT PO BOX) (City) (State) (Zip)

Daytime Phone # _____ Evening Phone # _____

Social Security Number: _____

Date of Birth: _____

Categories of Examination: Everyone is required to take the core module. Also check the categories applied for on your Temporary License Application.

        Core Module   [ ] **All applicants must take and pass Core**
        Chest Module   [ ]
        Extremities Module [ ]
        Skull/Sinus Module [ ]
        Spine Module   [ ]
        Podiatry Module   [ ]

I, hereby release the State Department of Health, Division of Radiation Control to submit the information contained on this application to the testing center.

_____
(Signature)   (Date)

This form and your $100.00 check or money order must be mailed to:

State Department of Health
Radiation Control Section
Radiologic Technology Licensure Program
Broadway Medical Building
5000 E. 3rd Street, Suite 500
Our Town, US 10000

FIGURE 1-4 Application for the limited scope of practice in radiography examination
Source: Delmar, Cengage Learning.

Continuing Education and Professional Organizations

Continuing education is encouraged for all allied health professionals and may be obtained by attending professional meetings, seminars, and conventions at county, state, regional, and national levels. Some states have mandatory continuing education policies and require that radiographers show evidence of a certain number of continuing education units (CEUs) in order to renew a certificate or license.

Continuing education is aimed at improving the quality of work performed by radiographers and increasing their value to the employer and to everyone seeking medical attention. In addition, by taking part in a professional organization, radiographers have an opportunity to develop valuable job networks, enhance technical knowledge and skills, and have a feeling of professional fellowship within the whole occupation of radiology.

Continuing education (CE) became mandatory for renewal or reinstatement of the ARRT registration in 1995 (ARRT, 2008a). The ARRT suggests that all technologists should select CE topics that are related to their area of practice and that address the needs of the patient and the radiographer. According to the ASRT Code of Ethics, "the radiologic technologist continually strives to improve knowledge and skills by participating in continuing education and professional activities, sharing with colleagues and investigating new aspects of professional practice" (ARRT, 2008a).

Many states that have licensure or certification for the limited radiography scope of practice also require continuing education for renewal or reinstatement of the credential. Figure 1-5 provides an examples of the scope of continuing education that may be required for continued practice in limited radiography (Connecticut Department of Public Health, 2008). Figure 1-6 provides an example of a state form requiring licensees to submit evidence of earned approved continuing education during a renewal cycle (California Department of Public Health, 2008).

Research studies reveal a correlation between success and continuing education, confirming the significance of continuous training for today's work force. As medical technology advances, transfer of training through continuing education plays a major role in the health care setting. Limited radiographers will find various ways to fulfill continuing education requirements, such as attending in-service programs, conferences, completing self-study or online courses.

Professional growth often results from experiences encountered in the day-to-day medical arena; however, by participating in an organized radiography association, members make a conscious decision about professional growth. The ASRT, established in 1920, has affiliate societies in each of the fifty states and the

Department of Public Health

Radiographer Continuing Education Requirements

Number of Hours

Commencing on the first date of license renewal after October 1, 2008, licensed radiographers shall either maintain registration as a radiographer or radiation therapy technologist issued by the American Registry of Radiologic Technologists (ARRT) or earn a minimum of twenty-four hours of qualifying continuing education within the previous twenty-four month period. One contact hour is a minimum of fifty minutes of continuing education activity.

Qualifying Continuing Education

The Connecticut Department of Public Health does not review and approve CE courses. It is incumbent on the provider and the practitioner to ensure that the continuing education activities meet the following requirements:

Qualifying continuing education activities include, but are not limited to, courses, including on-line courses, offered or approved by the American College of Radiology, American Healthcare Radiology Administrators, American Institute of Ultrasound in Medicine, American Society of Radiologic Technologists, Canadian Association of Medical Radiation Technologists, Radiological Society of North America, Society of Diagnostic Medical Sonography, Society of Nuclear Medicine Technologist Section, Society for Vascular Ultrasound, Section for Magnetic Resonance Technologists, a hospital or other health care institution, regionally accredited schools of higher education or a state or local health department.

Documentation/Record Retention

Each licensee must obtain a certificate of completion from the provider of the continuing education and retain records of attendance for all continuing education hours and shall retain such documentation for a minimum of three years following the year in which the continuing education activities were completed. Only upon a request by the Department should the licensee submit such certificates to the Department.

Each licensee applying for license renewal will be asked to attest that the licensee satisfies the continuing education requirements. Certificates of completion should not be mailed to the Department at the time of license renewal unless a licensee is specifically directed to do so.

Exemptions

A licensee who is applying for license renewal for the first time is exempt from continuing education requirements.

The Department may, for a licensee who is not engaged in active practice or who has a medical disability or illness, grant a waiver of the continuing education requirements for a specified period of time or may grant the licensee an extension of time in which to fulfill the requirements. Licensees may request a waiver by filing an *application* with the Department.

Return to Active Practice Following Exemption

Individuals who have received an exemption or waiver may not return to active practice until the licensee has met the continuing education requirements as outlined above.

FIGURE 1-5 Radiographer continuing education requirements. Connecticut Department of Public Health Source: http://www.ct.gov. Accessed November 11, 2008.

State Health and Human Services Agency

State Department of Public Health
Radiologic Health Branch

Earned Approved Continuing Education Credits for Renewing
State X-Ray Technician Limited Permits

This list can only be accepted when submitted with a completed RENEWAL APPLICATION form and fees.

Number (shown on your Permit)	Expiration Date	This box for RHB use only

An approved continuing education credit is one hour of instruction received in subjects related to the application of X-ray to the human body and accepted for purposes of credentialing, assigning professional status, or certification, by any of the following **groups**:

Code	Group
A.	American Registry of Radiologic Technologists;
B.	State Medical Board;
C.	State Osteopathic Medical Board;
D.	Board of Podiatric Medicine;
E.	State Board of Chiropractic Examiners;
F.	Board of Dental Examiners.

Course Title				
Provider or Sponsor	Location (City, State)	Date	Code	Hours
Course Title				
Provider or Sponsor	Location (City, State)	Date	Code	Hours
Course Title				
Provider or Sponsor	Location (City, State)	Date	Code	Hours
Course Title				
Provider or Sponsor	Location (City, State)	Date	Code	Hours
Course Title				
Provider or Sponsor	Location (City, State)	Date	Code	Hours

Do not send us copies of your Continuing Education documents. You are required to maintain these documents for five years so that you can make them available to the Department upon request.

I certify that I have earned the approved continuing education credits listed on this form. I understand that the State Department of Public Health may cancel permits that are procured by fraud, misrepresentation, or mistake.

Signature	Date

FIGURE 1-6 Earned approved continuing education credits for renewing x-ray technician limited permits
Source: Delmar, Cengage Learning.

Commonwealth of Puerto Rico as well as district groups within the state societies. The ASRT state and district groups provide regular opportunities for radiographers to meet, network and share ideas, hear speakers, and obtain current medical and scientific information.

The national society and some state affiliates publish journals containing timely information for radiographers. Membership in these groups provides continuing education, professional growth, and an opportunity to develop leadership skills. For additional information about the ASRT affiliate in a particular state, contact the national office (American Society of Radiologic Technologists, 15000 Central Avenue, Albuquerque, NM 87123-4605) or online at www.asrt.org.

Occupational Progress and Professionalization

Since 1981, significant progress has been made toward credentialing operators of ionizing radiation equipment and establishing guidelines for educational programs. However, the next decade will determine if limited radiography will be accepted as a vital and necessary level of practice across the United States.

A new profession within radiology may be emerging; the ingredients certainly exist including mandated initial training and continuing education for limited radiographers in many states. The following events are signs that professionalization of limited radiography has occurred.

- In 2008, the U.S. House of Representatives and U.S. Senate approved a Medicare bill (H.R. 6331) that included a section directing the Secretary of Health and Human Services to establish standards for personnel who perform CT, MRI, nuclear medicine, and PET procedures. The radiography community suggested that passage of CARE bill (H.R. 583 and S. 1042) legislation be approved, which will ensure that all medical imaging and radiation therapy patients have procedures performed by qualified personnel. To keep track of details regarding the passage of this legislation, go to the ASRT website www.asrt.org.
- In 2007, the ASRT published *The Practice Standards for Medical Imaging and Radiation Therapy: Limited X-ray Machine Operator Standards.*
- In 1981, the Consumer-Patient Radiation Health and Safety Act set forth mandates for training and credentialing.
- The scope and practice of limited radiography has been defined by many states. A task inventory outlining the scope of practice for limited radiographers has been developed by the American Registry of Radiologic Technologists (ARRT).

These manifestations reflect professional outlook and behavior.

The Future

It is a certainty that the demand for radiographers will grow in the future. There is also the possibility that the limited radiography scope of practice will increase as the radiologic technologist is called upon to conduct new procedures using sophisticated imaging modalities. As limited radiographers become better educated and more capable, medical professionals may see an opportunity to utilize a multiskilled person.

The future may also bring professional recognition and full acceptance by established radiography associations, accreditation agencies, and other allied health professions. Another future option includes geographic employment flexibility as more states adopt reciprocity guidelines for licensed or certified limited radiographers. Career advancement and mobility are also future possibilities as career ladders, articulation agreements, and competency challenge examinations are developed to allow limited radiographers to advance into radiologic technology and specialized radiography areas.

REVIEW QUESTIONS

1. Wilhelm Conrad Roentgen announced his discovery of x-rays in November:
   a. 1975
   b. 1955
   c. 1925
   d. 1895

2. **All** of the following are true regarding the American Registry of Radiologic Technologists (ARRT), **except**:
   a. the ARRT is the largest certifying body in the radiological profession
   b. the ARRT is the world's largest and oldest membership association for medical imaging technologists and radiation therapists
   c. the ARRT promotes a high standard of patient care by recognizing qualified individuals in medical imaging, interventional procedures, and radiation therapy
   d. one of the ARRT's roles is to test and certify technologists

3. The ARRT offers certification in _____ primary pathways.
   a. two
   b. five
   c. seven
   d. twelve

4. **All** of the following are true regarding the limited radiography scope of practice, **except**:
   a. in most states limited radiographers may perform x-ray examinations requiring contrast media
   b. includes performance of basic noncontrast x-ray examinations
   c. limited radiographers are usually employed in medical offices and outpatient and ambulatory care clinics
   d. limited radiographers may also be called practical technologists, basic x-ray machine operators, or limited permittees

5. The intent of the 1981 Public Law 97-35 (the Consumer-Patient Radiation Health and Safety Act) was to give Congress the power to:
   a. impose a tax on medical imaging procedures
   b. regulate nuclear energy production
   c. protect consumers and patients from unnecessary or excessive radiation exposure
   d. oversee interstate transport of medical-nuclear waste

6. The intent of the 2003 Consumer-Assurance of Radiologic Excellence (RadCARE) bill was to establish minimum educational and credentialing standards for those who plan and deliver radiation therapy and perform and those who perform all types of diagnostic imaging procedures, except medical ultrasonography.
   a. True
   b. False

7. In 2008, Medicare bill (H.R. 6331), excludes those who perform:
   a. x-ray and fluoroscopy
   b. ultrasonography
   c. radiation therapy
   d. all of the above

8. A one-time process of initially recognizing individuals who have satisfied certain standards with a profession is referred to as:
   a. registration
   b. certification
   c. licensing
   d. permitting

9. Registration is a procedure required to maintain active status of certification.
   a. True
   b. False

10. The limited scope of practice in radiography examination has _____ test questions in the core module.
    a. 25
    b. 50
    c. 75
    d. 100

11. In the core module of the limited scope of practice in radiography examination, 35 test questions pertain to:
    a. patient care and education
    b. radiation protection
    c. image production and evaluation
    d. equipment operation and quality control

12. In the radiographic procedure module section of the limited scope of practice in radiography examination, the spine section contains _____ test questions.
    a. 75
    b. 50
    c. 25
    d. 15

13. The ARRT's examination for bone densitometry equipment operators contains a total of _____ test questions.
    a. 100
    b. 80
    c. 60
    d. 40

14. All test questions on the limited scope of practice in radiography and the bone densitometry equipment operators' examination are in a discussion or true and false type format.
    a. True
    b. False

15. According to the Connecticut Department of Public Health statement concerning radiographers continuing education requirements, one contact hour is a minimum of _____ of continuing education activity.
    a. 3 hours
    b. 1.5 hours
    c. 50 minutes
    d. 15 minutes

REFERENCES

American Registry of Radiologic Technologists. (2008a). *Annual report to registered technologists.* St. Paul, MN: American Registry of Radiologic Technologists.

American Registry of Radiologic Technologists. (2008b). *Certification vs registration. What's the difference.* Retrieved from http://www.arrt.org

American Registry of Radiologic Technologists. (2008c). *Certifications offered.* Retrieved from http://www.arrt.org

American Registry of Radiologic Technologists. (2008d). *Content specifications for the bone densitometry equipment operator examination.* Retrieved from http://www.arrt.org

American Registry of Radiologic Technologists. (2008e). *Content specifications for the examination for the limited scope of practice in radiography.* Retrieved from http://www.arrt.org

American Registry of Radiologic Technologists. (2008f). Licensing vs certification and registration. Retrieved from http://www.arrt.org

American Registry of Radiologic Technologists. (2008g). *Limited scope examination; Format of the examination.* Retrieved from http://www.arrt.org

American Registry of Radiologic Technologists. (2008h). *Supporting discipline required.* Retrieved from http://www.arrt.org

American Society of Radiologic Technologists. (1995) *The shadowmakers: A history of radiologic technology.* Albuquerque, NM: American Society of Radiologic Technologists.

American Society of Radiologic Technologists. (2007). *The practice standards for medical imaging and radiation therapy: Limited x-ray machine operator standards.* Retrieved from http://www.asrt.org

American Society of Radiologic Technologists. (2008). *Support the CARE bill.* Retrieved from http://www.asrt.org

American Society of Radiologic Technologists. (2009). *About our profession.* Retrieved from www.asrt.org

California Department of Public Health, Radiologic Health Branch. (2008). *Earned approved continuing education credits for renewing California x-ray technician limited permits.* Retrieved from http://www.dhs.ca.gov

Chang, S. (December 26, 2005). Not everyone cares. *Advance for Imaging and Radiation Therapy Professionals:* 10.

Chang, S. (2005). Licensure: A state by state guide for radiologic technologists. *Advance for Imaging and Radiation Therapy Professionals, 19*(4), 18–35.

Clements, R. (2003, July 28). Limited permit x-ray operators. [Letter to the editor.] *RT Image, 16*(30), 8.

Connecticut Department of Public Health. (2008). *Radiographer continuing education requirements, number of hours.* Retrieved from http:www.ct.gov

Joint Review Committee on Education in Radiologic Technology. (2008). Retrieved from http://www.jrcert.org

Kollmer, J. (2005). Completing the puzzle: Reviewing the roles and responsibilities of the three major organizations that rule the RT's career. *RT-Image,* 26–29.

McElveny, C. (2005). Why LXMOS are included in the CARE bill. *Advance for Imaging and Radiation Therapy Professionals, 18*(23), 11.

McElveny, C. & Olmstead, D. (2003). Inside the ASRT: Practice spurs 14 house resolutions. *ASRT Scanner, 25*(7), 11–18.

Tuggle, N. (2002). Inside the ASRT: Defining the profession one resolution at a time. *ASRT Scanner, 34*(7), 11–15.

SUGGESTED READINGS

American Registry of Radiologic Technologists. (2008). *Certifications offered.* Retrieved from http://www.arrt.org

American Registry of Radiologic Technologists. (2008). *Certification vs registration. What's the difference.* Retrieved from http://www.arrt/org

American Registry of Radiologic Technologists. (2008). *Content specifications for the examination for the limited scope of practice in radiography.* (2008) Retrieved from http://www.arrt.org

American Registry of Radiologic Technologists. (2008). *Content specifications for the bone densitometry equipment operator examination.* Retrieved from http://www.arrt.org

American Registry of Radiologic Technologists. (2008). *Limited scope examination; Format of the examination.* Retrieved from http://www.arrt.org

American Society of Radiologic Technologists. (1995). *The shadowmakers: A history of radiologic technology.* Albuquerque, NM. American Society of Radiologic Technologists.

American Society of Radiologic Technologists. (2007). *The practice standards for medical imaging and radiation therapy. Limited x-ray machine operator standards.* Retrieved from http://www.asrt.org

American Society of Radiologic Technologists. (2009). *About our profession.* Retrieved from www.asrt.org

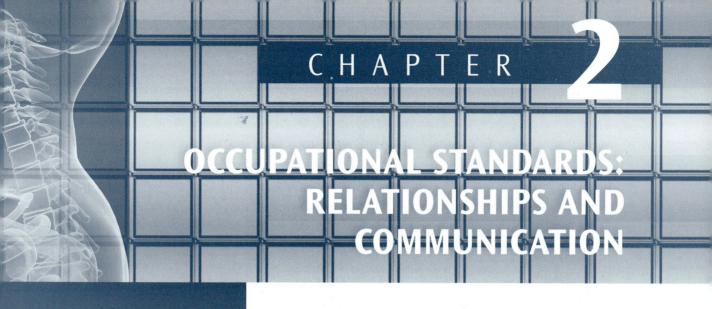

CHAPTER 2

OCCUPATIONAL STANDARDS: RELATIONSHIPS AND COMMUNICATION

Key Terms

Asymptomatic Patient
Caring
Chain of Command
Communication (verbal/ nonverbal)
Cultural Diversity
Empathy
Hierachy of Human Needs
Patient Advocate
Rapport
Sympathy
Symptomatic Patient

Chapter Outline

Taking Patient Information
Explaining Radiography Procedures to Patients
Reporting to Coworkers, Physicians, and Supervisors
Recognizing Common Barriers to Communication

Objectives

Upon completion of the chapter, the student will meet the following objectives by verifying knowledge of the facts and principles presented through oral and written communication at a level deemed competent.

- Describe in a written paragraph the importance of positive interpersonal relationships in health care settings.
- Discuss why there may be differences between how patients with symptoms and those without symptoms may perceive the medical environment and suggest ways to avoid miscommunication as a result of these differences.
- Explain how Abraham Maslow's hierarchy of human needs relates to the limited radiographer.
- Recognize examples of actions that exemplify empathy, sympathy, and caring within the limited radiographer's role and scope of practice.
- List three suggestions for creating positive interactions with patients.
- List and explain five negative barriers to establishing positive relationships with others.
- Define the term patient advocate and list two examples of ways that the limited radiographer may serve as a patient advocate.
- List three suggestions for improving relationships with coworkers, doctors, and supervisors.
- Describe what is meant by "chain of command" and discuss how it promotes effective communication and team efforts.
- List five ways the limited radiographer uses communication in the health care setting.
- Define the term cultural diversity and give two examples on how differences in culture impact the delivery of medical care.
- Recall and state an appropriate method of introducing yourself to others.
- Given sample verbal messages; change them into "I" messages.
- List five important tips for communicating with referring physicians and agencies.
- Given sample patient questions, concerns, or statements; use paraphrasing techniques to form a written response.
- Identify five keys to becoming an effective listener.
- List five barriers to communication and give suggestions on how to overcome them.

PART I Relationships

Introduction

Health care is service oriented and requires constant interaction and communication with others. A limited radiographer's typical day involves talking with patients and their families, doctors, other medical personnel, and people in outside agencies and businesses. One must be able to interact and communicate with a variety of personalities and also be able to observe and listen in order to interpret verbal and nonverbal messages.

From the moment patients and visitors enter a medical facility, they begin to form opinions about the facility and the staff who provide services. Patient and visitor satisfaction often determines whether they will return to use a facility's services and often influences their recommendations about the facility to others (Pinette, 2003). If the limited radiographer, as well as other members of the health care team, adopts a policy of consumer satisfaction as a daily responsibility, everyone who has contact with the medical facility should have a positive image of the medical facility and staff. In the medical environment, professional image is reflected through individual and group behavior. In today's fast-paced medical setting, one may wonder if projecting a positive image and achieving consumer satisfaction are attainable on a daily basis. Why are these goals a challenge in health care settings? One explanation may be that the nature of the health care environment itself creates a stressful, demanding situation that poses threats and fosters fears, anxieties, and apprehensions.

Interpersonal Relationships with Patients

Limited radiographers generally serve two classifications of patients: those who are not ill or do not have any disease symptoms (asymptomatic patients) and those who exhibit disease symptoms (symptomatic patients). Asymptomatic patients may be in the medical facility to undergo a routine diagnostic examination. These patients may react and communicate differently from patients who are symptomatic and experiencing pain or discomfort. Differences between patients and their reasons for seeking medical care are key elements in the way patients perceive the medical environment. Most people will have some anxiety, apprehension, and fear of the unknown, yet the degree to which individuals experience these feelings is closely linked to their reason(s) for being a patient. Try to recall or imagine your personal feelings in the following situations:

- You are a patient for an annual checkup. You are in excellent physical condition and feel healthy.

- You are a patient for an examination. You have found a lump in your right breast during self-examination.
- You have smoked one pack of cigarettes every day since you were fourteen years old and have suddenly developed a cough.

The relationship of needs, perceptions, and behaviors can be further explained by considering the hierarchy of human needs.

Hierarchy of Human Needs. All humans have needs that must be met for both physiological and psychological survival and growth. Physiological needs are related to survival (food, water, air, shelter), whereas psychological needs relate to requirements for love, belonging, and self-esteem. Abraham Maslow, a famous psychologist, described these needs and ranked them in order of importance. Maslow's hierarchy of needs is usually illustrated in a pyramid form with fundamental physiological survival needs having priority over the psychological needs (Figure 2-1).

Maslow believed that people seek to satisfy their physiological needs first. Once these needs are met, people may proceed to fulfill higher-order psychological needs related to emotional and spiritual growth.

Maslow and other psychologists also found that if individuals are confronted with a life-threatening situation, they will defer their psychological needs to only those physiologic needs related to survival. This regression or letting go is linked to the primitive survival instinct. In the face of such events, the needs associated with survival generally take precedence over all other needs.

It is important to remember that a person's sense of belonging and feelings of well-being, security, and self-control may be compromised because of an illness. Showing concern—which can be as simple as being courteous—can help in such situations. Using friendly and encouraging words may help others to cope with stressful circumstances. "How are you feeling today?" "May I help you with your coat and umbrella?" "Please," and "Thank you" are all verbal indicators that you want to help and that you value the other person. A smile helps to show caring and a desire to help others.

All people, and especially patients, seek comfort, reassurance, and answers to their questions. They seek to restore balance to their lives by regaining control. Limited radiographers can meet such patient needs by simply taking time to be understanding.

Suggestions for Relating to Patients

- *Show Concern.* Provide a welcoming environment. Show concern by being an empathetic, nonjudgmental person. Concern can be expressed by a touch that

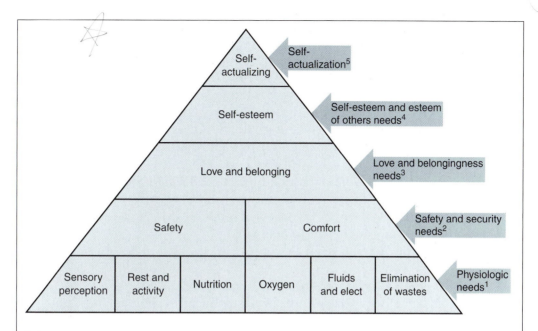

1. **Physiologic needs:** Basic life needs for food, shelter, air, water, sleep, and sexual fulfillment. Once these basic needs are satisfied, a person may pursue other needs.

2. **Safety and security needs:** After a person meets his/her physiologic needs, he/she begins to seek a safe place that is sheltered from harm.

3. **Love and belongingness needs:** Once the basic physiologic and safety and security needs are met, the person begins to seek someone to share life and acceptance in a social group.

4. **Self-esteem and the esteem of others needs:** Regard for self comes from positive feedback from others in society. Many emotional and physiological factors impact on self-regard and self-esteem. Before a person can grow and reach a higher level on the pyramid, the lower-level needs must be met and the person must feel a sense of stability and security.

5. **Self-actualization:** After all prior levels of needs have been met, the person begins to grow intellectually and spiritually. Human beings begin to question the nature of life and often seek to fulfill this question by performing humanitarian acts.

FIGURE 2-1 Hierarchy of basic needs according to Maslow
Source: Delmar, Cengage Learning.

shows support and encouragement. Don't hurry the patient or appear rushed to get to the next patient.

- *Show Empathy.* "Empathy is defined as the capacity to recognize or understand another's state of mind or emotion" (Webster's, 1994). "It is often characterized as the ability to 'put oneself into another's shoes,' or to in some way experience the outlook or emotions of another being within oneself" (Webster's, 1994). Empathy should not be confused with sympathy. Sympathy is expressed when one has a strong concern for the other person, whereas empathy is actually sharing another's suffering, if only briefly (Webster's, 1994).

- *Show Respect.* Showing respect to others is another way of providing a welcoming "We Care" environment. All sexes, races, religions, and socioeconomic levels are represented in any patient population. Respect can be verbalized in the way one talks to this diverse population and can be nonverbal via attitude and attention.
- *Show Caring.* Caring is demonstrated when the limited radiographer listens, provides information, helps, communicates, shows respect, touches, and protects (Church, 2004).
- Treat others as you would want to be treated.
- Treat all patients equally regardless of their sex, race, religion, or socioeconomic level.
- Remember children are people too.
- React professionally to what you see or hear while providing patient care.

Respect and concern can be shown by paying attention to detail. Details, often insignificant in a nonmedical environment, can take on great significance when a person is in a threatening or fearful situation. Loss of identity as an individual (Figure 2-2) and lack of privacy can threaten basic human needs. Use the patient's name and provide personal privacy whenever possible.

A person's needs and perceptions can predict the outcome of relationships and communication. Such needs and perceptions influence whether people are open to positive interpersonal relationships or unconsciously set up barriers. Table 2-1 shows positive and negative styles that have such influences.

Patient Advocacy

The limited radiographer is in a unique position to serve as a patient advocate. "Patient advocacy refers to speaking on behalf of a patient in order to protect their rights and help them obtain needed information and services" (Webster's, 1994). Limited radiographers serve as an advocate when they are acting in the patient's "best interest," whatever that might be, and are concerned with doing "good" for the patient (Ingram, 2008).

Advocacy in action takes many forms and includes such activities as respecting a person's privacy and ensuring patient safety during examinations. The limited radiographer serves as a patient advocate when proper radiation protection is applied and quality control procedures are observed (Church, 2004). Effective quality control

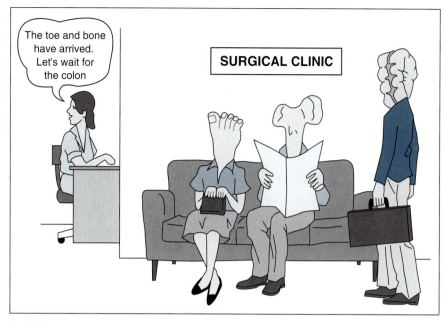

FIGURE 2-2 Professionals' view of patients. Using patients' names instead of calling them by a number, body part, or procedure shows respect and caring for them as individuals. (*From Purtilo, R.* (1990). Health Professional/Patient Interactions, *4th ed. Philadephia: W.B. Saunders Company, p. 169.*)

TABLE 2-1 Establishing Interpersonal Relationships

Positive Style (Open to Interpersonal Relationships)	Negative Style (Barriers to Interpersonal Relationships)
Silence	Commanding
Open-ended acknowledgment	Threatening
Listening	Advising
Feedback	Lecturing
Assertiveness	Criticizing
Problem-solving approach	Shaming
	Interpreting
	Sympathizing
	Interrogating
	Humoring

improves image quality, reduces retake examination, and provides diagnostic-quality radiographs for interpretation.

Limited radiographers also may serve as an advocate for special patient populations such as the elderly, pediatric, memory impaired, and the handicapped. Additional information about special needs patients is provided in Chapter 8, Basic Positioning and Special Needs Patients. Further information may be obtained about patient advocacy from the National Patient Advocate Foundation's website http://www.npaf.org.

Interpersonal Relationships with Physicians and Supervisors

A positive work relationship with physicians and immediate supervisors is important. To reach the medical team's objectives, everyone must be able to communicate effectively and be supportive of each other. This cannot occur when there is disrespect or even dislike for one another.

Suggestions:
- Provide positive feedback. Physicians and especially supervisors need to hear that they have done something right or good instead of wrong or bad. If you notice something that physicians or supervisors do that you consider right or good, tell them so. Encouragement and praise can be contagious.
- Address physicians by their title—"Doctor." This helps maintain a professional atmosphere.
- Give and expect common courtesy.
- In conversations with coworkers, patients, or others, reflect an attitude of confidence and support for the physician's professional integrity and ability.

Interpersonal Relationships with Others

Radiographers interact with a variety of people; these include company sales and service representatives, hospital/clinic or medical office staff, service workers, and visitors or patient family members. Everyone should be acknowledged and treated in a pleasant, agreeable manner. Visitors who do not accompany a patient should identify themselves and state the nature of their business. Generally, sales and service representatives or other business people will present a business card and explain the purpose of their visit. Every medical facility will operate differently, so it is necessary to find out how to greet and handle regular business callers and those who are unsolicited.

The key to effective interpersonal relationships with others is to treat each person as a valuable individual and to treat others as you would like to be treated.

PART II Communication

Introduction

In daily life, family members, coworkers, friends, and acquaintances may be able to communicate in loose, imprecise, and familiar ways because the social-personal history between the communicators in known and the circumstances surrounding the message mutually understood. However, in medical care settings, communication must be precise and results in understanding and agreement on what is wrong and what must be done as quickly and accurately as possible. The skill with which communication is accomplished may tilt a delicate relationship or attitude in one crucial direction or another.

Concepts of Communication

Communication may be defined as the exchange of information between two persons. The information is called a *message*. The person who communicates first is the *sender*, and the person to whom the communication is sent is called the *receiver*. The roles of sender and receiver may constantly change during the course of the interchange. This process is one form of communication and the receiver is more likely to interpret the information of the message correctly if the message is simple and precise. The sending and receiving process can become complicated and information misinterpreted because a person's tone, voice modulation, pauses, and nonverbal cues can express attitudes and emotions that the words do not convey. For example, consider the simple message "Close the window." Repeat this message several times, altering your tone of voice, pauses, and body language. Note how methods of expression and tone can confuse understanding of the real message. Imagine how a simple message like "Good morning" can be interpreted if the greeter slams a door immediately after the words are said!

Cultural Diversity

Culture, rather than genetics or biological differences, creates unique human societies (Pinette, 2003). Cultural diversity is a term used to express the cultural differences that exist between people, such as language, dress and traditions, and the way societies organize themselves (Webster's, 1994). It also refers to moral concepts and religious tenants and the way societies interact with the environment

(Webster's, 1994). For example, the Muslim culture dictates that no alcoholic beverages may be consumed, while the Japanese consume fish and soybeans as their main protein sources.

The United States has long been called a "melting pot," a phrase coined to describe the assimilation of large-scale immigration of peoples from many different countries. The U.S. Census Bureau estimates that in 2007, the foreign-born population reached an all-time high of 38.1 million, representing 12.6% of the U.S. population. Of these, about 12 million people, or 31% of all foreign-born, were born in Mexico (U.S. Census, 2008). In 2007, about 19.7% of the population age 5 and over spoke a language other than English at home. At least one-in-five residents of Arizona, California, New Mexico, and Texas spoke Spanish at home in 2007 (U.S. Census, 2008).

The first step in serving patients with dignity and respect is to acknowledge the differences that exist among various cultures. This will enable the limited radiographer to effectively provide services to patients and visitors of all cultures. Limited radiographers should continually strive to become knowledgeable of the belief practices, nutritional preferences, communication styles, and mode of dress requirements of different cultures that represent the population demographics served by the medical facility where they work.

Nonverbal Communication

In this type of communication the message is sent by facial gestures and body motions. A major issue with nonverbal communication is that these messages can be misinterpreted by others. One of the most important nonverbal techniques is eye contact or avoidance of eye contact. In America, looking the other person "straight in the eye" is considered to be the sign of an honest, truthful, sincere person. In Japan, eye contact during a conversation, especially between a subordinate and supervisor, would be considered an insult.

Visual messages such as facial expressions, are a factor in nonverbal communication and also in self-esteem. For example, facial expressions with a smile and the eyebrows raised can show happiness and offer reassurance; likewise, facial expressions with a frown and the head down can express fear and appear evasive or angry.

In addition to considering appropriate facial expressions for the medical environment, it is necessary to think about the radiographer's general verbal attitude. Is it too casual? Is there too much familiarity with patients or team workers (e.g., "Hi, Honey" or "Turn over, Honey.")? This type of familiarity can embarrass patients undergoing radiography procedures. Socializing with coworkers while performing procedures changes the tone of the encounter.

Communication for the Limited Radiographer

Physicians and their staff are increasingly challenged to provide high-quality care in the limited amount of time allotted for patient visits and examinations. Insufficient time with patients and staff shortages to handle the volume of patients are frequently cited as major causes of poor communication. Researchers report that building rapport and acknowledging the social and emotional concerns of patients can improve quality of care and efficiency, irrespective of the contact time (Nelson, 2008).

Communication, verbal and nonverbal, is how we present ourselves to others. The combination of what you say, how you say it, and your nonverbal cues while you are saying it form the basis of communication and the impression you make on others. The following are examples of everyday work activities that have such impact:

- Introducing yourself to others
- Giving and receiving messages
- Placing and receiving telephone calls
- Using the intercom system
- Consulting with coworkers, physicians, and supervisors
- Consulting with referring physicians and agencies
- Scheduling patients for radiographs
- Responding to patient concerns, questions, and statements
- Giving patients instructions
- Taking patient information
- Explaining radiographic procedures to patients
- Reporting to coworkers, supervisors, and physicians

A radiographer's most important tool is the ability to really observe what is happening when interacting with others. The words *look, hear,* and *feel* are very important when dealing with others. One does not have to ask, "How are you?" Observe the other person's complexion, posture, movement, etc.

Introducing Yourself to Others

In the medical environment, you are like a host or hostess. It is part of your job to greet others and introduce yourself. A usual introduction consists of the verbal exchange and nonthreatening body language.

An example of a verbal exchange is "Hello (Good morning, Good afternoon). I am Susan Spencer." Most facilities require that employees wear a name tag that lists name and job title so patients and others can quickly recall the name.

Body language should vary according to the age (or physical condition) of the person to whom you are introducing yourself. Greet adults face to face with an arm's-length distance between yourself and the other person. Distance is important in communication—if you are too close, you may threaten the other person's private space; if you are too far, you may convey a feeling of unfriendliness. Keep your arms and hands down by your side in a relaxed position. Extend your hand if the other person offers to shake hands. When you greet children, get down to the child's height. This technique can also be used for wheelchair patients.

Taking Messages

Health care providers should always have a pen and pad of paper handy so that oral messages can be written down. Commercial message pads are available that list all the essential parts of a message so a critical part will not be omitted—time, date, message content, name, and follow-up directions. Tips for writing messages are:

- Write the message.
- Repeat the message you have just written to check the accuracy of its content.
- Relay or act on the message.

Are you forgetful? If so, keep a bulletin board near your work area. Section off a small area and label messages "To Act On." Check this area several times a day.

Failure to promptly process messages or correctly communicate information contributes to an interruption of care and services, often causing patients to undergo additional treatments and testing. Medical errors often have fatal consequences that have been associated with ineffective communication between medical staff.

Talking with Coworkers, Physicians, and Supervisors

Limited radiographers will talk with coworkers, physicians, and supervisors about many things. It is important to remember that if you have a question about a radiography request or any aspect of a procedure, *never* proceed until you seek assistance. There are situations in which the limited radiographer must seek assistance from the supervisor. Knowing when this is necessary comes from recognizing and understanding the chain of command.

A chain of command, formal or informal, exists in every work environment. The physician is usually the leader and may employ a supervisor to direct and manage the health care team. The physician or supervisor leads the team in providing services and meeting objectives. Limited radiographers may be surrounded by authorities who have varying priorities and time-line expectations. The chain of command concept helps address this confusing situation in a positive way by designating one person as supervisor. The supervisor, who knows the overall goals and objectives, focuses the team's efforts on the priorities to be accomplished. For the chain-of-command concept to work and for all team members to be a functioning part of the group, effective communication and relay of information between and among members must be maintained in a systematic way. A chain of command provides a network system and prevents details and important tasks from being overlooked.

If at any time grievances, complaints, or suggestions need to be discussed, the limited radiographer should take these matters to the immediate supervisor. It is okay to have a grievance or complaint, but the chain of command, not an open public arena, should be used to communicate such issues. Employee, coworker, and supervisor communication, if conducted with candor and a problem-solving attitude (identifying what may be unsatisfactory and correcting it if possible), can be very helpful in improving work relationships. This type of interchange tends to identify and solve problems before they become unsolvable.

Using "I" messages is effective when you are giving criticism, explaining a problem, making a suggestion, or expressing an opinion. "I" messages do not make others feel offended or put them in a defensive position. There are two parts to the "I" message: the first part describes your feelings and the second part describes the desired change. The example shown in Table 2-2 illustrates how an "I" message is more effective in communicating a problem than a "You" message.

Talking with Referring Physicians and Agencies

Limited radiographers may have to talk with referring physicians and persons from agencies such as hospitals, nursing homes, or radiology clinics. The following tips should help you perform such tasks efficiently:

- Organize information and questions before contacting the referring physician or agency.
- Gather all facts and needed documents.

TABLE 2-2   "I" Messages

"You" Message (Blames Others)	"I" Message (First Part) Describes Feelings	"I" Message (Second Part) Describes Desired Change
"You really make me mad."	"I'm feeling upset about this."	"I would like to talk with you and see if we can't work this out."

- Briefly write down key points.
- Make telephone contact.
- Identify yourself, facility, and reasons for the contact.
- Make notes of necessary information. Review with contact.
- Thank contact for his/her time.
- Chart information if necessary.

Scheduling and Preparation Considerations

Often a patient must be scheduled for multiple x-ray examinations. If contrast media is used, the x-ray examinations must be scheduled in the correct sequence so that residual barium will not be present to obscure anatomic structures of clinical interest. A common rule is: those x-ray examinations whose contrast media is excreted quickly and completely should be scheduled first. The following provides a sequence for scheduling x-ray examinations and those exams that can be performed together.

Sequence: Intravenous Pyleogram (IVP), Gallbladder, Barium Enema, and Upper Gastro-intestinal (UGI)

Exams that can be performed together: Gallbladder and IVP, IVP and Barium Enema, and Gallbladder and UGI

Responding to Patient Concerns, Questions, and Statements

Limited radiographers are not expected to know all the answers and many times may not be able to release certain information because of confidentiality. However, it is important to always acknowledge patient questions and statements and be perceptive regarding concerns and fears. Effective listening and paraphrasing techniques allow you to respond verbally to patients without appearing curt or that you are withholding the information requested.

Paraphrasing means repeating what a person has said to you but using slightly different words. Paraphrasing a statement helps to determine whether the message has been understood as it was intended (Table 2-3).

TABLE 2-3 Paraphrasing

Patient's Statement	Radiographer's Paraphrase
"You know, when I fell I hit my knee rather hard and it hurts more than the ankle you are x-raying."	"Are you saying that your knee hurts more than your ankle?"

Giving Patient Instructions

Limited radiographers often find themselves giving instructions to patients. These instructions may be as simple as where to find the restroom or as complex as how to take self-administered medication for an outpatient examination. Patients suffer the consequences when instructions are not given clearly or when they do not fully understand directions. The following tips should help you give patients instructions clearly and accurately:

1. Speak slowly.
2. In case of complex instructions, have a written copy of the instructions for the patient. Instructions you give repeatedly to patients should be printed to save time. This also gives patients a handy reference source if they have questions after they leave the facility.
3. Repeat instructions if necessary.
4. Ask the patient to repeat instructions back to you.
5. Ask for questions. Don't appear hurried. Wait. Answer all questions.
6. Never assume that everyone can read.

Taking Patient Information

Patient information is personal and confidential. Provide for privacy. If you must take patient information in an area where others are waiting, be discreet and use a soft voice. Use simple words and double check information. Often, limited radiographers ask questions of a very personal nature, such as (to a female patient), "Could you be pregnant? When was your last menstrual period?" Avoid an unpleasant communication interchange, keep your voice tone low, move closer to the patient to indicate that a question is private. Go further than just the question. You may want to explain briefly how the question relates to radiographic examinations.

Explaining Radiography Procedures to Patients

Limited radiographers need to be able to explain to the patient the nature of the radiography procedures. This usually consists of simple factual information. After identifying the patient as the correct patient, the radiographer may say, "Hello, my name is Elana Brown. I'm going to take the x-rays of your right arm that Dr. Christopher ordered." If the patient shows concern over radiation exposure, you will be able to explain briefly how collimation works and give assurance when you place the protective lead apron across the patient's lap.

If at any time the patient indicates an error, such as "It's not my right arm that needs the x-ray, it's my left arm," or refuses to have the x-ray examination, STOP and check with your supervisor or the physician. Never proceed with a radiographic procedure if there is a question about the exact nature of the procedure or if the patient refuses.

Mistakes are often made because of miscommunication. Often, this results from not listening to what others are saying. Listening skills are a critical key to effective communication. Limited radiographers need good listening skills not only when receiving directions from physicians and supervisors but also when gathering information and facts from patients and coworkers. Good listeners do not interrupt when others are talking. Also, good listeners use paraphrasing techniques (see Table 2-3) in order to determine if they understand the message.

Reporting to Coworkers, Physicians, and Supervisors

Limited radiographers and other health care providers may be with a patient longer than the physician is and may detect things that need to be reported. If a patient's condition changes during a radiographic procedure, report the change immediately to the physician. Reporting is usually oral but may require written documentation in the patient record. Reporting tips follow.

- Think first. Be specific. What needs to be reported?
- Report to the appropriate person. (*Never* leave a patient unattended while reporting a change in condition.)

Recognizing Common Barriers to Communication

Ideally, if everyone recognized common barriers to communication, everyday tasks could be achieved with greater understanding and less effort. However, that is not often the case. Limited radiographers especially need to overcome such barriers, not only when barriers originate in the patient, but also when they are self-initiated. A few common barriers to communication are:

- Poor eye contact
- Interrupting the other person before s/he is finished speaking
- Poor listening skills
    Thinking ahead instead of listening
    Pretending to listen
    Misunderstanding
    Ignoring what is said
- Poor oral-verbal skills
    Fear of speaking up
    Rudely disagreeing
    Criticizing instead of explaining

REVIEW QUESTIONS

1. Asymptomatic patients are those who are not ill or do not have any disease symptoms.
   a. True
   b. False

2. Psychological needs relate to requirements for:
   1. self-esteem
   2. food and water
   3. love and belonging
   4. air and shelter

   Possible Responses
   a. 1 and 4
   b. 1 and 3
   c. 2 and 3
   d. 1, 2, & 3

3. Abraham Maslow described the:
   a. structure of cells
   b. planetary orbitals
   c. x-ray interaction with matter
   d. hierarchy of human needs

4. The outcome of relationships and communication is often influenced by a person's:
   a. needs
   b. perceptions
   c. expectations
   d. all of the above

5. The capacity to recognize or understand another's state of mind or emotion is:
   a. projection
   b. illusion
   c. empathy
   d. sympathy

6. A patient advocate is someone who speaks on behalf of a patient in order to protect the patient's rights and help them obtain needed information and services.
   a. True
   b. False

7. **All** of the following are examples of a positive communication style, **except**:
   a. listening
   b. shaming
   c. giving feedback
   d. problem solving

8. The U.S. Census Bureau estimates that in 2007, the foreign-born population was ___ million.
   a. 1.5
   b. 28.3
   c. 38.1
   d. 45

9. Examinations that can be performed together include:
   a. gallbladder (GB) and intravenous pyleogram (IVP)
   b. IVP and barium enema (BE)
   c. gallbladder (GB) and upper gastro-intestinal (UGI)
   d. All of the above

10. Common barriers to communication include:
    1. poor eye contact
    2. active listening
    3. interruption
    4. criticizing instead of explaining

    Possible Responses
    a. 1 and 3
    b. 2 and 4
    c. 3 and 4
    d. 1, 3, & 4

REFERENCES

Church, E. (2004) Patient advocacy: the technologist's role. *Radiologic Technology, 75*(4), 272–289.

Ingram, R. (1998). The nurse as the patient's advocate. Retrieved, from http://www.richard.ingram.nhspeople.net 1–7.

Nelson, R. (2008) Improving communication skills enhances efficiency and patient-clinician relationships. *Medscape Medical News.* Retrieved, from http://www.medscape.com

Pinette, S. (2003). Productivity and quality patient care. *Radiologic Technology, 74*(55), 413–423.

U.S. Census Bureau. Newsroom. (2008) *One-in-five speak Spanish in four states: New census bureau data show how America lives.* Retrieved from http://www.census.gov

Webster's II New Riverside University Dictionary. (1994). Boston: Houghton Mifflin Company.

SUGGESTED READINGS

Anderson, K. (2005). On the cutting edge of cultural competency. *ASRT Scanner 38*(3).

Ater, J. (2001). Communication breakdown hidden hazards that could jeopardize healthcare. *RT-Image 14*(15).

Brewner, M. M., McMahon, W. C., & Roche, M. P. (1984). *Job Survival Skills.* New York: Educational Designs, Inc.

Casanas, J. (2004). Navigating the cultural divide. *RT-Image 17*(13).

Chenevert, M. (1978). *Special Techniques in Assertiveness Training for Women in the Health Professions.* St. Louis: C.V. Mosby Co.

Goldstein, L. (1998). Tailoring care to patient's needs. *Radiologic Technology 70*(3).

Newman, J. (1998). Managing cultural diversity: the art of communication. *Radiologic Techechnology 69*(3).

Purtilo, R. (1984). *Health Professional/Patient Interactions* (3d ed.). Philadelphia: W.B. Saunders Company.

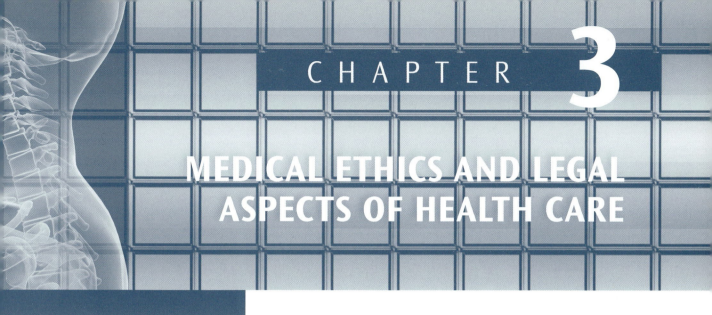

CHAPTER 3

MEDICAL ETHICS AND LEGAL ASPECTS OF HEALTH CARE

Key Terms

Administrative Regulations
Americans With Disabilities Act (ADA)
Assault
Autonomy
Battery
Beneficence
Bioethics
Biomedical Ethics
Code of Ethics
Confidentiality
Common Law
Constitutional Law
Defamation
Ethics
False Imprisonment
Gross Negligence
Health Insurance Portability and Accountability Act (HIPAA)
Implied Consent
Informed Consent
Justice
Mental Capacity
Negligence
Nonmaleficence
Philosophy
Professional Ethics
Re Ipsa Loquitur
Statutes
Torts

Chapter Outline

Radiographs as Permanent Records
Releasing Films
Informed Consent Forms
Radiation Safety

Objectives

Upon completion of the chapter, the student will meet the following objectives by verifying knowledge of the facts and principles presented through oral and written communication at a level deemed competent.

⊃ Briefly define professional education according to views based on educational philosophy.
⊃ Identify criteria of a true profession and the relationship of a true profession to ethics and medical ethics.
⊃ Briefly define philosophy.
⊃ Define moral ethics, biomedical ethics, and professional ethics.
⊃ Differentiate between legal/moral concepts.
⊃ Define given terms applicable to legal radiography issues.
⊃ Explain the radiographer's code of ethics.
⊃ Identify and discuss the AHA Patient's Bill of Rights.
⊃ Describe certain policies and procedures that must be established for performing radiographic procedures.
⊃ Identify and discuss compliance with health care laws.

Introduction

Some ideas are merely timely whereas others are timeless. The views of McGlothlin (1960) and Pellegrino (1983) expressed in the following paragraphs belong in the latter category. Neither their philosophies nor their definitions are obsolete; rather, they are as applicable today as when they were written and continue to represent the charge of health professional practice, the description of true professions, and identification of ethical considerations related to medical professional practice.

In his book *Patterns of Professional Education*, McGlothlin identified the major focus of professional education in medicine, nursing, law, teaching, social work, and clinical psychology as direct contact with people—people who are patients, students, or clients and who need help solving their problems. He called these professions, very simply, "helping professions." He said that professional education had two aims: (1) to supply enough professional people to help (quantity) and (2) to assure society that they (professionals) are competent (quality).

In 1983 (23 years later), Edmund Pellegrino, in *"What is a Profession?" Journal of Allied Health*, described true professions as those that deal with humans when they are most vulnerable and when they lack the knowledge to make their own decisions. Thus the professional-patient relationship is not of equal power, because generally all the knowledge is on the side of the professional and the need for help is on the patient's side.

Pellegrino further described true professions as being set apart from sociological structures by philosophical definitions. Relatedly, many occupations that were once regarded as crafts, arts, trades, and commerce have developed many elements associated with traditional professions:

- setting standards for entry
- defining specific skills or knowledge
- establishing educational requirements and curriculum
- forming national organizations
- publishing journals
- setting fees and standards for performance
- setting codes of ethics

All of these elements arise from social accountability. The article points out other elements, however, that constitute higher moral and ethical codes. These evolve from philosophical definitions created by the special nature of human relations when people are vulnerable (sick) and in need. It is clear that the fundamental concepts of health professionals and their ethical education change very little in terms of purpose. Before we consider the philosophy that constitutes medical ethics, let us first look at radiography in the professional perspective.

Development of a Profession

Professions deal with people and are bound both by sociological structures and by the need to have a higher moral and ethical code that addresses two additional components: (1) ethics and (2) behavior (or manners). Irvin M. Borish states that a true profession evolves in stages and comes to possess three criteria: (1) developed specialized skills, (2) a humane code of ethics, and (3) ethical respect from society as an honorable vocation (Borish, 1983).

In light of what Borish holds to be criteria for a true profession, does radiography measure up to the definition? With many clinical specialties, administrators, and educators, radiographers form a highly diverse and specialized group. Compared to some other codes of ethics, the code adopted by the radiography profession is very humane and addresses standards of conduct. With regard to respect from society, does society value radiography as an honorable profession? Do people know who radiographers are and what they do? Who communicates that message? Radiographers must communicate the message, each of us, in whatever role we play—general or limited radiographer, specialist, administrator, or educator. No one else will carry the message for us.

Definitions of Philosophy and Ethics

Philosophy

Most of us assume that we practice appropriate behavior and that we understand what ethical behavior is. This is generally true in a society that attempts to philosophically understand all behavior and also attempts to teach that understanding. Philosophy deals with the search for truth, the general understanding of values and reality. Many areas are included in philosophy: aesthetics (nature of beauty), epistemology (how knowledge is gained), ethics (what is good and bad; moral duty and obligation), and metaphysics (study of what really exists).

Ethics is the area concerned with the examination of human behavior. There are good and bad behaviors and there are times when we are bound by a certain duty or obligation. From the time we are old enough to understand, we begin to learn the difference between right and wrong and that we all are expected to use reasonable care in our behavior toward others.

Ethics

By definition, ethics refers to the study of human behavior which involves the study of various cultures, religions, groups, and individuals in a systematic way. It is important to try to understand that all persons who require health care will not have the same attitude toward the health care delivery system.

Biomedical ethics, or bioethics, involves the knowledge and application of modern medical technologies. Professional ethics relates to standards of conduct, dealing with duties, and the rights and obligations of practitioners. It requires that moral judgments and values be based on reason and that individuals carefully consider and take responsibility for their own actions.

Medical Ethics

If we consider professional codes of ethics as "a systematic collection of regulations and rules of procedure or conduct" (*The American Heritage Dictionary*, 1991, p. 287) and then think in terms of those members being in the medical profession, we find that many of the rules and regulations are general to all disciplines and specialty areas that comprise the medical profession. Although the following discussion does not pretend to address all the rules or standards relevant to ethical behavior for the health care provider, let us look at several elements relevant to medical ethics.

First, a trusting relationship must be established between the patient and the health care provider (radiographer). Some essential elements in building trust are protecting patients' rights at all times, recognizing the psychological state of patients, realizing that each patient is unique, and exhibiting respect and cooperation in interpersonal relationships with patients and other health care providers.

There are four principles on which trusting relationships are based: (1) autonomy, (2) beneficence, (3) nonmaleficence, and (4) justice. These four principles largely record the basis for developing various forms and writing health policies and documents, certain rules and regulations, and privacy policies that are required by all health care facilities. Students and/or health care professionals may review these forms and documents at a health care facility upon appropriate request.

Autonomy

Autonomy is the freedom to govern self and to make one's own decisions according to one's own moral principles. Individual reasons for actions are personal. If we look at each person as an end in himself/herself, then we see that that person has an inherent right to be respected or treated as an autonomous or self-governing individual. In medical ethics, autonomy is viewed as the right of patients to determine what will be done with their own bodies. Two critical elements that arise out of autonomy are informed consent and confidentiality.

Informed Consent. This is recognized as an individual's right to autonomy. Informed consent means that certain standards of disclosure must be followed to assure a patient's full understanding about a medical procedure or treatment. Standards of disclosure include the following, but may vary with facilities:

1. The patient must receive sufficient information in terms he or she can understand.
2. Details of the procedure or treatment must be outlined and discussed.
3. Potential risks and benefits of the procedure or treatment must be disclosed.
4. All available alternatives must be considered and discussed.

Valid informed consent may be determined when:

1. All information according to standards of disclosure has been adequately communicated.
2. The patient has the **mental capacity** to understand all information and can make a fair informed decision.
3. Consent for the treatment or procedure is given voluntarily.

Even though the duty of obtaining an informed consent may be delegated to other trained personnel, the physician who is performing the procedure is ultimately responsible for obtaining and assessing that informed consent has been correctly conducted and completed.

Consent of Minors.   Factors that determine whether a minor's consent to a medical or surgical procedure is legally effective are maturity, age of minor, and emancipation. Consent for performing a procedure on a minor must be obtained from a parent or parents or from someone acting in *loco parentis*, i.e., a supervisor or guardian. Emancipation describes a minor who is married or lives independent of a parent or parents (emancipated from his or her parents). Most states do not require parental consent for medical or surgical procedures if the minor is emancipated.

Mental Capacity.   Generally, a person may not be judged competent for reasons of age, mental illness, debilitating disease, or for any other reason that results in diminished capacity to make a rational decision. A person may be declared legally incompetent through a judicial proceeding and a legal guardian appointed where no legal guardian exists and the physician determines the person to be incompetent. Even though the person may give consent, consent from the spouse or nearest relative should also be obtained.

Implied Consent.   **Implied consent** is an exception to the rule of informed consent. Implied consent refers to a situation in which a person is unconscious or when a life-threatening emergency exists and no one is available to provide legal permission. It may be assumed in such a situation that because it is an emergency, under normal conditions the patient would give consent to save his or her life or to prevent permanent health impairment. If the patient, however, has previously refused treatment prior to the existence of the situation at issue, implied consent is not valid.

Confidentiality.   **Confidentiality** is the patient's basic right to privacy. Confidentiality involves legal as well as ethical considerations. Although not deliberate in many cases, confidentiality is generally the most commonly abused aspect of ethics. Health care providers have a tendency to discuss among themselves what they see and hear. However, they are not expected to discuss any disease or condition or its prognosis with the patient or anyone else. If asked such questions by the patient, the radiographer should explain, "I don't know the answer to that, but your doctor will be happy to discuss it with you."

Confidentiality is the basis for development and implementation of the Health Insurance Portability and Accountability Act (HIPAA), which will be discussed later in this chapter.

Beneficence and Nonmaleficence

Beneficence relates to duty of others to provide or improve conditions that promote physical and emotional well-being. Nonmaleficence refers to preventing or not causing harm intentionally (i.e., physical assault) or not subjecting another to harm. To illustrate how medical decisions sometimes involve issues of beneficence or nonmaleficence, let us consider the medical professional confronted with the situation of a terminally ill patient. Can/should enough drugs to reduce the severity of pain to a comfortable stage be given when, if given, the drugs may hasten death or cause drug addiction? Is it more important that the patient be made comfortable by reducing her/his pain (beneficence) or be put at risk of being harmfully subjected to drug addiction or even early death (nonmaleficence—do no harm)?

Justice

Justice deals with the balancing and fair distribution of medical care, facilities, and resources for society. Simply stated, justice in this sense refers to distributive justice and requires that all economic goods and services be equally distributed unless an unequal distribution would be of greater benefit to all. In some situations, institutions may consider the needs of the poor or those who have less before they consider the needs of more fortunate groups.

To be sure, the poor, the imprisoned, the lonely, and the rejected are also deprived of the full expression of their humanity, so much so, that men in these conditions may long for death to liberate them. But none save saints seeks illness as a road to liberation. The poor man can still hope for a change of fortune, the prisoner for a reprieve, the lonely for a friend. But the ill person remains impaired even when freed of these other constraints and the free exercise of his humanity (Pellegrino quoted in Kestenbaum, 1982, p. 159).

Law for the Radiographer

The intent of this chapter is to deal with some legal concepts as they generally apply to health care delivery. To attempt a wide-scale, in-depth explanation of the law as it specifically applies to limited radiography in all states would be a major project and beyond the scope of this book. Also, ethical and legal concepts must be situationally applied, according to a particular incident, location, persons involved, and many other elements.

The past several years have seen a steadily increasing need for health care professionals to become knowledgeable about the legal implications of medical practice. In most allied health disciplines, students participating in clinical area learning activities must provide proof of malpractice insurance. Issues relating to malpractice are critical to the health worker. Therefore, it is important to have some general knowledge of the structure of law.

Four Types of Law

There are four types of law: (1) *statutes,* (2) *administrative regulations,* (3) *common law,* and (4) *constitutional law.*

Statutes are laws. They are the principles and rules that are enacted by legislative bodies, such as the Congress of the United States or state legislative bodies. Statutory laws may be amended, expanded, or repealed by the legislative bodies.

Administrative regulations are written by boards or agencies that have been established by legislative bodies for areas where certain kinds of expertise are required to develop specific regulations. Licensing of hospitals, nursing homes, physicians, nurses, and radiographers are some areas where legislators rely on administrative agencies. The regulations are as legally binding as any law the legislators enact.

Common law is a system of applied law and usually develops in the absence of codified written laws or laws enacted through legislation (pertinent statutes). Common law is based on court (i.e., judges') decisions and legal principles and opinion-set precedents considered in those decisions; judges' written opinions often reflect the doctrines of common law. Much common law has evolved over the years and serves to help make decisions in subsequent cases. Common law is legally binding when it is not in conflict with other laws.

Constitutional law is the highest order of law; it is the branch of public law of a nation or state. In matters of constitutional law, the courts do not make law, rather they determine whether a law agrees or is consistent with the constitution of a nation or particular state. If a law is determined to be unconstitutional, it is declared invalid.

Ethical/Legal Behavior

By definition, ethical behavior relates to moral or good conduct (i.e., what is right to do). Legal behavior is what the law or government says we have to do. There are distinctly legal and distinctly moral issues involved in providing medical services. Sometimes what must be done and what should be done become entangled. For example, take the case of a hospital refusing to accept a child who later dies. The hospital had no legal obligation to accept the child, but few people would dispute it may have had a moral obligation to do so. Also consider the case of the physician who has to make the decision to assist or not to assist an injured motorist on the highway.

If the physician decides to assist, he or she assumes the legal obligation of reasonable care and personal liability. However, even under Good Samaritan laws, which vary from state to state, the physician has no legal obligation to assist. The nature or purpose of a Good Samaritan statute is to encourage voluntary medical assistance to strangers in an emergency situation. Thus, the doctor's decision may depend on ethical or moral values. When health care professionals perform their duties, their actions do have an effect on such issues as patients' autonomy, beneficence, nonmaleficence, and justice; because these actions involve moral behavior, they sometimes result in problems that require legal answers.

Professional disciplines, such as radiography, are expected to establish their own moral standards of behavior based on common thinking. In light of so much litigation regarding medical procedures, complex modern medical technology, and patients' rights, the trend is that law is becoming more concretely intermingled with codes of ethics.

Codes of Ethics

Two examples of professional codes of ethics are frequently used to illustrate specific standards of professional conduct: the American Medical Association Principles of Medical Ethics and the American Nurses' Association Code. The American Society of Radiologic Technologists Code of Ethics is another specifically written document. All three of these documents are good examples of how aspects of duties, ideals, values, and goals of the professional can be expressed. Historically, professional codes have not been utilized and/or may not have contained appropriate language. Such terms as *fairness*, *justice*, *equality*, *duties*, and *rights* have not been used or their meaning has been only vaguely defined. Written codes of ethics are important because they may help bring about professional autonomy, which is appropriate as long as the intent is to better serve and improve the health care delivery system, not to be self-serving.

Currently, there is no code of ethics specifically written for limited radiographers. It would therefore be prudent for limited radiographers to recognize and follow the existing code of ethics written and adopted by the American Society of Radiologic Technologists.

The Code of Ethics for the Profession of Radiologic Technology was developed and adopted by the American Society of Radiologic Technologists and the American Registry of Radiologic Technologists (Figure 3-1). As you read the Code of Ethics, you should recognize some areas that reflect the previous discussion on the theory of ethics.

CODE OF ETHICS

1. The radiologic technologist conducts herself or himself in a professional manner, responds to patient needs, and supports colleagues and associates in providing quality patient care.

2. The radiologic technologist acts to advance the principal objective of the profession to provide services to humanity with full respect for the dignity of mankind.

3. The radiologic technologist delivers patient care and service unrestricted by the concerns of personal attributes or the nature of the disease or illness, and without discrimination on the basis of sex, race, creed, religion, or socio-economic status.

4. The radiologic technologist practices technology founded upon theoretical knowledge and concepts, uses equipment and accessories consistent with the purposes for which they were designed, and employs procedures and techniques appropriately.

5. The radiologic technologist assesses situations; exercises care, discretion, and judgment; assumes responsibility for professional decisions; and acts in the best interest of the patient.

6. The radiologic technologist acts as an agent through observation and communication to obtain pertinent information for the physician to aid in the diagnosis and treatment of the patient and recognizes that interpretation and diagnosis are outside the scope of practice for the profession.

7. The radiologic technologist uses equipment and accessories, employs techniques and procedures, performs services in accordance with an accepted standard of practice, and demonstrates expertise in minimizing radiation exposure to the patient, self, and other members of the healthcare team.

8. The radiologic technologist practices ethical conduct appropriate to the profession and protects the patient's right to quality radiologic technology care.

9. The radiologic technologist respects confidences entrusted in the course of professional practice, respects the patient's right to privacy, and reveals confidential information only as required by law or to protect the welfare of the individual or the community.

10. The radiologic technologist continually strives to improve knowledge and skills by participating in continuing education and professional activities, sharing knowledge with colleagues, and investigating new aspects of professional practice.

FIGURE 3-1 ASRT code of ethics

Revised and Adopted by the American Society of Radiologic Technologists and the American Registry of Radiologic Technologists, February 2003.

Legal/Ethical Definitions

Before briefly discussing the procedural aspects of radiology, some ethical/legal definitions pertinent to limited radiographer interaction with patients and limited radiographer/patient relationships need to be clarified.

Assault. Assault is any willful attempt or threat to inflict injury upon the person of another, when coupled with an apparent present ability to do so, and any intentional display of force such as would give the victim reason to fear or expect immediate bodily harm.

Battery. Battery is any unlawful touching of another that is without justification or excuse.

The ethical concept related to assault and battery is autonomy. Patients must be given full disclosure (informed consent) about what procedure is going to be performed on their bodies. Otherwise, actions toward them could be perceived as intending harm or as touching their bodies without permission.

False Imprisonment. False imprisonment is the conscious restraint of the freedom of another without proper authorization, privilege, or consent of that individual.

The ethical concept related to false imprisonment is again autonomy. No one has the right to physically restrain another against his/her will or without permission. The best approach to immobilizing or restraining a patient who may move during exposure is to discuss the procedure directly with the patient. In the case of children, seek parental permission. The two occasions where restraint is justified are (1) when the patient may pose a physical threat to the limited radiographer and (2) when the patient may pose a physical threat to himself/herself.

Negligence. Negligence is the omission to do something that a reasonable person (guided by those considerations which ordinarily regulate human affairs) would do, or the doing of something that a reasonable and prudent person would not do.

The related ethical concept deals with the basic duty or obligation to do that which is correct or to behave in a reasonable manner. Negligence is probably the most common cause of litigation. But to prove negligence, the plaintiff must establish four facts: (1) that a duty existed, (2) that a duty was breached, (3) that an injury occurred, and (4) that the breach of duty was the proximate cause of the injury. Negligence is usually determined by assessing how something is customarily done by persons (for example, radiographers) in a similar situation performing a similar procedure (radiographic procedures).

Gross Negligence. Gross negligence involves a stronger case of duty. It is intentional failure to perform a manifest duty in reckless disregard of the consequences as affecting the life or property of another.

The related ethical concept is to do no harm (i.e., nonmaleficence). Possibly the strongest determinant for gross negligence is foreseeability. If a situation is clearly a threat or is dangerous to others, and no action is taken to correct the hazard or risk, then one may be held personally accountable for disregard of how others may be affected by a foreseeable hazard. Negligence may be unintentional or gross, which is intentional. Both are wrongful acts and are legally classified as torts.

Defamation. Defamation is the act of bringing harm to another person's reputation through libel (written word) or slander (spoken word).

Defamation is related ethically to confidentiality and is probably the most commonly abused rule of professional conduct. Respecting and protecting the patient's right to privacy (autonomy) is the responsibility of all health care providers. Discussing a patient's medical condition (e.g., AIDS) unnecessarily with another person could be determined as a defamation of character.

Res Ipsa Loquitur. Res ipsa loquitur or "the thing speaks for itself" is a situation where the injured person in no way contributed to her/his injury. That is, the whole incident was under the control of the offender or defendant. Again, negligence becomes obvious. The ethical concept of nonmaleficence is related to res ipsa loquitur, which is not to cause harm intentionally (negligence) or not to subject another to harm.

Patients' Rights

One of the most important documents to become familiar with in today's health care delivery is the Patient's Bill of Rights. The document is based on both the ethical and legal concepts of autonomy and most of its principles deal with confidentiality and informed consent.

The following eight principal areas of patients' rights and responsibilities were identified by the Advisory Commission on Consumer Protection and Quality in the Health Care Industry appointed by the President in 1997.

    I. Information Disclosure
   II. Choice of Providers and Plans
  III. Access to Emergency Services

A full copy of the document (Consumer Bill of Rights and Responsibilities) can be accessed at http://www.opm.gov/insure/health/billrights/asp.

Compliance with Health Laws

All radiography departments, medical offices, or other health care facilities must comply with health care laws . Two of the most important applicable laws are the **Americans with Disabilities Act (ADA)** and the **Health Insurance Portability and Accountability Act (HIPAA).**

ADA. This law, enacted in 1990, is intended to protect persons with disabilities. It guarantees the civil rights of persons with disabilities in the United States. Information regarding federal disability legislation may be accessed at "A Guide to Disability Rights Laws" at the Department of Justice web page www.ada.gov/cguide.htm.

The ADA prohibits discrimination on the basis of disability in employment, state and local government, public accommodations, commercial facilities, transportation, and telecommunications. It also applies to the United States Congress.

To be protected by the ADA, one must have a disability or association with an individual with a disability. An individual with a disability is defined by the ADA as a person who has a physical or mental impairment that substantially limits one or more major life activities, a person who has a history or record of such impairment, or a person who is perceived by others as having such an impairment. The ADA does not specifically name all impairments that may be covered.

Some impairments are more easily recognized than others, such as the loss of sight or physical mobility. The ADA omitted definitions and examples of three need-to-know terms—significant/insignificant, major/minor, and reasonable/unreasonable—leaving it to the legal system to determine these boundaries.

Regardless of the exact definitions of the need-to-know terms, the first responsibility of the medical radiographer in caring for patients is to determine whether the patient has any special needs that require attention during diagnostic imaging procedures. The ADA requires only reasonable accommodations, which are those that do not impose an undue hardship on the medical facility. The radiographer should make a commitment to providing appropriate care for disabled patients to the extent possible during every radiographic procedure.

In many cases, accommodating a disabled patient requires only spending a little more time and making a higher-level effort than providing the same service to a patient who is not disabled. Asking patients when they make an appointment if they need any type of special assistance or determining the nature of any disability prior to the office visit usually allows the radiographer to plan for the additional assistance required. The following are examples of what might be required to accommodate ADA-covered patients.

Effective communication is the key to providing quality care to patients. Accommodating a hearing-impaired patient for a radiographic procedure may involve writing down instructions, asking and answering questions in writing, and communicating with gestures and pointing. A medical care facility may employ an interpreter or train at least one staff member to communicate in sign language. Also, many hearing-impaired persons may have a health care advocate who communicates in sign language and accompanies them on medical care visits.

A vision-impaired patient will need to have written instructions and information read aloud or have access to Braille versions. The radiographer may be required to fill in any paper forms the patient must submit. The radiographer may also need to lead the patient through unfamiliar rooms, halls, and corridors. Ensuring patient safety is of the utmost importance and the radiographer has a key responsibility during the diagnostic imaging procedure.

Accommodating wheelchair-bound patients may be difficult because of stairs and doorways and negotiating space in the diagnostic imaging room. Several accommodations may be workable for the wheelchair-bound patient. The radiographer will have to use judgment in choosing an accommodation consistent with the individual patient's needs without presenting a safety or health risk to the patient or anyone else. Variable ADA-covered patient circumstances may result in a radiographer taking much longer to perform an examination; such variables may include but not be limited to:

- the complexity of the directions or information the radiographer has to read to, write for, or sign to a vision- or hearing-impaired patient;
- the degree of difficulty associated with the positioning of the body required for the procedure; or
- the amount of cooperation provided by the patient and his/her caregivers.

The ADA does not require a medical facility to make unreasonable accommodations—ones that would cause the facility an undue hardship. The cost of accommodations relative to how much the facility makes is a consideration when assessing a particular facility's obligations under the ADA. The purpose of the ADA is to ensure that disabled Americans receive fair treatment from all members of society, including health care professionals and organizations. Compliance is not only legally necessary, it also gives the radiographer the opportunity to provide quality patient care and customer satisfaction. Taking special care of disabled persons has always been a part of health care providers' responsibility. Enactment of the ADA provided recourse for disabled persons who are not provided reasonable assistance and accommodations when they seek health care.

HIPAA. The federal law known as the Health Insurance Portability and Accountability Act (HIPAA), enacted in 1996, was written and implemented to provide (a) health insurance reform (Title I) and (b) administrative simplification (Title II), that is, establishment of national standards for collection and documentation of health information or privacy of information, known as protected health information (PHI). The health reform provisions principally affect radiographers as consumers—ability to get health coverage for self and family, maintenance of existing health coverage through employer or individual health insurance, and maintenance of continuous health coverage during a job change as well as protection in areas related to pre-existing condition exclusions, discrimination related to past or present poor health, right to purchase health insurance, and renewal of coverage regardless of health conditions.

Regardless of HIPAA provisions, health insurance coverage varies widely under state and federal law, including whether it is even offered. It may or may not be mandated. However, all employer group health plans with two or more employees, including self-insured, must comply with HIPAA regulations. States can apply the option of requiring group rules to apply to one employee. As practitioners, radiographers are not called upon to deal with HIPAA-related health insurance issues; however, practicing radiographers are affected by HIPAA-related security and privacy of health data issues.

Historically, confidentiality has been taught as part of the radiography curriculum. Radiographers have visual access to patients' private information. Depending on the type of imaging examination being done, the information provided to radiology may be extensive. Moreover, health care providers work with persons when they are most vulnerable and in need of help, that is, when they are ill. These concerns are familiar to the radiographer. Even so, provisions in Title II of HIPAA have made it necessary for radiographers to pay even closer attention to patient-related security and privacy issues.

In an *ASRT Scanner* article, "HIPAA Unlocked, Key Facts You Need to Know," the author points out that the intent of the administrative simplification provisions "is to improve health care by facilitating the use of medical information while lowering costs by streamlining administrative transactions" (Ford, 2003). Succinctly, this involves moving medical information, including medical records, from a paper to an electronic format. This change brings with it the need for regulations regarding privacy of patients' identifiable electronic health data to prevent misuse of sensitive personal information.

National standards for PHI collection and documentation address how information is gathered about health care plans, providers, and agencies collecting and distributing information or clearinghouses (i.e., banks or businesses where checks and bills are exchanged). "PHI encompasses demographic data that can identify a patient, including name, address, birth date and Social Security number, as it relates to the patient's past, present, or future health condition; health care; or payment for health care" (Ford, 2003). In this article, the author makes the following suggestions to help radiographers meet HIPAA privacy standards (Ford, 2003).

- Snap off view boxes in areas accessible to unauthorized people and return film to its original jacket after use; turn over the film jacket to hide the patient's name; pick up films quickly.
- Remove all patient-identifying information from the envelope and check-out label when sending films; create and save logs showing to whom the film was sent, and how and when it was returned.
- Remove patient's identifying information before using a film in a training session or workshop.
- Control access to ultrasound, x-ray and computer imaging rooms.
- Blank your ultrasound or computer screen or use a screen saver so no image shows if someone enters the room; remove previous images before the next patient enters.
- Lock file cabinets or storage rooms for films, back up disks and other information; control and record access to them; save the log.
- Control access to printers and fax machines that handle PHI; shred, don't just throw away your slip-ups and extra copies.

A computer specialist probably has installed software to address electronic privacy. Firewalls and virus protection should be in place. You should change your password regularly, you should be allowed access to data only on a "need to know" basis, your system should be compatible with those you need to "talk" to, and you should have had training on how it all works. Here are some other things you can do to maintain privacy on your system.

- Keep your password confidential and be sure only you use it.
- After signing on, ensure no unauthorized person uses your system.
- When transmitting electronic images, check that the image and all information are correct, ensure the recipient is authorized to receive the PHI; record who received it and when; save the log.
- Control access to e-mails containing PHI; set your e-mail program to request a "Return Receipt" for all messages you send; use of encryption is required for PHI (effective April 2005).

Caution should also be exercised in the reception and waiting room areas so that personal patient information is not inadvertently revealed to others; for example, having patients sign in on a sign-in sheet seems harmless but reveals the names of patients who have signed in before them.

Finally, it is important to use discretion in what you say in conversations and the circumstances in which you have a conversation. Remember PHI is private and belongs to the person to whom it pertains. It is privileged information. Any discussion of confidential patient information with inappropriate personnel is unacceptable. In social arenas, it is considered gossip to expose or discuss anyone's private information. Be sure that when you discuss medical information with or about another person to do so in privacy and out of hearing distance of others.

Procedural Aspects of Radiology

Uppermost in the radiographer's mind is producing not only high-quality diagnostic images but also images of human anatomy that are pleasing to the eye. However, we must take all aspects of the image into consideration. Although not limited to this discussion, some of the most important aspects deal with how we produce images from beginning to end and what could happen during the performance relevant to (1) the examination request, (2) film labeling, (3) film identification, (4) records, (5) retention of records, (6) informed consent forms, (7) radiation safety, (8) equipment safety (refer to compliance regulations and technologist certification), (9) procedure complications, and (10) film release. Some of these elements have relevance to our discussion in the earlier part of the chapter, particularly some elements related to autonomy (informed consent and confidentiality), beneficence, and nonmaleficence. Most radiology facilities are already adapted or are in the process of adapting to relevant computerized procedural and policy forms. It is therefore suggested that these forms be examined in clinical facilities where students are assigned. This will provide personal examination of how these forms are written by different facilities in compliance with appropriate and current regulations.

Examination Request

Before ever seeing the patient, the radiographer receives an examination request that has been ordered by the patient's attending physician. Items included on the requisition include the patient's name and vital statistics, the type of radiographic procedure to be performed (e.g., chest), why it needs to be done (history), and the doctor's signature.

A common practice is for the radiographer to ask the female patient who is of appropriate (childbearing) age when she had her last menstrual period (LMP). The information should be written on the request; some practitioners prefer to have the patient's personal signature in the LMP area of request. Where this is the policy and a patient is unable to sign her name, the attending physician or a guardian may sign for her.

The limited radiographer is clearly placed in a decision-making position when reading the examination request (1) to make sure signatures are appropriate, (2) to ensure that critical questions have been asked, and (3) to determine that the patient's medical history relating to the radiographic examination is stated on the request. The information included on an examination request is critical to making sure that the proper examination is done and that the radiologist has sufficient background information to aid in interpreting the radiographic image.

Film Labeling/Identification

Film labeling, using lead letters to indicate the patient's identification and that the correct side of the body has been marked, is crucial. If a radiograph has no markings on it, it really belongs to no one and therefore has no value and should be discarded. If for some reason, a radiograph was not labeled at the time it was taken, it must be marked immediately after processing. Legally, the markings should be put on the film in a permanent manner (e.g., a black felt pen). This shows there was no intent of deception and that the one who marked the film can demonstrate that the markings are clearly correct.

Radiographs as Permanent Records

Radiographs and other images are permanent records. Although the information contained in records is subject to the patient's use, the records belong to the office or institution where they were made. It is therefore important that these records be accurately maintained for future purposes. Some important reasons are: (1) follow-up for certain diseases or conditions (e.g., cancer, emphysema); (2) annual physical (e.g., chest examinations); (3) legal procedures, such as in trauma cases; and (4) research and teaching. Appropriate policies and procedures must be established for not losing records when they are loaned to doctors or other persons (e.g., lawyers). There also must be policies established regarding records subpoenaed for litigation. These kinds of policies are a protection for everyone involved. Keep in mind that records provide continuity for a patient's medical history. Electronic medical records have changed the way records are maintained and have increased accessibility to patient records. HIPAA provides complete rules for access and security for medical records. The patient and the health care provider directly involved in delivery of the patient's health care have the right to view the records. The patient may, however, grant permission for other persons to view the records.

Releasing Films

The following procedures are suggested for releasing films from the office or department to other physicians, the patient, or other than medical personnel.

1. *Other physicians*—a release form must be filled out by the patient. The films may be transferred to a different film jacket to be sent out. (Until the films are returned, the original film jacket and reports are refiled.) The jacket for sending out should be stamped *Please Return* to with your office name and address provided (like a self-addressed reply envelope).
2. *The patient*—the patient must fill out a release form and sign it. The doctor to whom the patient is taking the film should be notified. When the films have served the intended purpose, they must be returned to the proper office or department.
3. *Other than medical personnel*—this category includes such persons as lawyers and insurance company personnel. A release/consent form must be filled out by the patient and/or the physician. Generally, a fee is charged to attorneys or insurance agencies for release of a patient's film.

The best method for record keeping today is through computerized programs so that standard procedures and accuracy may be ensured. The length of time that medical records must be kept depends on state regulations regarding medical records. Generally five years of current records are kept on file and then purged for storage or discard. If records are of minors, the length of time they must be kept may be longer than five years. Radiology records also provide information for administrative reports. A daily log of appointments and procedures is generally maintained; billing is indicated for examinations completed. Quality control reports are generated to show film usage and numbers and types of procedures completed.

Informed Consent Forms

Informed consent forms must always be available and limited radiographers must be educated in their appropriate use. Informed consents should be written so that persons from all levels of education may understand them. The forms should indicate that the patient has been appropriately informed about the risks, benefits, and alternatives with regard to the procedure to be performed on the patient's body. If the duty has been delegated by the physician, the limited radiographer should make sure the consent form has been signed and is in the patient's record for review by the physician prior to doing the radiographic procedure. If the form is not appropriately completed, medical personnel and the office or institution involved in performing the procedure may be subject to legal action should any mistakes or unexpected events occur. (See the sample consent form in Figure 3-2.) Figure 3-2 is not intended to show an informed consent form currently used in

PATIENT'S CONSENT STATEMENT FOR RADIOGRAPHIC PROCEDURE

I, _____, understand that my doctor, _____
(physician performing procedure)

has ordered a _____ which requires the injection or introduction of
(type of procedure)

_____ into my body for diagnostic purposes.
(contrast medium)

I have answered the following questions as far as I know them to be true according to my personal knowledge.

Are you allergic to any types of: medication ☐   food ☐   shellfish ☐   other ☐

If so, what? _____

_____

Have you ever had any of the following? (Check all that apply)

☐ Asthma   ☐ Diabetes   ☐ Neurological Problems

☐ Cardiac (Heart) Disease   ☐ Renal (Kidney) Disease   ☐ Do not know

If you have had this radiographic procedure before or any similar type procedure that included an injection, did you have any problems after the injection?

_____

_____

After reading and discussing this form, and having my questions answered satisfactorily by the physician performing the procedure, I voluntarily consent to the injection of contrast medium for the following procedure: _____

_____   Date: _____
(Signature of Patient)

Witness: _____

Patient is unable to consent because: _____

_____

_____   Date: _____
(Signature of legal guardian or
closest available relative)

Witness: _____   Witness: _____

_____

Note. This is a sample only. Consent forms are designed for specific use and must be checked with legal counsel before use. Consent forms should be obtained by the performing physician or other qualified persons trained in managing such procedures.

FIGURE 3-2 Sample radiographic informed consent form

Source: Delmar, Cengage Learning.

any given radiology department. It is included to suggest information that may be requested on consent forms; however, additional information may also be requested. All forms must be written to comply with current health laws, which are discussed in this chapter.

Radiation Safety

Radiation safety must be in compliance with (1) the National Council on Radiation Protection and Measurements (NCRP), which is a regulatory agency for evaluating the relationship between radiation exposure and biological effects; and (2) the Consumer-Patient Radiation Health and Safety Act of 1981 (refer to Chapter 1), which deals with the establishment of minimum standards for accreditation of radiologic technology programs for persons who administer radiographic procedures. Radiation safety procedures must be written and documentation of equipment inspections must be kept on file at the office or facility.

REVIEW QUESTIONS

1. Ethics is concerned with:
    a. nature of beauty
    b. what really exists
    c. human behavior
    d. knowledge gained

2. Professional ethics relates to:
    a. modern technology
    b. standards of conduct
    c. metaphysics
    d. truth

3. The freedom to govern self is based on:
    a. justice
    b. autonomy
    c. confidentiality
    d. beneficence

4. The person legally responsible for obtaining and assessing correct informed consent is the:
   a. limited radiographer
   b. patient
   c. physician performing the procedure
   d. referring physician

5. The patient's basic right to privacy is based on:
   a. type of illness
   b. informed decision
   c. confidentiality
   d. beneficence

6. Nonmaleficence refers to:
   a. disclosing information
   b. doing duty toward others
   c. distributing fairly
   d. doing no harm

7. Principles and rules enacted by legislative bodies are:
   a. common law
   b. statutes
   c. administrative regulations
   d. none of the above

8. Fairness, justice, duties, rights, and equality are terms that should be used to develop:
   a. administrative regulations
   b. disclosure of information
   c. codes of ethics
   d. all of the above

9. Unlawful touching of another without permission is:
   a. battery
   b. assault
   c. negligence
   d. false imprisonment

10. Conscious restraint of freedom is:
    a. negligence
    b. defamation
    c. false imprisonment
    d. battery

11. True professionals are said to be individuals involved in human relations in health care delivery, drafts, trades, and commerce.
    a. True
    b. False

12. True professions deal with humans when they are vulnerable; thus, practitioners of those professions are held to a higher standard of conduct.
    a. True
    b. False

13. A true profession may be associated with the following element(s):
    a. humane codes of ethics
    b. specialized skills
    c. society's respect as an honorable vocation
    d. a and b only
    e. a, b, and c

14. There are four general types of law.
    a. True
    b. False

15. Administrative regulations that are written by agencies or boards established by legislative bodies are as legally binding as statutes.
    a. True
    b. False

16. The patient's bill of rights is based on:
    a. autonomy
    b. informed consent
    c. confidentiality
    d. a and c
    e. a, b, and c

17. Unmarked films that are marked after processing may be marked with a black marker so long as there is no apparent intent of deception and the radiographer who produced the films can demonstrate that the markings are clearly correct.
    a. True
    b. False

18. Radiographs as permanent records belong to the:
    a. patient
    b. physician's office
    c. hospital
    d. b and c
    e. a, b, and c

19. Films may be released under specific conditions to the following:
    a. other physicians
    b. the patient
    c. lawyers and insurance companies
    d. a and c
    e. a, b, and c

20. The regulatory agency established for evaluation of the relationship between radiation exposure and biological effects is:
    a. Consumer-Patient Health and Safety Act 1981
    b. National Council on Radiation Protection and Measurements
    c. a and b
    d. none of the above

21. The American Disabilities Act (ADA) is a protective law for persons with disabilities in the United States. It was enacted into law in:
    a. 1999
    b. 1993
    c. 1990
    d. 1992

22. ADA prohibits discrimination based on:
    1. state and local government employment
    2. public accommodations
    3. commercial facilities
    4. transportation and telecommunications

    Possible Responses
    a. 1 only
    b. 2 and 3
    c. 1, 2, and 3
    d. 1, 2, 3, and 4

23. The ADA requires reasonable accommodations for caring for disabled persons. One of the most accommodating and key elements in providing care is:
    a. good personality
    b. using patient's first name
    c. effective communication
    d. speedy work

24. ADA-covered patient circumstances may require a radiographer to take more time to perform an examination. Such variables may include:
    1. complexity of directions to the patient
    2. patient cooperation
    3. degree of difficulty associated with the procedure

    Possible Responses
    a. 1 and 2
    b. 1 and 3
    c. 2 and 3
    d. 1, 2, and 3

25. The Health Insurance Portability and Accountability Act (HIPAA) was enacted in:
    a. 1986
    b. 1991
    c. 1996
    d. 1994

26. HIPAA reinforces a practice that radiographers have historically known as:
    a. being sympathetic
    b. confidentiality
    c. being empathetic
    d. patient flow

27. The implementation of HIPAA provided for:
    1. establishment of national standards for collection and documentation of health information
    2. health insurance reform
    3. protected health information (PHI)

    Possible Responses
    a. 1 and 2
    b. 1 and 3
    c. 2 and 3
    d. 1, 2, and 3

28. National standards for PHI collection and documentation focus on how information is gathered by:
1. health care plans
2. providers
3. agencies collecting and distributing information
4. banks and businesses where checks and bills are exchanged

Possible Responses

a. 1 and 2
b. 2 and 3
c. 3 and 4
d. 1, 2, 3, and 4

29. PHI information includes data that identify the patient's:
1. birth date
2. social security number
3. name and address

Possible Responses

a. 1 and 2
b. 1 and 3
c. 2 and 3
d. 1, 2, and 3

30. E-mails regarding patient information required a return receipt or had to be encrypted after:
a. May 2005
b. October 2005
c. April 2005
d. November 2005

REFERENCES

The American Heritage Dictionary (2nd college ed.). (1991). Boston: Houghton Mifflin Company.

Borish, I. M. (1983). The academy and professionalism. *The American Journal of Optometry & Physiological Optics, 57* (2), 18–23.

Ford, J. (2003). HIPAA unlocked, key facts you need to know. *ASRT Scanner, 36* (3), 8–11.

Kestenbaum, V. (Ed.). (1982). *The Humanity of the Ill.* Knoxville: University of Tennessee Press.

McGlothlin, W. (1960). *Patterns of Professional Education*. New York: Putnam.

Pellegrino, E. (1983). *What is a profession? Journal of Allied Health, 12* (3), 168–176.

United States Department of Justice. (2005). *1990 A guide to disability rights laws*. Retrieved from http://www.ada.gov

United States Office of Personnel Management. (2008). *Patients' bill of rights*. Retrieved from http://www.opm.gov

SUGGESTED READINGS

Engelhardt, H. T., Jr. (1996). *The Foundations of Bioethics* (2nd ed.) New York: Oxford University Press.

Obergfell, A. (1995). *Law and Ethics in Diagnostic Imaging and Therapeutic Radiology*. Philadelphia: W. B. Saunders Company.

Pozgar, G. D. (1996). *Legal Aspects of Health Care Administration* (6th ed.). Rockville, MD: Aspen Publications.

Weston, A. (1977). *A Practical Companion to Ethics*. New York: Oxford University Press.

Wilson, B. G. (1997). *Ethics and Basic Law for Medical Imaging Professionals*. Philadelphia: F. A. Davis Company.

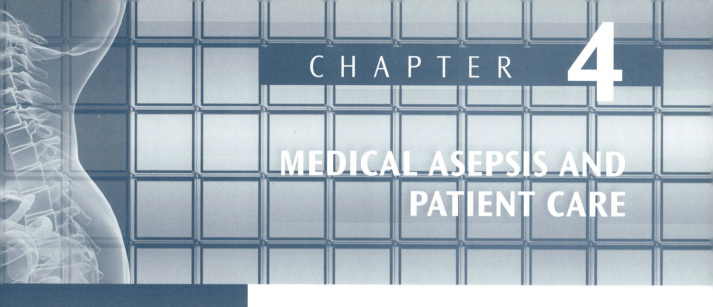

CHAPTER 4

MEDICAL ASEPSIS AND PATIENT CARE

Key Terms

Airborne Pathogens
Asepsis
Bacteria
Blood Pressure
Disinfection
Epistaxis
Ergonomics
Fomite
Fungi
Germs
Host
Hypertension
Hypotension
Infection Control
Microorganisms
No Manual Lift Policy
Nonpathogenic
Nosocomial Infections
Pathogenic Organisms
Prehypertension
Protozoa
Pulse
Respiration
Rickettsiae
Surgical Asepsis
Transmission-Based Precautions
Universal Precautions
Vector
Viruses
Vital Signs

Chapter Outline

Introduction
Infection Control
Microorganisms
  Bacteria
  Fungi
  Protozoa
  Rickettsiae
  Viruses
Nosocomial Infections
Microbial Growth and Infection
Levels of Infection Control
  Asepsis
  Disinfection
  Surgical Asepsis
  Exposure
Recommendations for the Management of Health Care
Personnel Potentially Exposed to HBV, HVC, or HIV
  Management of Occupational Blood Exposure
Safety Measures
  Preventing Falls

Objectives

Upon completion of the chapter, the student will meet the following objectives by verifying knowledge of the facts and principles presented through oral and written communication at a level deemed competent.

⊃ Describe the limited radiographer's role in preventing the spread of microorganisms.

⊃ Recall and outline the requirements for microbial growth.

⊃ Differentiate between the levels of infection control by comparing and contrasting methods and uses of medical asepsis, disinfection, and surgical asepsis.

⊃ Recall facts concerning universal and transmission based precautions.

⊃ Select correct responses regarding ergonomics and body mechanics when assisting, moving, and transporting patients.

⊃ Select appropriate responses related to making entries on the patient record.

⊃ Identify the common vital signs and describe their importance in the assessment of patient conditions.

⊃ Identify normal vital sign ranges for adults and children, to include temperature, pulse, respiration, and blood pressure.

⊃ Discriminate between appropriate and inappropriate procedures and techniques related to taking and recording vital signs, administering oxygen, responding to emergencies, and handling trauma patients.

⊃ Define what constitutes a medical emergency and identify the limited radiographer's role.

Introduction

Today, health care is provided in a variety of settings, from hospitals offering a wide range of services to those providing specialized care, such as community health agencies, private medical offices, mobile van care units, ambulatory emergency clinics, nursing homes, hospices, and self-help organizations. Home health care is becoming a vital service in the health care industry; so are health maintenance organizations, which stress a holistic wellness approach. Rehabilitation is also very important today to help people return to an active life after an accident or illness. The traditional objectives of medical science—prevention, detection, and treatment of disease—remain the foundations for delivery of health care. However, ethical, moral, and legal debates are taking issue with procedures used to initiate, prolong, and redesign the life process. As scientific advances continue to expand the role and scope of health care, these and other ethical and legal questions concerning rights and responsibilities will continue to be addressed.

Despite these unanswered questions and the turmoil they bring to the entire health care community, the everyday needs of patients seeking health care must be served. The limited radiographer's primary responsibility is to provide diagnostic-quality radiographs as requested by a licensed independent practitioner. Because of the nature of the work, limited radiographers also give basic patient care and have an important role in the entire process of health care delivery.

The ASRT *Practice Standards for Medical Imaging and Radiation Therapy: Limited X-ray Machine Operators* that specifically address the information presented in this chapter include the following standards and rationale (2008).

- **Standard One-Assessment**
  The limited x-ray machine operator collects pertinent data about the patient and the procedure.
  Rationale: The planning and provision of safe and effective medical services relies on the collection of pertinent information about equipment, procedures, and the work environment.
- **Standard Three-Patient Education**
  The limited x-ray machine operator informs the patient, public, and other health care providers about procedures, equipment, and facilities
  Rationale: Open communication prommotes safe practices.
- **Standard Eight-Documentation**
  The limited x-ray machine operator documents quality assurance activities and results.
  Rationale: Documentation provides evidence of quality assurance activities designed to enhance safety.

Infection Control

Medical institutions, clinics, doctors' offices, and others provide services to many people. Infection control (i.e., the prevention of the spread of infectious conditions and diseases) is an important responsibility and goal for everyone. Consider the unlimited possibilities for disease transmission and cross infection between and among the many people who enter a medical facility. Infection can spread from a single focal point or person of contamination to many other parts of the medical care chain and the general public (Figure 4-1).

Limited radiographers are responsible for preventing the spread of microorganisms to others and for protecting themselves from contamination. By consistent application of basic techniques of hand washing, proper disinfection, and disposal of contaminated items, the total number of infectious organisms can be reduced or diluted to a harmless level.

The goal then becomes to protect self, patient, and others from becoming infected and from serving as a source of infectious organisms to others.

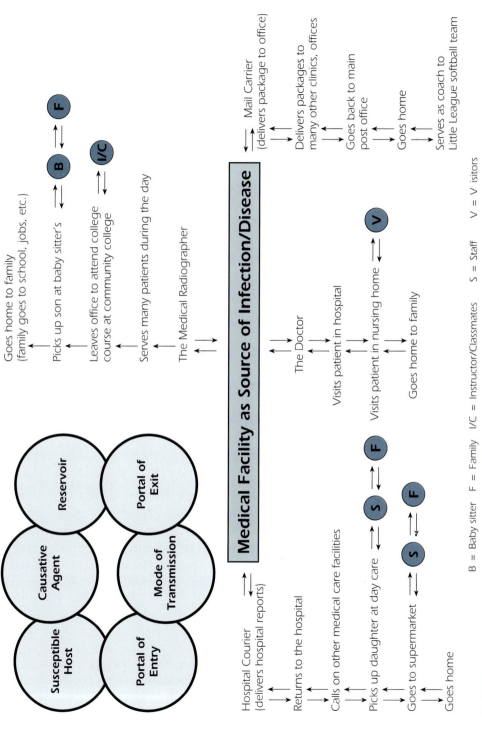

FIGURE 4-1 Cycle of infection
Source: Delmar, Cengage Learning.

B = Baby sitter   F = Family   I/C = Instructor/Classmates   S = Staff   V = Visitors

Medical Facility as Source of Infection/Disease

Susceptible Host

Causative Agent

Reservoir

Portal of Entry

Mode of Transmission

Portal of Exit

Hospital Courier
(delivers hospital reports)

Returns to the hospital

Calls on other medical care facilities

Picks up daughter at day care → S → F

Goes to supermarket → S

Goes home

The Doctor

Visits patient in hospital

Visits patient in nursing home → V

Goes home to family

Goes home to family
(family goes to school, jobs, etc.)

Picks up son at baby sitter's → B → F

Leaves office to attend college course at community college → I/C

Serves many patients during the day

The Medical Radiographer

Mail Carrier
(delivers package to office)

Delivers packages to many other clinics, offices

Goes back to main post office

Goes home

Serves as coach to Little League softball team

Microorganisms

The environment is teeming with microorganisms, which are extremely small and invisible except by microscope. Microorganisms also reside on all skin surfaces of the body and are especially numerous in the respiratory passages, mouth, and entire length of the digestive system. Not all microorganisms are harmful; microorganisms that are not harmful are called nonpathogenic. Those that are harmful and capable of causing diseases are referred to as germs or pathogenic organisms. The five general classifications of microorganisms are *bacteria, fungi, protozoa, rickettsiae,* and *viruses.*

Bacteria

Bacteria are one-celled organisms, both pathogenic and nonpathogenic, and are identified and classified according to their morphology (shape) and structure.

Bacteria are further described as Gram-positive, Gram-negative, or acid fast which refer to the chemical composition of the bacterial cell wall. Composition of the bacterial cell wall plays an important role in antibiotic sensitivity (Shagam, 1999).

Bacteria, unlike viruses, are not dependent on the host for replication and growth. This fact allows drug treatments, which target the particular bacteria but have low toxicity to the host (Shagam, 1999).

Diseases and conditions caused by bacteria include urinary tract infections, pneumonia, septic shock, Legionnaires disease, endocarditis, and skin and wound infections (Shagam, 1999).

Fungi

Fungi exist in two forms, yeasts and molds. Yeasts are one-celled organisms, whereas molds are multicelled. Approximately 50% of all fungi may cause disease in humans. Fungi require moisture and darkness to survive and are often called opportunistic because they are not particularly pathogenic until they encounter a compromised host. Fungi infections occur under numerous conditions and may be a symptom of a more serious disease or infection. Common fungal diseases are thrush, moniliasis, and histoplasmosis.

Protozoa

Protozoa are microscopic one-celled organisms. Infection occurs as a result of ingestion of the parasite or from an insect/animal bite. Examples of protozoal diseases are amebiasis, malaria, and toxoplasmosis.

Rickettsiae

Rickettsiae are microscopic life forms found in tissues of fleas, lice, ticks, and other insects. Rickettsial infections are transmitted to humans by the bite of infected insects, which are called a **vector** or the carrier of disease. Common examples of rickettsial diseases are typhus and Rocky Mountain spotted fever.

Viruses

Viruses are the smallest known organisms. Viruses cannot exist outside a living organism cell but use the host's cells for replication (Shagam, 1999). Humans are susceptible to several hundred different viruses. Common virus infections are influenza, measles, German measles, mumps, chicken pox, herpes simplex, and smallpox. Because of their prevalence, viruses are an important consideration in infection control. They are spread primarily by humans via respiratory and intestinal excretions.

Nosocomial Infections

Nosocomial infections occur as a result of treatment in a hospital or medical care facility, but secondary to the patient's original condition (Tabor's Cyclopedic Medical Dictionary, 1985). Infections are considered to be nosocomial if they first appear 48 hours or more after hospital admission or within 30 days after discharge. Nosocomial infections are often referred to as opportunistic infections because they mainly affect those with compromised immune status.

Nosocomial infections have a significant impact on the length of hospital stay and medical care costs (Centers for Disease Control and Prevention [CDC], 2006a). In the United States, nosocomial infections annually affect 2 million acute-care patients, cost $4.5 billion, and contribute to thousands of deaths (Shagam, 1999). The reasons why nosocomial infections are so common and often deadly include:

- Hospitals, nursing homes, and medical facilities house large numbers of people who are sick and who may have compromised immune status;
- Increased use of outpatient treatment means that people who are in the hospital are sicker than in the past;
- Medical staff move from patient to patient, providing a conduit for the spread of pathogens;
- Many diagnostic procedures and treatments are invasive, allowing easy entry for pathogens; and
- Sanitation protocols may be either unheeded by hospital staff or too lax to sufficiently isolate patients from infectious agents (Taber's, 1985).

The types of microbes most often involved in nosocomial infections are viruses, bacteria, and fungi. The most common nosocomial infections are of the urinary tract, surgical sites, and pneumonia. Other known diseases in the nosocomial classification include gastroenteritis, ventilator associated pneumonia, *Pseudomonas aerugionsa*, and *Staphylococcus aureus* (Taber's, 1985).

Overuse of prescribed antibiotics has set the stage for the emergence of antibiotic resistant pathogens. Bacteria has the ability to evolve and become resistant to known available antibiotics.

The United States Centers for Disease Control and Prevention (CDC) link the increasing bacterial threat to the overuse of antibiotics. For example, before the 1950s, penicillin was effective against *Staphyloccus aureus* (*Staph*) but by the early 1960s scientists found bacteria that had developed resistance (CDC, 2006a).

Thorough hand washing and/or use of alcohol rub by all medical personnel before each patient contact is one of the most effective ways to combat nosocomial infections (Association for Professionals in Infection Control and Epidemiology, Inc. [APICE], 2008; CDC, 2008).

Microbial Growth and Infection

Microorganisms have certain specific requirements for growth. Knowing these requirements will help the radiographer recognize and eliminate conditions conducive to microbial growth. In this way, the spread of infection to others can be inhibited.

Requirements for Growth:
1. **Host** or reservoir in which to live and grow. The host can be a human being, animal, soil, water, or food. Hosts must provide water and nourishment for the microorganisms.
2. Warm and dark environment. Most microorganisms grow best at body temperature (98.6 degrees Fahrenheit) and prefer a dark environment.

Microorganisms can be spread by a number of methods (Figure 4-2). Infection is caused when microorganisms enter a susceptible host and grow in the body. An infection can be localized or affect the entire body. The factors involved in the process of infection are:

- source of infection (reservoir)
- the microorganisms (causative agent)
- a portal of exit from the reservoir
- a host with a level of susceptibility and a portal of entry

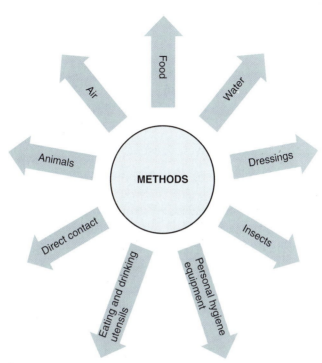

FIGURE 4-2 Methods of spreading microorganisms
Source: Delmar, Cengage Learning.

Direct spread of microorganisms occurs when the microorganisms are passed from one person to another by touching or contact. Indirect spread of microorganisms involves the transmission of pathogens by one of three means:

1. Fomites: A fomite is an object that has been contaminated with the pathogen. Common examples are a limited radiographer's uniform or the radiographic table. Common fomites are doors, examination tables, equipment, and hypodermic needles.
2. Vector: A vector is an animal or insect whose body serves as host to the pathogen. The bite of the infected vector spreads the disease.

Disease	Vector
Rabies	Bats, dogs, etc.
Bubonic Plague	Fleas
Rat bite fevers	Rats
Malaria	Mosquitoes

3. Airborne: Airborne pathogens are spread by dust or droplet contamination. This occurs when infected individuals sneeze or cough toward a susceptible host.

Remember the following important facts about microorganisms as they relate to the spread of infection:

- Microorganisms are everywhere in our environment.
- Microorganisms cannot move by themselves, but must be transported from one host to another.
- Microorganisms are opportunistic.
- Severity of infection depends on:
    number of pathogenic organisms present
    virulence (strength) of organisms
    resistance of infected person

The human body's defenses are usually strong enough to protect against invading opportunistic microorganisms. However, those seeking health care may have a medical condition or a compromised immune system that leaves them with reduced defenses against the attack. Table 4-1 provides an overview of transmission routes and suggested precautions.

Levels of Infection Control

Infection control includes various actions and procedures that reduce or eliminate the number of pathogenic organisms present. There are three levels of infection control: asepsis, disinfection, and surgical asepsis.

TABLE 4-1 Transmission of Pathogens and Suggested Personnel Precautions

Transmission	Suggested Precautions
Airborne	Personnel should wear appropriate respiratory protection. The mode of patient transport through the facility should minimize spread of microorganisms to others. The patient should be placed in an isolation room that prevents transmission of airborne droplets through the ventilation system.
Droplet	Minimize dispersal of droplets by having the patient wear a mask. Personnel should wear a mask when working within 3 feet of the patient and the patient should be placed in a private room.
Contact	Personnel should wear gloves and change gloves after contact with infective material. The patient should be placed in a private room. If contact with the patient is likely, personnel should wear a clean, nonsterile gown.

Source: Shagam, Janet Yagoda, Ph.D. The Radiology Department and Nosocomial Infections. *Radiologic Technology* Vol.70, No.5 May/June 1999 pp. 418–433.

Asepsis

Asepsis is defined as the absence of all disease-producing microorganisms and is very important to breaking the infection cycle. Aseptic techniques physically eliminate pathogens and the conditions that promote their growth and spread. Such techniques include proper hand washing, handling and disposing of contaminated linens, and housekeeping.

Hand Washing.   The hands are a limited radiographer's tools. Radiographers constantly use their hands to prepare the examination room and equipment, to assist and position the patient, and to perform all the tasks associated with providing radiographs. During these tasks, the hands are exposed to pathogens that can infect the limited radiographer, who, in turn, can become a reservoir of infection passed on to others. According to the Centers for Disease Control and Prevention (CDC), the single most important measure that health care workers can use to reduce the risk of transmitting pathogens is handwashing (CDC, 2006a, 2008; APICE, 2008; CDC, 2008).

The purpose of handwashing is to remove dirt, organic material and microorganisms (APICE, 2008). To be effective, handwashing should be of sufficient duration for mechanical action to allow antimicrobial products enough contact time to achieve the desired results (APICE, 2008). There are three methods of handwashing, and the most effective method depends upon the purpose. For example, handwashing for the purpose of removing soil and microorganisms is best accomplished using soap or detergent and scrubbing for at least 10 to 15 seconds. For hand antisepsis to remove or destroy microorganisms, the use of an antimicrobial soap or detergent or alcohol-based hand rub used for at least 10 to 15 seconds is recommended (APICE, 2008). When decontaminating hands with an alcohol-based hand rub, the product should be applied to the palm of one hand and then the hands rubbed together, covering all surfaces of hands and fingers, until the hands are dry (CDC, 2008). The manufacturer's recommendations regarding the volume of product to use should be followed. Antimicrobial-impregnated wipes (i.e., towelettes) may be considered as an alternative to washing hands with non-anitmicrobial soap and water (CDC, 2008). Because they are not as effective as alcohol-based hand rubs or washing hands with an antimicrobial soap and water for reducing bacterial counts on the hands, they are not a substitute (CDC, 2008).

The surgical hand scrub intended to reduce, remove, or destroy microorganisms and reduce resistant flora requires a more intense method. Antimicrobial soap or detergent preparation and brushing to create friction for at least 120 seconds, or alcohol-based preparation for at least 120 seconds is required for the surgical hand scrub.

Any handwashing product can be contaminated or support growth of microorganisms (APICE, 2008). Bar soap should be changed frequently (APICE, 2008; CDC, 2008). Small bars and soap racks are recommended. Liquid products should be stored in closed containers and dispensed from disposal containers or containers that can be thoroughly washed and dried before refilling (APICE, 2008; CDC, 2008).

Whether artificial nails contribute to transmission of microorganisms is unknown. However, research has shown that health care workers who wear artificial nails are more likely to harbor gram-negative pathogens on their fingertips than those who have natural nails, both before and after hand washing (CDC, 2008).

Use of lotions or creams to minimize the occurrence of irritant contact dermatitis associated with hand antisepsis or handwashing is recommended (APICE, 2008; CDC, 2008). Information should be solicited from manufacturers regarding any effects that hand lotions, creams, or alcohol-based hand antiseptics may have on the persistent effects of antimicrobial soaps being used in the health care setting (CDC, 2008).

To prevent the spread of infectious microorganisms hands must be washed frequently, such as before and after working with each patient. It may be necessary to wash hands several times during the period of patient contact for a specific radiographic procedure. In addition to frequent hand washing, any cut or break in the skin should be covered with a sterile dressing. Since dry, chapped, or abraded skin also serves as a portal of entry for microorganisms, care should be taken to keep the skin smooth and intact.

Handling and Disposing of Linens.   All used linen should be considered soiled and a source of pathogenic microorganisms. The use of disposable gowns, sheets, drapes, and pillow covers eliminates risks associated with cleaning and reuse of linens. Used linen, whether disposable or nondisposable, should be handled as little as possible and with minimum movement to prevent contamination of the air and of persons handling the linen (Figure 4-3).

All used linen should be bagged at the location where it is used. Do not sort or rinse linens in the patient care area. Linens soiled with blood or body fluids should be placed and transported in bags that prevent leakage.

Housekeeping.   Housekeeping activities include cleaning environmental surfaces such as walls, floors, and other surfaces. Because these surfaces are not directly associated with the transmission of microorganisms to patients or others, attempts to disinfect or sterilize are not necessary; however, regular cleaning and soil removal must be performed.

Cleaning schedules and methods vary according to the type of medical facility, the particular service area, and the amount and type of soil present. Furniture and hard-surfaced floors should be cleaned on a regular basis and when soiling or spills occur. Walls, window coverings, and blinds should be cleaned when they are visibly

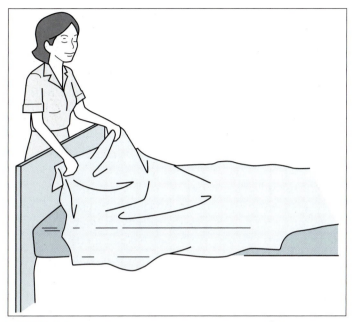

FIGURE 4-3 Handling linens. Linens should be unfolded, never flipped or fanned, because brisk movement stirs air currents that carry microorganisms into the air.
Source: Delmar, Cengage Learning.

soiled. Vigorous cleaning and scrubbing with a disinfectant-detergent formula is considered effective against growth of microorganisms.

Disinfection

Disinfection is the destruction of microorganisms by using chemical methods. In radiography, disinfection methods are used on the radiographic table and certain equipment, accessories, and noninvasive articles. Commercially available disinfectant solutions may be used, but a solution of sodium hypochlorite (household bleach) is an inexpensive and effective germicide. Concentrations ranging from 1:100 dilution of household bleach to water are effective depending on the amount of organic material present on the surface. Regardless of the type or brand of disinfectant solution used, the following recommendations apply. Information on specific label claims of commercial germicides can be obtained from the Environmental Protection Agency (EPA) website http://www.epa.gov/EPA_PEST.

1. Read the directions provided for preparing and using disinfectants.
2. In patient-care areas, visible material should first be removed and then the area should be decontaminated. With large spills of cultured or concentrated

infectious agents, the contaminated area should be flooded with a liquid germicide before cleaning, then decontaminated with a fresh germicidal chemical. Gloves should be worn during all cleaning and decontaminating procedures.

Common radiography items that require disinfection are the radiography table top as well as calipers, cassette surfaces, and immobilization aids.

Surgical Asepsis

Certain areas of the human body are free of microorganisms—"sterile"—and during invasive procedures, the use of sterile technique is required. These areas include the internal tissues and organs such as the muscles, glands, bone marrow, brain, spinal cord, and circulatory system. Body fluids such as blood, urine in the kidney and bladder, and cerebrospinal fluid are also normally free of microbes but can become infected when disease-causing microbes bypass natural protective barriers (Shagam, 1999).

Surgical asepsis includes procedures and techniques used to destroy microorganisms before they enter the body. Such aseptic techniques are used whenever a surgical incision is made in the body. They are also used with invasive procedures, such as urinary catheterization, and when sterile instruments are handled and dressings are changed.

Surgical asepsis means that everything coming in contact with the patient is sterile. If an article is touched by an unsterile item, or if there is any question about the sterility of an item, it must be considered contaminated. Surgical asepsis is not generally used in procedures related to limited radiography procedures. For further information on surgical asepsis procedures, consult available nursing, health, and health assistant textbooks.

Universal and transmission-based precautions are two-tiered. The first level of precautions, known as Standard Precautions (SP), is designed for the care of all patients regardless of their diagnosis or presumed infection status. Standard precautions include the major features of universal precautions (UP), which are used to limit the risk of transmission of blood-borne pathogens and pathogens from wet body substances (urine, saliva, mucous, semen, and tears). Universal precautions applies to blood, all body fluids, secretions, and excretions (except sweat), regardless of whether they contain blood (Shagam, 1999).

The second tier of precautions is designed for the care of patients infected with transmittable pathogens. When there is a known or presumed infection, transmission-based precautions (TBP) are necessary. There are three types of TBPs: airborne precautions, droplet precautions, and contact precautions (Shagam, 1999).

HIV/AIDS and hepatitis B are just two of the many diseases that health care personnel encounter in their daily work. The following suggestions include effective infection control measures for most other pathogens as well as HIV/AIDS and hepatitis B. The recommendations are taken from *"Preventing Occupational HIV Transmission to Healthcare Personnel,"* published by the Centers for Disease Control & Prevention, National Center for HIV, STD, and TB Prevention, Divisions of HIV/AIDS Prevention, and the *Morbidity and Mortality Weekly Report* (MMWR) (CDC, 2006b; 2006c). It is important to review the most recent recommendations on a regular basis. These are available on the CDC's website http://www.cdc.gov.

Exposure

An exposure that might place health care personnel at risk for hepatitis B virus (HBV), hepatitis C virus (HCV), or human immunodeficiency virus (HIV) is defined as a percutaneous injury (e.g., a needlestick or cut with a sharp object), or contact of mucous membrane, or nonintact skin (e.g., exposed skin that is chapped, abraded, or afflicted with dermatitis) with blood, tissue, or other body fluids that are potentially infectious (CDC, 2006b; 2006c).

In addition to blood and body fluids containing visible blood, semen and vaginal secretions also are considered potentially infectious. Although semen and vaginal secretions have been implicated in the sexual transmission of HBV, HCV, and HIV, they have not been implicated in occupational transmission from patients to health care personnel. The following fluids also are considered potentially infectious: cerebrospinal fluid, synovial fluid, pleural fluid, peritoneal fluid, pericardial fluid, and amniotic fluid. The risk for transmission of HBV, HCV, and HIV infection from these fluids is unknown; the potential risk to health care personnel from occupational exposures has not been assessed by epidemiologic studies in health care settings. Feces, nasal secretions, saliva, sputum, sweat, tears, urine, and vomitus are not considered potentially infectious unless they contain blood. The risk for transmission of HBV, HVC, and HIV infection from these fluids and materials is extremely low.

Any direct contact (i.e., contact without barrier protection) to concentrated virus in a research laboratory production facility is considered an exposure that requires clinical evaluation. For human bites, the clinical evaluation must include the possibility that both the person bitten and the person who inflicted the bite were exposed to bloodborne pathogens. Transmission of HBV or HIV infection only rarely has been reported by this route (CDC, 2006b; 2006c).

Recommendations for the Management of Health Care Personnel Potentially Exposed to HBV, HCV, or HIV

Exposure prevention remains the primary strategy for reducing occupational blood-borne pathogen infections; however, occupational exposures will continue to occur. Health care facilities should make available to their personnel a system that includes written protocols for prompt reporting, evaluation, counseling, treatment, and follow-up of occupational exposures that might place health care personnel at risk for acquiring a bloodborne infection. Refer to Table 4-2 for CDC recommendations for the contents of the occupational exposure report. Health care personnel should be educated concerning the risk for and prevention of bloodborne infections, including the need to be vaccinated against hepatitis B (CDC, 2006b; 2006c).

Employers are required to establish exposure-control plans that include post-exposure follow-up for their employees and to comply with incident reporting requirements mandated in 1992 bloodborne pathogen standard issued by the Occupational Safety and Health Administration (OSHA). Access to clinicians who can provide post-exposure care should be available during all working hours, including nights and weekends. HBIG, hepatitis B vaccine, and antiretroviral agents for HIV PEP should be available for timely administration.

Health care personnel should report occupational exposures immediately after they occur. Any person who performs tasks involving contact with blood, blood-contaminated body fluids, other body fluids, or sharps should be vaccinated against

TABLE 4-2   Recommendations for the Contents of the Occupational Exposure Report Based on Information from the Centers for Disease Control and Prevention

- Date and time of exposure;
- Details of the procedure being performed, including where and how the exposure occurred; if related to a sharp device, the type and brand of device, and how and when in the course of handling the device the exposure occurred;
- Details of the exposure, including the type and amount of fluid or material and the severity of the exposure, e.g., for a percutaneous exposure, depth of injury and whether fluid was injected; for a skin or mucous membrane exposure, the estimated volume of material and the condition of the skin (e.g., chapped, abraded, intact);
- Details about the exposure source (e.g., whether the source material contained HBV, HCV, or HIV; if the source is HIV-infected, the stage of disease, history of antiretroviral therapy, viral load, and antiretroviral resistance information, if known);
- Details about the exposed person (e.g., hepatitis B vaccination and vaccine-response status); and
- Details about counseling, post-exposure management, and follow-up.

hepatitis B. Prevaccination serologic screening for previous infection is not indicated for persons being vaccinated because of occupational risk.

Management of Occupational Blood Exposure

Provide immediate care to the exposure site.

- Wash wounds and skin with soap and water.
- Flush mucous membranes with water.

Determine risk associated with exposure by

- Type of fluid (e.g., blood, visibly bloody fluid, other potentially infectious fluid or tissue, and concentrated virus) and
- Type of exposure (e.g., percutaneous injury, mucous membrane or nonintact skin exposure, and bites resulting in blood exposure).

Evaluate exposure source.

- Assess the risk of infection using available information.
- Test unknown sources, assess risk of exposure to HBV, HCV, or HIV infection.
- Do not test discarded needles or syringes for virus contamination.

Evaluate the exposed person.

- Assess immune status for HBV infection (e.g., by history of hepatitis B vaccination and vaccine response).

Give post exposure prophylaxis (PEP). As mentioned previously, the CDC recommendations may change as new information becomes available and can be accessed at the CDC's website http://www.cdc.gov.

- Follow CDC recommendations for post-exposure treatment.
- Perform follow-up testing and provide counseling. Exposed persons should seek medical evaluation for any acute illness occurring during follow-up.
  HBV exposures: Follow-up anti-HBs testing in persons who receive hepatitis B vaccine. Test for anti HBs 1–2 months after last dose of vaccine.
  HCV exposures: Perform baseline and follow-up testing for anti-HCV and alanine aminotransferase (ALT) 4-6 months after exposures. Perform HCV RNA at 4-6 weeks if earlier diagnosis of HCV infection desired. Confirm repeatedly reactive anti-HCV enzyme immunoassays (EIAs) with supplemental tests. HIV exposures: Perform HIV-antibody testing for at least 6-month post exposure (e.g., at baseline, 6 weeks, 3 months, and 6 months). Perform HIV antibody testing if illness compatible with an acute retroviral syndrome occurs. Advise exposed persons to use precautions to prevent secondary transmission

during the follow-up period. Evaluate exposed persons taking PEP within 72 hours after exposure and monitor for drug toxicity for at least 2 weeks.

Worldwide more than two billion people are infected with mycobacterium tuberculosis (TB). TB most commonly invades the respiratory system via airborne transmission but can also infect the nervous system, kidney, spleen, or other tissues (CDC, 2006b).

Those working in health care professions are three times more likely to contract TB than the general population (CDC, 2006b). At highest risk are those who give care and provide diagnostic imaging services to patients who are HIV positive, homeless, or who were born outside the United States. Only those patients with active TB disease are contagious, but two key factors must be considered in transmission of TB. These factors include total contact time with a TB contagious patient and the ventilation where the contact occurs.

In 1994, the Centers for Disease Control and Prevention (CDC) recommended special precautions for radiology departments in regions of the country with a high prevalence of TB. The recommendations included separated, well-ventilated areas for patients with TB. The precautions also suggested that patients with TB should wear surgical masks and minimize the length of time in the radiology area where others might be waiting.

To protect themselves, radiographers should be informed about the transmission routes of TB and aware if the area where they work is considered to be a high prevalence TB area. Steps that radiographers can take to protect themselves include periodic TB testing and being vigilant about identifying personal risk and by taking precautions to minimize risk.

Safety Measures

Safety is the responsibility of everyone and must be an integral part of health care services. This concern includes not only the patient, but extends to everyone entering the health care facility. Accidents involving patients and staff can be reduced if simple safety measures are followed.

Preventing Falls

Patients may misjudge the distance from the radiographic examination table to the floor and fall as they attempt to get on and/or off the table. To reduce the likelihood of patient falls, you should always be at the table and provide a foot stool. Provide assistance also when the patient is getting on and off the table.

Tripping and falling account for numerous accidents. Protruding objects, loose scatter rugs, electrical cords, etc., should be removed or secured to prevent injuries.

Fire Safety

Fire safety begins with a fire safety plan that includes learning the location of fire doors, escape routes, and fire extinguishers, and knowing the evacuation procedure to follow during drills or the real thing. For further information, ask your supervisor about the facility's fire safety plan and participate in fire safety classes and evacuation drills.

Effective fire safety measures also include:

1. Smoking only in designated smoking areas
2. Fire inspections that try to uncover potential fire hazards before they cause fires
3. Annual preventative maintenance inspections on the heating and cooling units and other major electrical appliances/equipment
4. Installing smoke detectors and posting fire evacuation routes and fire exit signs
5. Regular checks on smoke detectors and fire extinguishers
6. Health care workers who are constantly alert to potential fire hazards

Electrical Safety

Electrical safety involves proper use of electrical equipment and basic maintenance of the cords and circuits. Electrical equipment should be located away from sinks and other water reservoirs to avoid the possibility of electric shock. Electrical cords should be routinely inspected and broken or frayed cords replaced. Extension cords are a potential hazard and should not be overloaded with multiple appliances connected. Electric cords should not be draped around other items. A three-prong or safety plug provides added electrical grounding and is generally provided with heavy duty equipment or equipment that is in constant use, such as the electrocardiograph and laboratory centrifuge machines.

Accidents

Accidents do not just happen, they result from someone's inattention to details. Common sources of accidents are:

- Loose area rugs or torn carpet
- Unstable furniture or broken furniture
- Dangling electrical cords
- Young children or confused/disoriented person left alone/unattended
- Wet floors or highly waxed floors

The key to avoiding accidents is prevention. Each health worker should carefully look at his/her work environment and reduce or eliminate potential accident conditions.

Reporting Accidents.   Accidents should be reported immediately to the staff supervisor. Each medical facility will have a procedure for reporting and recording accidents. Remember prevention is better than a cure.

Ergonomics and Principles of Body Mechanics

Ergonomics

Ergonomics is the science of fitting the job to the worker (Occupational Safety & Health Administration [OSHA], 2008). When there is a mismatch between the physical requirements of the job and the physical capacity of the worker, work-related musculoskeletal disorders (MSDs) can result. Ergonomics is the practice of designing equipment and work tasks to conform to the capability of the worker; it provides a means for adjusting the work environment and work practices to prevent injuries before they occur (OSHA, 2008). Medical imaging facilities have been identified as an environment where ergonomic stressors exist (OSHA, 2008). These stressors result in acute and chronic injuries to radiographers and support staff while attempting to move patients (OSHA, 2008; Radiology's big challenge, 2007). In a research study performed at Massachusetts General Hospital in Boston between 1989 and 2003, approximately 83% of radiographers reported some pain when moving obese patients (Radiology's, 2007).

Health care workers consistently rank among top occupations with disabling back injuries, primarily from manually lifting patients (OSHA, 2008; Radiology's, 2007). A national health care policy for safe patient handling and a no manual lift policy is urgently needed to address this crisis (OSHA, 2008; Radiology's, 2007). Under workers' compensation law, health care workers injured lifting patients may not sue their employer for not providing mechanical life equipment (Radiology's, 2007). The safety of imaging staff resides with regulations established by the U.S. Department of Labor, OSHA.

> OSHA's OSH Act of 1970 strives to: "...*assure safe and healthful working conditions for working men and women...*" and mandates that "...*each employer shall furnish to each of his/her employees a place of employment which are free from recognized hazards that are causing or are likely to cause death or serious physical harm to his/her employees*" (OSHA, 2008).

OSHA recommends minimizing manual lifting of patients in all cases and eliminating lifting when possible (2008). OSHA recommends that employers identify and address ergonomic issues in their facility's safety and health plan that should include at least the following areas:

- Management/leadership/employee participation;
- Workplace analysis;
- Accident and record analysis;
- Hazard prevention and control;
- Medical management; and,
- Training (2008).

Assisting the ambulatory patient or transporting the non-ambulatory patient to the imaging area via wheelchair or gurney can pose significant risk to the limited radiographer and support staff. The safety of limited radiographers and patients is at risk during transport to and from the imaging area and during positioning for imaging procedures. According to the Bureau of Labor Statistics employees in nursing and personal care facilities suffer over 200,000 work-related injuries and illnesses a year (OSHA, 2008). Many of these are serious injuries and more than half require time away from work (OSHA, 2008). Such injuries may include musculoskeletal injuries such as muscle and ligament strain and tears, joint and tendon inflammation, pinched nerves, and herniated discs (OSHA, 2008).

Workday tasks pose an increased ergonomic risk to radiographers and staff when they are:

- Repetitive;
- Done in awkward postures (e.g., reaching across gurneys and tables to lift patients);
- Done using a great deal of force (e.g., pushing wheelchairs or gurneys across elevation changes or up ramps);
- Lifting heavy objects (e.g., manually lifting immobile patients); or,
- Combining these factors (OSHA, 2008).

Other potential hazards for radiographers and staff include:

- Overexertion; trying to stop a patient from falling or picking a patient up from floor or bed;
- Multiple lifts per shift (more than 20);
- Lifting alone, no available staff to help;
- Lifting non-cooperative, confused patients;
- Lifting patients that cannot support their own weight;
- Expecting employees to perform work beyond their physical capabilities;
- Distance to be moved, and the distance the patient is from the staff;
- Awkward postures required by the activity; and,

- Ineffective training of employees in body mechanics and proper lifting techniques (OSHA, 2008).

Possible solutions to the risks posed by transporting and positioning patients for imaging procedures include continually identifying the most hazardous tasks and implementing engineering and work practice controls to help reduce or prevent injuries in those tasks (OSHA, 2008). Limited radiographers who consistently perform imaging tasks using proper body mechanics report fewer work-related injuries. The principles of body mechanics will be discussed later in this chapter.

OSHA recommends minimizing manual lifting of patients in all cases and eliminating lifting when possible (OSHA, 2008). It is suggested that when possible let the transport equipment and imaging system do the work. Imaging systems with tilting tables allow the patient to stand, lean, and be lowered into position, and footsteps and handrails should be available for the patient and radiographer to use. Imaging tables which move up, down, forward, and back also provide additional assistance to the radiographer during patient positioning. Additional equipment and supplies that may be used to avoid strain and injury when transporting and positioning the patient include:

- Mechanical lift equipment to help lift patients who cannot support their own weight;
- Overhead track mounted patient lifters, which is a system built into the ceiling to allow for patient mobility without manual lifting;
- Sliding board used under the patient to reduce the need for lifting during transfer;
- Slip sheets/roller sheets that help to reduce friction while laterally transferring and positioning patients;
- Height adjustable gurneys to allow for easy transfer from bed height to imaging table height;
- Trapeze lifts which allow patients with upper muscle strength to help reposition themselves;
- Walking belts or gait belts (with handles) that provide stabilization for ambulatory patients by allowing staff to hold onto the belt and support the patient; and,
- Wheelchairs with removable arms to allow for easier lateral transfers (OSHA, 2008).

The following is a review of additional measures that should be addressed in imaging facilities to prevent injuries and accidents.

- Trips, slips, and falls may occur from spills or environmental hazards. To prevent such occurrences, attention should be given to slippery or wet floors and floors surfaces that are uneven. Cluttered or obstructed work areas and passageways, poorly maintained walkway, or broken equipment pose potential hazards to all staff.

- Awkward postures accompanied by twisted, hyper-extended, or flexed back position increase the potential for injury. Good work practice recommends avoiding awkward postures while lifting or moving patients. Use recommended assist devices whenever possible, and team lifting based on patient assessment.
- Improper transfer of equipment like intravenous poles, wheelchairs, oxygen canisters, respiratory equipment, dialysis equipment, portable imaging equipment, or multiple items at the same time can result in injuries. Staff should place equipment on a rolling device if possible to allow for easier transport and should push rather than pull equipment. Staff should also ensure that passageways are unobstructed before attempting to move or transfer equipment and should seek help in moving bulky equipment or multiple items.
- Staff should limit reaching or lifting hazards when lifting trash, laundry, or other kinds of bags (OSHA, 2008).

The term "body mechanics" refers to good posture, alignment of the body segments, and correct use of muscles or muscle groups. Good posture occurs when all parts of the body are in balance and each segment aligned (Figure 4-4). Good posture provides a balanced body that is steady and secure and less prone to improper muscle use, falls, and mishaps. In addition to a balanced stable body, good posture allows the internal organs to work with greater efficiency. The following are tips for good posture:

1. Stand with feet parallel and 4 to 8 inches apart.
2. Keep body weight equally distributed on both feet.
3. Hold head erect with chin held in.
4. Hold chest and shoulders up.
5. Keep knees slightly bent.

Good posture needs to be maintained during the performance of workday activities. Basic tips for good body mechanics during task performance are:

- Keep the body's line close to the center of gravity (the waistline) when moving or lifting patients or objects.
- Bend the knees when picking up an object from the floor. Do not bend from the waist.
- Pull weight with the upper arms using the biceps.
- Balance the load over both feet when lifting. Bring the patient or object close to the body, bend the knees, and set the spine to support the load. Use arm muscles to lift. Always keep body balanced. Do not twist the body to move with a load, rather change foot positions.
- Keep body balanced over feet and spread feet apart to provide a base of support.

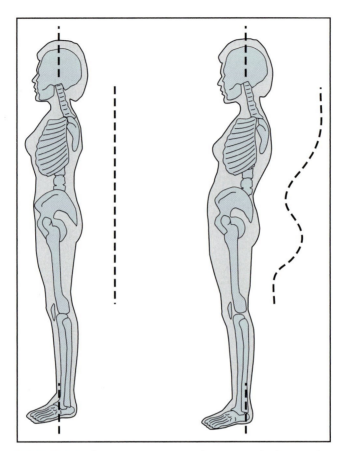

FIGURE 4-4 Correct posture, upright position. In the upright position, the center of gravity is the center of the pelvis.
Source: Delmar, Cengage Learning.

Moving and Transporting Patients

Limited radiographers work in a variety of settings and will encounter all kinds of patients. Examples of patient types follow.

Ambulatory patients—those who can walk and move. Ambulatory patients may require aides such as a walker, cane, or crutches.

Nonambulatory patients—those who cannot walk and move. Nonambulatory patients may arrive at the health care facility in an ambulance and be transported on a stretcher or a wheelchair. Ambulatory patients whose condition warrants may require transfer by wheelchair.

Before moving and transporting a patient, the radiographer must evaluate the patient's ability to aid in the process. Every patient must be considered in this evaluation since a patient's condition can change quickly. Generally, limited radiographers move and transport patients between a reception area or examination room to the radiography room and on and off the radiographic table. The following should be considered when assessing the patient:

- *General condition.* How does the patient appear? Is the patient alert, responsive, oriented, and functioning?
- *Mobility.* Did the patient walk into the facility without assistance? Are the patient's motions restricted in any way?
- *Strength and endurance.* Can the patient stand and walk without assistance? If so, will the patient become fatigued and be unable to complete the transfer without resting or assistance?
- *Balance.* Can the patient maintain balance? If the radiography procedure requires prolonged sitting or standing can the patient maintain the position without assistance?
- *Understanding and acceptance.* Does the patient understand the need to move and be transported? Does the patient seem willing and accepting of the move and transfer, or is the patient fearful?

After the initial assessment, the limited radiographer must decide what is the best way to move the patient and how much help will be required to safely make the move and transport. Never attempt to move or transport a patient without adequate assistance; to do so may cause injury to self or patient. It is helpful to remember the following rules related to patient transport:

- Move and transfer a patient over the shortest distance.
- Inform the patient about the move and ask for cooperation and help.
- Give short, simple commands.
- Give only the help the patient needs for safety and comfort.
- For standing and walking transfers, the patient should wear shoes.
- Lock all wheels on stretchers and wheelchairs before assisting the patient to move.

Trauma Radiography Guidelines

Patients who have experienced trauma may be unable to move and assume a position normally used for routine radiographic examinations. After the patient has been medically evaluated, it is the responsibility of the radiographer performing the examination to move the radiographic and accessory equipment around the patient so it will not cause the patient additional injury and discomfort. Each patient requires special attention and the following general trauma positions guidelines may be adapted to each situation.

1. Do not move the patient unless absolutely necessary.
2. A minimum of two radiographs should be taken for each anatomic area. Try to obtain two radiographs at 90 degree angles to each other.
3. If the patient is conscious and coherent, explain exactly what is happening before beginning the radiographic examination.
4. Maintain the routine central ray entrance and exit point to as close to usual entrance and exit as possible.
5. Place the cassette adjacent to the part being radiographed to avoid magnification of the image.
6. Include both joints when possible on radiographs of long bones. If this is not possible, include the joint closest to the injury.
7. Do not remove splints or bandages unless instructed to do so.
8. Maintain intravenous fluid bottles above the level of the needle site.
9. Remove clothing from the unaffected side first.

Methods of Transfer

Patient transfer can be divided into ambulatory and nonambulatory methods and the skills and safety precautions associated with each.

Although a patient is ambulatory, an initial assessment should be conducted. It is the limited radiographer's responsibility to remain alert and observant of any change in status of the ambulatory patient and give assistance as needed.

The ambulatory patient should be provided with a footstool when getting on and off the radiography table. Also, it is best to walk with the ambulatory patient instead of way ahead or behind, just in case assistance is required.

In transferring nonambulatory patients, the limited radiographer must take great care to prevent further injury and to protect the skin. These patients may be handicapped, paralyzed, seriously injured, and/or unconscious. The body, head, and neck will require support during the move. Common methods of transfer include using a three-carrier lift, sheet transfer, and logrolling the patient.

Patients may use a walking aid to support their body. Patients with walking aids will require the greatest assistance when moving through heavy doors, narrow hallways, and especially in small dressing areas and in getting on and off the radiographic table.

Canes are used to provide balance and support when there is a weakness on one side of the body. A walker provides more support than a cane because it has four points of support. Limited radiographers should be alert to potential falls and loss of balance in the patient with a cane or walker. Should such an incident occur, the limited radiographer should provide support to the patient's weak side until she/he has regained support and balance on the cane or walker.

Crutches are used when one lower extremity is injured or when both extremities need strength. Patients with crutches are always at risk of falling because they must rest the upper arm weight on the crutches. When assisting the patient with crutches on and off the radiographic table, it is best to seek assistance and have support on both sides of the patient.

Patient History and Assessment

The patient history assists the radiographer in knowing the extent of the injury, disease process, and ability of the patient to cooperate. The patient history also assists in the medical interpretation of the radiographs (Figure 4-5).

Certain disease processes or conditions require more or less radiation than the same healthy anatomic area. Some examples requiring a decrease in x-ray exposure are emphysema, osteoporosis, atrophy, and demineralization. Those requiring an increase in x-ray exposure are ascites, acromegaly, lung abscess, Paget's disease, pleural effusion, pneumonia, and an increase in bone mineralization.

Assessment of the patient means communicating with the patient about the procedure. Gaining the patient's confidence and trust though verbal and non-verbal communication is essential in the production of a high-quality radiograph. From the moment a patient is greeted and their identification is established, the radiographer begins to develop a rapport with the patient but also begins to assess the patient (Figure 4-6). Assessment of the patient includes determining how much the patient will be able to assist during the radiographic procedure and whether modification of the routine is needed.

Often a patient's condition may not allow him or her to assume or maintain the routine or usual position for a particular x-ray examination. In these cases, the radiographer may be required to modify the usual procedure to provide the information requested. This may require different projections or central ray entrance, etc., however, the limited radiographer may not supply additional, unrequested positions without a medical request. The radiographer may consult with the attending physician to determine if additional positions, projections, or views are necessary.

1. **Have you experienced any of the following problems:**
   a. Significant weight change   ☐ YES   ☐ NO
   b. Increased thirst or urination   ☐ YES   ☐ NO
   c. Bothersome joint pains   ☐ YES   ☐ NO
   d. Change in size/firmness of stool   ☐ YES   ☐ NO
   e. Change in size/color of mole   ☐ YES   ☐ NO
   f. Trouble falling or staying asleep   ☐ YES   ☐ NO
   g. Chest pain, shortness of breath   ☐ YES   ☐ NO
   h. Stomach problems or heartburn   ☐ YES   ☐ NO
   i. Problems with maintaing balance doing routine tasks at home   ☐ YES   ☐ NO
   j. Periods of weakness, numbness or inability to talk   ☐ YES   ☐ NO
   k. Severe headaches   ☐ YES   ☐ NO
   l. Painful urination   ☐ YES   ☐ NO
   m. Blood in urine   ☐ YES   ☐ NO
2. **Prevention:**
   a. Exercise:
      Activity_____
      Days per week_____
      Time/duration_____minutes
      Exertion: ○ stroll   ○ mild   ○ heavy
   b. If over 30 years, have you had your cholesterol checked in last 5 years?   ☐ YES   ☐ NO
   c. Have you had a tetanus shot in past 10 years?   ☐ YES   ☐ NO
   d. How many sexual partners have you had
      In the last 12 months?_____ In your lifetime?_____
   e. When was your last dental check-up?_____
   f. If over 50, when was your last colonoscopy?_____
   g. WOMEN, please answer the following
      i. When was your last PAP Smear (female exam)?_____
      ii. If over 40, when was your last mammogram?_____
      iii. Last normal menstrual period_____
      iv. Birth control method_____
   h. MEN over 50, when was your last prostate exam?_____
3. **Do you drink alcohol?**
   If yes:
   a. Have you ever felt you should cut down on your drinking?   ☐ YES   ☐ NO
4. **Have you ever used tobacco?**
   If yes:
   Average number of packs/day:_____
   Number of years smoked:_____
   Year quit:_____
   When are you planning to quit?   ○ Now   ○ Next 6 months   ○ Sometime   ○ Never
5. **Social History**   ○ Married   ○ Single   ○ Divorced   ○ Widowed
   If married:
   Year's married_____
   Spouse's name_____
   Your place of employment_____
   If children:
   Number of children_____
   Ages and names_____
   Who lives in the home with you now?_____

Thank you for taking the time to fill this form out. This will be used as a guide to address concerns during today's visit, if time allows, or future visits as indicated.

FIGURE 4-5 Medical history questionnaire
Source: Delmar, Cengage Learning.

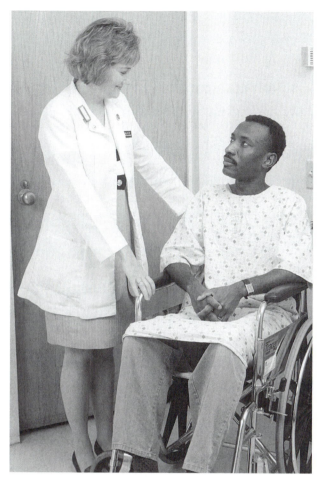

FIGURE 4-6 Greeting patient
Source: Delmar, Cengage Learning.

The Patient's Record: A Resource Document

Health care agencies use many types of forms for recording information about a patient. All of the forms used for a patient are placed in a folder and make up the patient's record. Charting is the process of making entries on the patient's record.

The patient's records serve many purposes:

- Guide to planning patient care
- Source of shared information that promotes continuity of the patient's care
- Source of information to keep all health personnel informed about the patient's care and condition

- Permanent summary of the patient's health status
- Research statistics
- Legal document

Making Entries on Patient Records

Each medical facility has certain guidelines about making entries on a patient's record. Such guidelines include who is responsible for writing on each form, the type of charting notations made, and what forms become part of the patient's permanent record.

Limited radiographers use patient records and make entries related to radiography procedures and basic patient care. Because limited radiographers generally function as a multiskilled professional, there may be many opportunities to refer to a patient's record and to make entries. Some examples are:

- The limited radiographer escorts a patient to the examination room, asks for the chief complaint, measures and records the vital signs, and enters the measurements on the patient record.
- The limited radiographer receives an oral telephone report on a special radiography procedure performed by a referral agency. The report is recorded and becomes part of the patient's record.
- The limited radiographer checks the chart to confirm the doctor's oral request for a radiograph.

Table 4-3 gives suggestions for making entries on a patient's medical record and Table 4-4 provides an example of an adult history form.

Meeting Patients' Needs

During any given day, a limited radiographer will provide care to a number of patients, each with a specific radiographic examination need. To complete the radiographs requested, patients may require assistance with meeting general and personal needs. Information related to meeting general and personal patient needs follows.

Physical Needs

Be aware of and provide for patients' privacy while they are dressing and undressing. Do not insist on staying with patients unless they ask for assistance or appear unable to help themselves. Knock on closed doors before entering, and close doors during procedures.

TABLE 4-3   The Patient's Record: A Resource Document

Suggestion	Explanation
Use a pen to make entries or retrieve electronic record from database.	The patient's record is a legal document and entries made in pencil can be too easily erased.
Make legible entries.	Write or print so others may read the penmanship. Illegible entries are useless.
Enter month, day, year.	Entries not properly dated lose their value as a source of information exchange and as a legal document. Many medical facilities also enter the time of day and AM or PM.
Follow facility policy concerning what should be recorded.	It is not necessary to record everything; follow facility policy.
Be brief and concise.	• Omit *a*, *an*, and *the*. • Omit writing patient name. • Use only standard common medical abbreviations.
Avoid personal judgment statements such as "seems like" or "appears to be." Quote the patient whenever possible. Record any adverse reactions, incidents, or mishaps the patient has.	If adverse reactions or unusual incidents are not recorded, it can be assumed they were not present. If the procedure or treatment requests are not documented as being carried out, it can be assumed they were not.
Some facilities require that documentation be made when ordered tests and procedures are completed. Describe instructions that a patient receives about examination preparation or self-administered contrast media. Do not rely on memory—record promptly.	Errors and omissions are likely if you rely on memory only.
Draw a line through an area left blank when not filled with information. Do not use ditto marks. Do not erase. Draw a single line through the error, write "error" near. Sign or initial all entries. Do not record for another person.	The line indicates that the area left blank was not intentionally omitted. Also, erasures may suggest falsification of information or facts.

Limited radiographers may not notice how cool the room temperature feels because they are busy working; however, to the patient who may be disrobed, the room may be very cool. Provide a light blanket or sheet for the patient to use if he or she feels chilled.

Other Needs

Patient valuables, such as a purse, wallet, watch, jewelry, eyeglasses, dentures, prostheses, or other such items, should never be left unattended. Ask patients to keep these items with them at all times. If a patient's valuables are stolen, report this immediately to the supervisor.

Patients may need assistance in finding or ambulating to the bathroom. Bathrooms should be kept stocked at all times with adequate toilet paper, paper towels, soap, and sanitary pads. Patients who cannot ambulate to the bathroom, may require assistance or a urinal or a bedpan. Limited radiographers may require additional assistance in positioning a patient on a bedpan.

IV Tubes, Urinary Catheters, Nasal Oxygen

Patients who have connecting IV tubes, urinary catheters, or nasal oxygen should be moved with care so as to not disturb these items. The limited radiographer's task is to take the required radiographs and to be observant of these items. If the IV tubing or urinary catheter becomes disconnected, it is important to report this immediately to the attending supervisor.

Limited radiographers often encounter patients who are receiving oxygen therapy. Without an adequate supply of oxygen in the body, metabolic activity decreases and life processes end. When individuals are unable to maintain a sufficient level of oxygen within their bodies, devices must be used to supplement their oxygen. It is safe to say that persons who require oxygen therapy are seriously ill and must be attended to carefully. An extremely important fact to remember is that *oxygen has properties that support combustion* and therefore becomes dangerous in the presence of sparks or flames. Although limited radiographers do not administer any type of oxygen therapy, it is important to recognize proper handling of patients receiving oxygen. Because oxygen is a highly combustible gas and radiographic equipment can cause sparks, the limited radiographer must always be extremely cautious and reduce the possibility of static electricity sparks when working where oxygen is being administered. Smoking is not allowed when oxygen is in use. Two common oxygen tanks are shown in Figure 4-7.

The amount of oxygen a patient is to receive is ordered by a physician. The various types of therapy devices are: (1) *nasal cannula* (Figure 4-8), (2) *nasal catheter*, (3) *face mask* (Figure 4-9), and (4) *oxygen tent*.

If an oxygen nasal cannula or face mask becomes dislodged or disconnected from the patient, the limited radiographer should put the nasal cannula or face mask back in place and ask the supervisor to check the equipment and the oxygen supply.

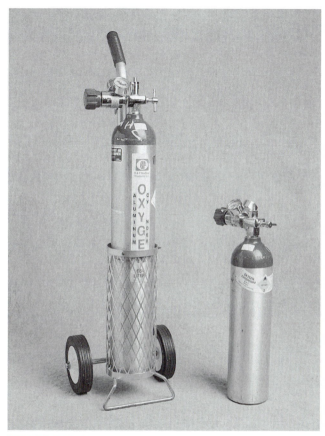

FIGURE 4-7 Oxygen tanks
Source: Delmar, Cengage Learning.

In most busy institutions where oxygen therapy is administered, experienced personnel are available to operate equipment and to provide assistance as needed.

Vital Signs

Limited radiographers must have knowledge of and be able to measure a patient's vital signs, i.e., those measures that let us know how a patient is doing on very basic levels of functioning—body temperature, pulse rate, blood pressure, and respiration rate. It is very important for limited radiographers to know the normal ranges of vital signs so that they can recognize deviations from the normal, which often indicate a medical emergency.

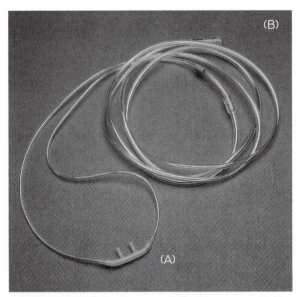

FIGURE 4-8 (A) Oxygen nasal cannula with (B) tubing
Source: Delmar, Cengage Learning.

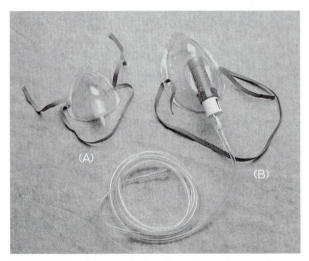

FIGURE 4-9 Oxygen masks (A) without tubing and
(B) with tubing
Source: Delmar, Cengage Learning.

The definition of a medical emergency is a sudden, unexpected change in a person's vital functions that demands immediate action. In the medical setting, emergencies may not be unexpected if the patient has had appropriate clinical assessment and is receiving medical treatment. Accordingly, there may be signs that

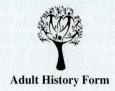

Adult History Form

TODAY'S DATE: **NAME**:

MEDICATION ALLERGIES: (such as penicillin), describe what happens when you take that medicine:

NON-MEDICATION ALLERGIES: (Latex, shellfish, bees):

MEDICATIONS: Prescription and Non-Prescription
        (including aspirin, vitamins, birth control, herbs, supplements, etc.)

Family History

Please check any family members who have the following health problems.

	Father	Mother	Brother	Sister	Grandparent	Other
Diabetes						
Glaucoma						
Cancer (List type)						
Heart attack						
Angina						
Stroke						
High blood pressure						
High cholesterol						
Alcoholism						
Drug Abuse						
Depression						
Mental Illness						
Suicide						
Other health problems						

PAST MEDICAL HISTORY

Please describe and give dates of any illnesses, injuries, hospitalizations, and surgeries:

TABLE 4-4   Example of an Adult History Form

all medical personnel who come in contact with the patient should recognize—signs that indicate trouble or a change in the patient's condition. For example, a patient's lips turning blue is a sign of a serious loss of oxygen to the brain and requires immediate action. *Immediate action* is probably the most critical aspect of any emergency; it is the required spontaneous reaction to the situation that actually constitutes the emergency.

Vital signs are important and useful because they provide the first signs of trouble for a patient; they also gauge a patient's return to a stable condition following physiological disturbances.

Temperature

Body temperature is a reflection of heat production and loss. The normal or average body temperature of a healthy person is 98.6 degrees F or 37 degrees centigrade. Average temperature may vary 1 to 2 degrees above or below 98.6 degrees F and still be within normal limits.

Body temperature is influenced by many factors. An increase in body temperature may be caused by a bacterial infection, physical activity, pregnancy, medication, and metabolism. A decrease in body temperature may be caused by a viral infection, exposure to cold, and fasting.

A person is said to have a fever when their body temperature increases beyond their average or baseline temperature. The term *pyrexia* is synonymous for fever. Afebrile means without a fever. Fevers may be classified into four categories: (1) continuous, (2) remittent, (3) intermittent, or (4) relapsing. A continuous fever is one that does not fluctuate but remains above the person's average temperature for a period of time. A fever that fluctuates, rising above average and returning, is termed intermittent. A remittent fever never returns to average temperature but remains above average. A relapsing fever is one that returns after a period of being at the average or baseline temperature.

Digital thermometers have largely replaced mercury thermometers. Regular digital thermometers use electronic heat sensors to record body temperatures, often in 30 seconds or less. Regular digital thermometers can be used in the mouth, armpit, or rectum. Digital ear thermometers, also called tympanic thermometers, use an infrared ray to measure temperature inside the ear canal (Figure 4-10).

The best type of thermometer or the best place to insert the thermometer depends on the patient's age and their ability to cooperate. From birth to 3 months, a regular digital thermometer is used to take a rectal temperature. For children from 3 months to 4 years, a digital ear thermometer or a digital pacifier thermometer is the recommended choice. For those 4 years and older, a digital thermometer can be held in place under the tongue.

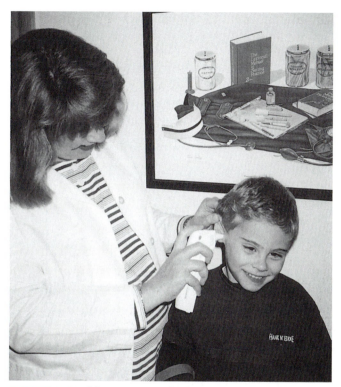

FIGURE 4-10   Measuring core body temperature with a tympanic thermometer
Source: Delmar, Cengage Learning.

Pulse

Each beat of the heart is a pulsation that occurs when the heart contracts (tightens) to send blood through the arterial system. The beat or pulse may be felt at certain places on the body starting at the head and moving downward to the feet, Figure 4-11. The name and location of the different pulses are:

- *Temporal*—in front of the ear at the temple
- *Carotid*—in the front of the neck over the carotid artery
- *Apical*—actual heartbeat over apex of the heart; heard with a stethoscope
- *Brachial*—over the brachial artery at the inner surface of the elbow
- *Radial*—at the wrist just above the base of the thumb
- *Femoral*—in the groin over the femoral artery
- *Popliteal*—posterior or just behind the knee joint
- *Pedal*—on the arch of the foot at the dorsal pedal (dorsalis pedis) artery

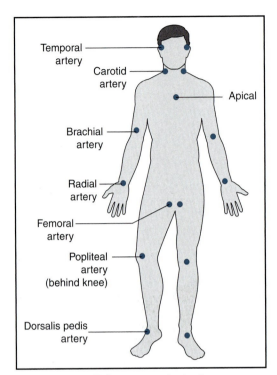

FIGURE 4-11 Pulse sites in the body
Source: Delmar, Cengage Learning.

The most common areas used to check pulse rate are (a) apical, with a stethoscope for accurate rate, and (b) radial, with the first two fingers placed on the inner side of the wrist at the depression just above the thumb. The farther away from the heart the pulse rate is taken, the more difficult it becomes to count because the pulse wave weakens.

Normal *pulse rates* range from 50 to 100 beats per minute for adults. Many activities and events will cause a change in the heart rate, thus resulting in a change in the pulse rate. Table 4-5 shows average pulse beats per minute according to age

TABLE 4-5   Average Pulse Beats per Minute According to Age Groups

| | Pulse Rate per Minute | | | | | | | |
| | | 2 | 4 | 6 | 8 | 10 | 12 | 16 |
	Newborn	Years	Years	Years	Years	Years	Years	Years
Female	115–130	110	100	100	90	90	90	90
Male	115–130	110	100	100	90	90	85	75

groups. Pulse rates are affected by age, body build, exercise, medications (drugs), blood pressure, body temperature, pain, and various foods and liquids.

There are several aspects to consider when checking pulse rates. A *regular* pulse has constant rhythm and equal time between pulses; this indicates good blood flow. An *irregular* pulse has inconsistent rhythm and may be felt as both strong and weak throbs. A *thready* pulse is weak, difficult to count, and irregular in rhythm; this pulse indicates poor blood flow. As stated earlier, when you are counting the radial pulse, place the tips of your first two fingers over the radial artery of the patient's wrist at the inner portion of the wrist just above the thumb and count the pulse beats for one minute. Do not apply your own thumb to the patient's wrist because the thumb has its own strong pulse. The procedure for pulse count is included with the procedure for counting respiration because pulse and respiration are generally checked together.

Respiration

The exchange of oxygen and carbon dioxide in the lungs is called respiration. Respiration occurs when a person takes in a breath (inhales) and lets out a breath (exhales). One such exchange is counted as one excursion of breathing. This exchange of gases is done at the rate of 16 to 20 times a minute by the average adult.

Changes that occur in the chest during inhalation and exhalation are important considerations for the limited radiographer when doing a chest film. During chest radiography, it is important that the limited radiographer allow the patient to breathe in and out a couple of times to ensure that the lungs are fully inflated and that the diaphragm has moved down, allowing more lung to be visualized.

To reduce possible patient anxiety, it is best to count respirations when the patient is unaware that the count is being taken. The rate of breathing, like pulse, can be affected by such common considerations as age (children breathe faster, older people slower), exercise, emotions, disease, temperature, and medications.

Respirations may be counted after a patient's pulse has been taken. To do so, it is best to continue holding the wrist so the patient will not realize you are counting breathing excursions (inhalations and exhalations). To count respiration, count the number of times the patient's chest moves up or rises. Count respirations for 60 seconds. When observing a child, breathe with the child; this technique is particularly useful when you are making a radiographic exposure of the chest on full inhalation. It is equally important to listen to the patient's breathing to determine if it is labored or unusual in sound. Normal breathing should be relaxed, even, and quiet. Respiration should be recorded as *regular, irregular, rapid, shallow,* or *labored.* Table 4-6 lists the medical term given to abnormal types of breathing and the characteristics of each.

TABLE 4-6 Abnormal Types of Breathing and Characteristics of Each Type

Apnea	Temporary cessation of breathing; suspended respiration
Cheyne-Stokes	An abnormal pattern of breathing where apnea occurs from 10 to 60 seconds followed by increased depth and frequency of breathing
Dyspnea	Audible labored or difficult breathing
Hyperventilation	Increased respiratory rate or breathing that is deeper than normal; forced respiration
Orthopnea	Difficulty breathing while recumbent
Otigopnea	A type of breathing that occurs in acute pulmonary disease when chest walls are thick; abnormally shallow or slow breathing
Rales	Abnormal sounds heard in the chest, caused by air passage in the bronchi that contains secretion
Spasmodic	Uneven
Stertorous	Labored
Stridor	Obstructed air passages that create a harsh sound during respiration; high-pitched sound like wind blowing
Tachypnea	An increase in respiration rate; as in hyperventilation; abnormally rapid breathing
Wheeze	Whistling sound as a result of narrowing of the lumen of respiratory passageway

Blood Pressure

Blood pressure (BP) is the force of the flow of blood exerted against the walls of the blood vessels. Blood pressure is measured by reading two numbers that register on an aneroid or mercury gauge called a sphygmomanometer, Figure 4-12.

Two numbers are read for blood pressure: (1) when the heart contracts or *systolic* pressure and (2) when the heart is relaxed or *diastolic* pressure. The average adult's blood pressure should be below 120/80 mm of mercury. The top number (120) is the systolic pressure and the bottom number (80) is the diastolic pressure. Blood pressure is crucial to good health and may vary with age and physical conditions.

The same activities and events that affect the pulse also affect blood pressure. Other important situations prevalent in our society today that cause blood pressure problems are (1) heart and kidney disease, (2) vascular disease in the brain, (3) emotional conditions, (4) drugs, and (5) higher blood pressure in men than women in the same age group.

Hypertension and hypotension are two conditions with which the health professional needs to be familiar. Hypertension is high blood pressure created and

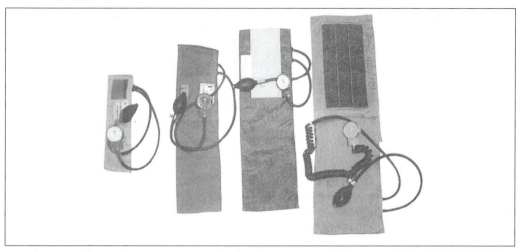

FIGURE 4-12 Aneroid manometer-type of sphygmomanometer for measuring blood pressure. Different size cuffs are shown. For an accurate measurement of blood pressure, it is important to use the proper size cuff on the patient. For example, a large adult cuff should not be used on a child. Source: Delmar, Cengage Learning.

exacerbated (made worse) by a variety of conditions including disease, emotional stress, and environmental stress. Hypotension is low blood pressure and is not necessarily an indication of illness unless the person has symptoms. However, low blood pressure related to shock or circulatory collapse is dangerous and can result in death if not treated.

A new classification of blood pressure, prehypertension, describes people with blood pressures between 120–130 millimeters of mercury systolic or 80–89 diastolic (American Heart Association [AHA], 2009).

The new prehypertension category focuses the physician, patient, and public attention on blood pressure in these ranges and encourages healthy lifestyles and in some instances treatment with blood-pressure lowering drugs (AHA, 2009).

To obtain an accurate blood pressure measurement, the limited radiographer must select the appropriate size cuff for the patient's arm. Cuff sizes range from newborn to obese and thigh cuffs are also available.

If the cuff size is too large, the measurement will produce a false low reading. A cuff too small will produce a false high reading. The size of the blood pressure cuff should should be based on the patient's arm size and not on their age. Proper sizing for an adult cuff should allow for at least one-third to one-half the arm circumference. The length of the bladder should cover approximately 80% of the arm for adults and two-thirds of the upper arm of a child.

To ensure accurate readings, these rules must be followed:

1. Select the appropriate cuff size to fit the patient.
2. Inflate and deflate the cuff gradually.
3. Palpate the pulse before placing the stethoscope firmly over the brachial artery.
4. Ask the patient to be absolutely still.

Medical Emergencies

Medical emergencies can and do occur in the office radiography environment. The limited radiographer must therefore have basic knowledge about medical emergencies and the immediate actions required.

Medical Emergencies Terminology

Anaphylactic shock: A serious form of shock due to extreme sensitivity to a drug or foreign substance.

Anaphylactic reactions: May result in death. Patient may flush, exhibit hives, nausea, and loss of breathing.

Antigen: A protein that when introduced into the body causes formation of antibodies against it.

Epilepsy: A sudden passing disturbance of brain function.

Fainting: Temporary loss of consciousness due to loss of blood to the brain.

Hyperventilation: Increase in the amount of air entering the alveolar or air sacs.

Cardiac Tampondae: A collection of fluid or blood in the sac surrounding the heart which causes compression and prevents the heart from beating normally.

Cyanosis: A bluish discoloration.

Pulmonary Embolus: Obstruction of the pulmonary artery or one of its branches by undissolved matter.

Diaphoresis: Profuse perspiration

Eclampsia: Convulsion and coma occurring in a pregnant or newly delivered woman; rising blood pressure and protein in the urine are warning signals.

Uremia: The retention of excessive by-products of protein metabolism in the blood and the toxic condition produced by it.

DNR: Do Not Resuscitate

Syncope: (dizzy)

Stroke: **(CVA)** Cerebrovascular accident is an interference with blood supplied to the brain **(TIA)** a partial vessel occlusion and usually mild and temporary.

(Thrombus) occurs when the cerebral vessel is totally occluded or ruptures, sudden loss of consciousness and one-sided paralysis (hemiparesis).

Vertigo: (sensation of having objects or the room spinning)

Shock

Shock is a life-threatening condition that occurs when the body is not getting enough blood flow. This can damage multiple organs and requires immediate medical treatment. There are several major classes of shock. These include:

- Cardiogenic shock which is generally associated with cardiovascular disease;
- Hypovolemic shock that is caused by inadequate blood volume;
- Anaphylactic shock which occurs due to an allergic reaction;
- Septic shock associated with infections; and
- Neurogenic shock caused by damage to the nervous system.

A person in shock will have extremely low blood pressure and depending on the specific cause and type of shock, symptoms will include one or more of the following:

- Anxiety or agitation;
- Confusion;
- Pale, cool, clammy skin;
- Low or no urine output;
- Bluish lips and fingernails;
- Dizziness, light-headedness, or faintness;
- Profuse sweating, moist skin;
- Rapid but weak pulse;
- Shallow breathing;
- Chest pain; and,
- Unconsciousness.

If the limited radiographer suspects that a patient is in shock, she/he should seek immediate help. The patient's airway should be checked, and if necessary rescue breathing and cardiopulmonary resuscitation should be started. Keep the patient warm and comfortable and loosen tight clothing. If the person vomits or drools, turn their head to one side. Do not give the person anything by mouth, do not attempt to move the patient, and seek immediate assistance.

Fainting

Fainting is probably the most common emergency that occurs in the radiography setting. The limited radiographer must constantly observe all patients for signs of dizziness, pallor, or cold, clammy skin. At the first sign of fainting, have the patient lie down or place the head between the legs lower than the body. Application of cool compresses on the face may also be effective. Seek assistance as soon as possible.

Seizures

Seizures are caused by medical problems ranging from emotion or anxiety reactions to brain tumors. Epilepsy, usually found in children or young adults, is probably the most common cause of seizures. The most important response to a seizure is to make sure that the patient does not injure his/her head or body during the convulsive phase or obstruct his/her airway with his/her tongue. It is best to simply stay with the patient and call for assistance.

A mild seizure (petit mal) may be of short duration or may go unnoticed. A more severe seizure (grand mal) always requires assistance. Some symptoms of grand mal are jerky movements, rapid breathing, a loud cry, muscle rigidity, incontinence of urine or stool, vomiting, and frothing (foaming at the mouth). All symptoms that occur before, during, and after a seizure should be reported to a supervisor. The limited radiographer should make no attempt to open the patient's mouth or to force a solid object (such as wrapped tongue blades) into the mouth or airway.

Vomiting

Provide patient with a basin, tissue, and water for rinsing their mouth. If the patient is recumbent, turn the head to the side to prevent choking from aspiration of vomitus. If the patient is feeling nauseous, ask them to breath slowly and deeply through the mouth.

Nosebleeds (Epistaxis)

Bleeding or hemorrhage from the nose is usually referred to as epistaxis. Universal Precautions should be used when attempting to control bleeding. Nosebleeds may be controlled by applying external pressure to the side of the bleeding nostril. Cold compresses to the face may also be of value. The patient's head should be elevated. Seek assistance from the supervisor or attending physician.

REVIEW QUESTIONS

1. Microscopic life forms found in tissues of fleas, lice, and ticks, and other insects is:
   a. bacteria
   b. fungi
   c. protozoa
   d. rickettsiae

2. One of the major differences between bacteria and viruses is that bacteria:
   a. cause malaria and toxoplasmosis
   b. are not dependent on the host for replication and growth
   c. exist in two forms; yeasts and molds
   d. are one-celled organisms

3. **All** of the following are true regarding nosocomial infections, **except**:
   a. generally acquired in hospitals and medical care facilities but secondary to the patient's original condition
   b. considered opportunistic
   c. are more common in healthy adults
   d. spread more by hands than any other method of transfer

4. Common fomites are:
   a. bats and dogs
   b. radiographic tables
   c. the radiographer's uniform
   d. both b and c

5. Asepsis is defined as the absence of all disease-producing microorganisms.
   a. True
   b. False

6. According to the Centers for Disease Control and Prevention (CDC), the single most important measure health care workers can use to reduce the risk of transmitting pathogens is:
   a. cleaning the x-ray equipment with an antiseptic solution
   b. increasing air ventilation rated in the radiography room
   c. handwashing
   d. wearing protective masks and eye shields

7. Effective hand washing for the purpose of removing soil and microorganisms includes the use of soap or detergent and scrubbing for at least ___ to ___.
   a. 1–2 seconds
   b. 10–15 seconds
   c. 1 minute
   d. 2 minutes

8. The x-ray table should be cleaned with:
   a. a disinfectant after every use
   b. water and a dry cloth once a day
   c. antiseptic twice a day
   d. disinfectant once a week

9. Universal precautions apply to:
   a. blood
   b. all bodily secretions
   c. excretions (except sweat)
   d. all of the above

10. Transmission-based precautions (TBP) are necessary in the care of patients infected with transmittable pathogens.
    a. True
    b. False

11. At highest risk for tuberculosis are those who give care and provide diagnostic imaging services to patients who:
    a. are HIV positive
    b. homeless
    c. born outside the United States
    d. all of the above

12. Ergonomics is the science of:
    a. studying microbial life forms
    b. balancing the daily financial records
    c. fitting the job to the worker
    d. measuring the heart's output

13. The body mechanics that the limited radiographer should use when lifting a patient include:
    1. keep the patient close to your body
    2. keep your back straight and do not twist at the trunk
    3. stand with your feet together

Possible Responses

a. 1 and 2
b. 1 and 3
c. 2 and 3
d. 1, 2, and 3

14. The benefits of computerized patient records include:
    1. legibility of entries
    2. communication among health care team members
    3. greater access to medical data for patient care
    4. education and quality improvement

Possible Responses

a. 1 and 2
b. 2 and 3
c. 3 and 4
d. 1, 2, 3, and 4

15. Congress passed the Health Insurance Portability and Accountability Act (HIPAA) to:
    a. reduce accidents in the radiology area
    b. increase accountability for radiation exposure to the general public
    c. protect patient's medical information and limit access to that information
    d. reduce nosocomial infection in health care facilities

16. **All** of the following are true regarding making entries on the patient medical record, **except**:
    a. all entries should be legible
    b. entries should be brief and concise and approved abbreviations used
    c. the month, date, and year should be included with all entries
    d. a number 2 lead pencil may be used to make entries

17. Normal adult body temperature when taken orally is ___ degrees Fahrenheit.
    a. 96.6
    b. 97.6
    c. 98.6
    d. 99.6

18. Normal adult pulse rate is within the range of:
    a. 50–100
    b. 50–70
    c. 80–100
    d. 115–130

19. The normal adult blood pressure range should be below:
    a. 60/100
    b. 80/120
    c. 85/125
    d. 90/130

20. A pulse which is weak, difficult to count, and irregular in rhythm is called:
    a. regular
    b. syncopated
    c. thready
    d. vascular

21. An abnormal breathing pattern where apnea occurs from 10 to 60 seconds followed by increased depth and frequency is:
    a. apnea
    b. dyspnea
    c. stridor
    d. Cheyne-Stokes

22. Difficult or labored breathing is called:
    a. apnea
    b. dyspnea
    c. stridor
    d. rales

23. Increased respiratory rate or breathing that is deeper than normal is:
    a. wheeze
    b. rales
    c. stridor
    d. hyperventilation

24. **All** of the following are true regarding intravenous (IV) tubes, urinary catheter, or nasal oxygen, **except**:
    a. if an oxygen nasal cannula or face mask becomes dislodged, the limited radiographer should not attempt to replace the cannula or face mask
    b. take all precautions to eliminate static electricity sparks in areas where oxygen is being administered
    c. take precautions not to dislodge IV tubes, urinary catheters, and oxygen tubes
    d. if IV tubing or a urinary catheter does become disconnected, the limited radiographer should report it immediately

25. Bleeding or hemorrhage from the nose is referred to as:
    a. epistaxis
    b. hemostasis
    c. hemoplysis
    d. none of the above

26. A serious form of shock due to extreme sensitivity to a drug or foreign substance is referred to as:
    a. antigen
    b. eclampsia
    c. anaphylactic
    d. cardiogenic

27. Cyanosis refers to:
    a. a bluish discoloration
    b. retention of excessive by-products of protein metabolism in the blood
    c. a serious form of shock
    d. an increase in the amount of air entering the alveolar or air sacs

28. If a patient vomits while lying on the x-ray table, the limited radiographer should:
    a. have the patient roll over and lie face down
    b. assist the patient to turn their head to the side to avoid aspiration
    c. give the patient an emesis basin and escort them to the bathroom
    d. give the patient a cold drink

REFERENCES

ACR Technical Standard for Electronic Practice of Medical Imaging. (2007). *American College of Radiology* Effective 10/01/07. Retrieved from http://www.acr.org

American Heart Association. (2009). Your high blood pressure questions answered: Guidelines lowered. Retrieved from http://www.americanheart.org

American Society of Radiologic Technologists. (2008). The practice standard for medical imaging and radiation therapy. Limited x-ray machine operator standards. Retrieved from http://www.asrt.org

Association for Professionals in Infection Control and Epidemiology, Inc. (2008). *Handwashing.* Retrieved from http://www.apic.org

Centers for Disease Control and Prevention. (2006a). Clinical syndromes or conditions warranting additional empiric precautions. Retrieved from http://www.cdc.gov.ncidod

Centers for Disease Control & Prevention. (2006b). Preventing occupational HIV transmission to healthcare personnel. Retrieved from the National Centers for HIV,

STD, and TB Prevention Divisions of HIV/AIDS Prevention website: http://www.cdc.gov.nchstp

Centers for Disease Control and Prevention. (2006c). U.S. Public Health Service Guidelines for the management of occupational exposures to HBV, HCV, and HIV recommendations for postexposure prophylasis. Retrieved from http://www.cdc.gov

Centers for Disease Control and Prevention. (2008). Guideline for hand hygiene in health-care settings. Retrieved from http://www.cdc.gov

Costal Family Medicine. (2008). Adult Patient History Form. Retrieved from http://costalfamilymedicine.com

Edlich, R.G., Hudson M.A., Buschbacher, R.M., & et al. (2005). Devastating injuries in healthcare workers: Description of the crisis and legislative solution to the epidemic of back injury from patient lifting. *Journal of Long-Term Effects of Medical Implants*. Retrieved from http://www.ncbi.nlm.nih.gov

Family Practice Management. (2008). *The HIPAA privacy rule: Three key forms*. Retrieved from http://www.aafp.org

Hendricks, M.M. (2007). Documentation for Mammography. *Radiologic Technology, 78*(5), 396–412.

Patterson-Neubert, A. (2004). Patient privacy at risk in hospital hallways, lobbies, cafeterias. Purdue News. Retrieved from http://news.UNS.Purdue.edu

Radiology's big challenge: Imaging the "morbidly obese." *Medicexchange.com*. August 21, 2007. Retrieved from http://www.mediexchange.com

Shagam, J. (1999). The radiology department and nosocomial infections. *Radiologic Technology, 70*(5), 418–433.

Shock. (2008). *Medline Plus*. Medical Encyclopedia. Retrieved from http://www.nlm.hih.gov

Taber's Cyclopedic Medical Dictionary (15th ed.). (1985). Philadelphia: F.A. Davis Company.

U.S. Department of Labor, Occupational Safety & Health Administration (OSHA). (2008). Ergonomics. Retrieved from http://www.osha.gov

SUGGESTED READINGS

Aberle, L. (2006). Exercise your skills in ergonomics. *Advance for Imaging and Radiation Therapy Professionals*. Merion Publications Inc. King of Prussia, PA.

Faguy, K. (2005). TB testing a must for R.T.'s. *ASRT Scanner, 38*(14).

Faguy, K. (2006). Hospital adopt safer patient-lifting policies. *ASRT Scanner, 28*(5), 14–15.

Leaper, C. (2004). Writing it down: The technologist's role in charting. *Radiology Today*. 15–16.

Moroney, M.A. (2003) Viral hepatitis. *Radiologic Techolnology, 75*(1), 35–43.

Palakow, N. (2005, January 31). All systems go: Maintaining safety in the diagnostic radiology suite. RT-*Image*, 26–29.

RADIOGRAPHIC PHYSICS

Key Terms

Alpha Particles
Anion
Atomic Mass Number
Atomic Number
Atom
Attenuation
Background Radiation
Beta Particles
Binding Energy
Cation
Characteristic Radiation
Chemically Stable
Compound
Coherent Scattering
Compton Effect
Coulomb per Kilogram
Electromagnetic Radiation
Electron
Element
Energy
Environmental Radiation
Gamma Radiation
Gray (Gy)
Hertz
Inert
Inertia
Ion

Chapter Outline

Introduction
  Natural Science Review
Units of Measurement
Concepts of Matter
Atomic Structure
  Basic Atomic Particles
Radiation
  Electromagnetic and Particulate Radiation
  Artificial Sources of Radiation
Ionization
X-Ray Interactions with Matter
  Coherent Scattering
  Photoelectric Absorption
  Compton Effect
  Photodisintegration
  Pair Production

Objectives

Upon completion of the chapter, the student will meet the following objectives by verifying knowledge of the facts and principles presented through oral and written communication at a level deemed competent.

⟳ Identify the common units of radiation measurement and atomic nomenclature.

⟳ Label an illustration of an atom with energy shells and the nucleus, proton, electron, and neutron.

⟳ State the electric charge of a proton, electron, and neutron.

⟳ Draw an illustration showing the atomic structure before and after ionization.

⟳ Identify the smallest unit of an atom, element, and compound.

⟳ List the origin and characteristics of electromagnetic radiation (gamma rays and x-ray) and particulate radiation.

Introduction

"Why must I study radiographic physics to be able to take a chest radiograph?" and "How does knowing about the production of x-rays relate to the everyday tasks of medical radiography?" are common questions asked by limited radiography students. Such questions express the students' need to understand how physics and related concepts apply to the everyday tasks performed by medical radiographers. One answer to these questions is that the basic laws and concepts of physics form the foundation of x-ray production, x-ray interactions with matter, and radiographic image formation.

This chapter presents the essential laws and concepts of physics that have a direct application to medical radiography and the production of diagnostic radiographs.

Natural Science Review

Physics is a branch of science that deals with matter and energy and their relation to each other. It includes heat, sound, light, mechanics, electricity, magnetism, and the basic structure and properties of matter. Physics, like chemistry, astronomy, and geology, is considered one of the physical sciences and is classified as a natural science.

Units of Measurement

Physics is a science, and uses a system of measurement to describe physical quantities such as length, mass, or time. In 1960, at the Eleventh General Conference of Weights and Measures, the Systèm Internationale d'Unites (SI) was defined and officially adopted (Table 5-1).

All scientific disciplines communicate using SI quantities and values. There are seven base SI units: mass, length, time, electric current, temperature, amount of substance, and luminous intensity. All other units are derived from the seven base units. The United States did not fully adopt the SI/metric units and continues to use standard or traditional measurements such as inches, feet, quarts, or pounds.

In the science of physics, the fundamental SI units include mass, length, and time. Mass is the amount or quantity of matter. The standard unit of mass is the kilogram (kg). The meter (m) is the unit of length. The meter, defined in 1983, is the distance that light travels in a vacuum in 1/299,792,485 second. The unit of time is the second, which is measured by the vibrations of 133 cesium atoms. This method is referred to as the atomic clock time. The SI/metric system uses prefixes to signify different order of magnitude of the units (Table 5-2).

Sometimes it may be easier to use very small or large units of measurement. In such cases, the following may be used in the conversion. To covert from grams to kilograms or micrograms, or to grams with any other prefix, the decimal point is moved. If the prefix moves up the table, the decimal point is moved to the left the number of exponent positions moved. If the prefix moves down the table, the decimal point is moved to the right the number of exponent positions moved.

TABLE 5-1   Base Units of the SI System of Measurement

Quantity	Unit	Symbol
Length	meter	m
Mass	kilogram	kg
Time	second	s
Electric current	ampere	A
Luminous intensity	candela	cd
Temperature	Kelvin	K
Amount of Substance	mole	mol

TABLE 5-2 Systems of Measurement

British System	Foot, pound, second
Metric System	Centimeter, gram, second, meter, kilogram
SI System (International System of Units)	A new system of measurement in science that provides for the interconversion of units among all branches of science. Based on the metric system.
Units of Measurement	
Length	The unit of length. The meter (m) is the basic unit of length in the metric system.
Mass	A measurement of the quantity of matter in a body. The kilogram (kg) is the SI unit of mass.
Time	Measurement of intervals between events. The standard unit of time is second (s).
Area	Measurement of a given surface dependent upon length of area; square meters (m^2).
Volume	Measurement of the capacity of a container, dependent upon length of container. Volume may be expressed in cubic meters (m^3), liters (l), milliliters (ml), or cubic centimeters (cc or cm^3).
Velocity	Speed in a given direction. Expressed in meters per second (m/s).
Temperature	Expressed as degrees Celsius or Fahrenheit. Celsius = 0°C freezing point of water 100°C boiling point of water Fahrenheit = 32°F freezing point of water 212°F boiling point of water

Example

25.2 g = 0.0252 kg	Move the decimal point three positions left
25.2 g = 25,200 mg	Move the decimal point three positions right
25.2 mg = 0.0000252	Move the decimal point six positions left

In recent years, the SI has been adopted for radiation protection; however, the traditional units of measuring radiation are still very much in use. In radiology, the important SI units and their traditional counterpart include the following: Coulomb per kilogram (C/kg), formerly the Roentgen (R); Gray (Gy) formerly the rad (radiation absorbed dose); and, Sievert (sv), formerly the rem (radiation equivalent man).

These and other units of radiation measurement will be discussed again in Chapter 15, Radiation Biology, and Chapter 16, Radiation Protection.

Table 5-3 provides a review of the SI units.

In the SI unit of measurement, the sievert has replaced the rem (radiation equivalent man). The sievert is the unit used when it is necessary to express the quantity of radiation received in an occupational exposure. The sievert is defined as the product of the absorbed dose in gray and the radiation-weighting factor (additional information may be found in Chapter 15, Radiation Biology. One sievert is equal to 100 rem, and 1 rem is equal to 10 mSv (Table 5-4).

One of the first units of measurement used for radiation was called the roentgen, after Professor Wilhelm Conrad Roentgen. The units of gray (Gy) and sievert (Sv) are used in measuring the effects of radiation on living matter. The gray is defined

TABLE 5-3 Derived Units Commonly Used in Radiography

Quantity	SI Unit	Symbol	Traditional Unit
Absorbed dose	gray	Gy	rad
Radioactivity (disintegrations/s)	becquerel	Bq	curie
Electric charge	coulomb	C	esu
Electrical potential (electromotive force) (potential difference)	volt	V	
Energy/work (quantity of heat)	joule	J	erg
Force	newton	N	
Magnetic flux	weber	Wb	
Magnetic flux density	tesla	T	gauss
Power	watt	W	
Frequency hertz	Hz (cycle/s)	cycles per sec	

TABLE 5-4 Conversions Between Conventional and SI Units

Conventional Unit (Column A)	Conversion Factor (Column B)	SI Unit (Column C)
roentgen	2.58×10^4	coulomb/kilogram
rod	0.01	gray
rem	0.01	sievert
curie	3.7×10^{10}	becquerel

Column A amount multiplied by Column B equals Column C amount.
Column C amount divided by Column B equals Column Amount.

as 1 joule (J) of energy absorbed in each kilogram (kg) of absorbing material. One gray is equivalent to 100 rads. The gray expresses the quantity of absorbed dose and is an important indicator when considering biologic effects resulting from radiation exposure. The gray replaces the rad (radiation absorbed dose), which is defined as 100 ergs of energy absorbed by 1 gram of absorbing material (Table 5-4).

Concepts of Matter

Matter is used to describe the substance that comprises all physical objects. Matter may be defined in terms of its properties, such as mass, volume, shape, and that it occupies space (Figure 5-1).

A principal characteristic of matter is mass, which is the quantity of matter contained in an object. In our world, matter is most commonly found as substances. A substance is defined as a material that has a definite and constant composition. When two or more substances are combined they form a mixture. For example, air is a mixture of oxygen, hydrogen, nitrogen, and a variety of other substances. Substances may be either simple or complex. Simple substances are known as elements and complex substances are known as compounds. An element is a substance that cannot be easily reduced (broken down) under normal conditions. There are ninety two naturally occurring elements identified on the Periodic Table of Elements. An additional 11 elements have been created in the laboratory through scientific investigations (Figure 5-2).

Many of the elements are commonly used in health care; such as calcium, sodium, and potassium. Elements that are commonly used in radiography include lead, tungsten, rhenium, copper, aluminum, iodine, and radium (Table 5-5).

The universe consists of matter and energy and there exists a unique interchangeable relationship between the two. In 1905, Albert Einstein (1879–1955) described this relationship in his well-known theory of relativity. Einstein mathematically described the relationship between matter and energy in the equation: $E = mc^2$.

Einstein's work in the area of matter and energy is best defined as the Law of Conservation. This law states that the sum total of all matter and energy in the universe is constant: matter and energy cannot be created or destroyed but can be converted from one form to another (Figure 5-3).

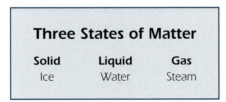

Three States of Matter

Solid	Liquid	Gas
Ice	Water	Steam

FIGURE 5-1 Three states of matter
Source: Delmar, Cengage Learning.

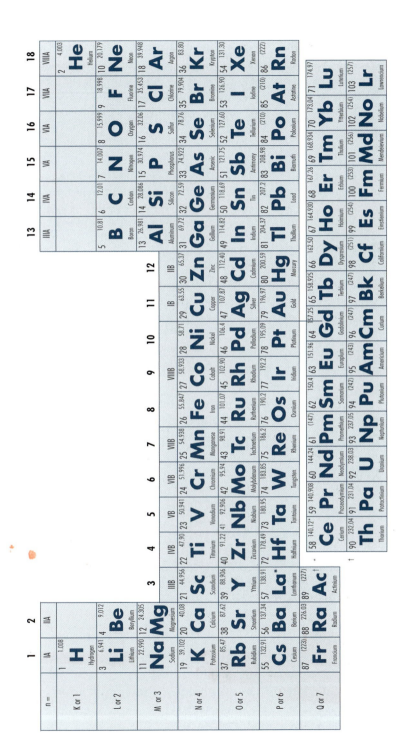

FIGURE 5-2 Periodic table of elements
Source: Delmar, Cengage Learning.

TABLE 5-5 Radiation Units of Measurement

Traditional Unit of Measurement	International Unit of Measurement	Definition
Roentgen (R)	Coulomb per kilogram (C/kg)	Quantity of charge released as x-rays or gamma rays pass through a specific quantity of dry air
RAD (r)	Gray (Gy) *defined as the energy transfer of 1 joule (J) per kilogram of irradiated object/ matter*	Radiation absorbed dose. Indicates the quantity of energy transferred to matter or an object by any type of ionizing radiation
REM (rad-equivalent man) *defined as the unit of the quantity, absorbed dose equivalent of any type of ionizing radiation that produces the same biological effect as 1 rad of radiation.*	Sievert (Sv) *One sievert equals one 100 rem.*	An absorbed dose in rad may be converted to a rem by use of the quality factor for the type of radiation. Sievert and rem are easily compared by taking the number of rem and dividing by hundred to find the sievert unit

Energy Transformation

Baking powder/yeast	Causes baking mixtures to rise.
Chemical battery	Coverts to electrical energy to power a flashlight or radio.
Sunlight	Captured in photosensitive solar cells for conversion to electricity.

FIGURE 5-3 Examples of matter and energy transformation
Source: Delmar, Cengage Learning.

Energy is the ability to do work, where work is defined as the application of force over a distance. The unit of energy is the joule (J). When energy is emitted and transferred through matter, it is called radiation. Kinetic energy is energy in motion. When an object is moving, it possesses kinetic energy. Examples of kinetic energy are a pitched baseball, a moving automobile, or a person walking. Because any moving object possesses two quantities, mass and velocity, kinetic energy is expressed in terms of mass and velocity.

Potential energy is stored energy. Potential energy exists because of an object's position. For this reason, potential energy is called energy of position. On the earth, an object's potential energy depends on its height above ground. Any object may possess either kinetic energy or potential energy or both. For example, if a person holds a ball above the ground, it will have potential energy by virtue of its height. However, it will have zero kinetic energy because it is not moving. If the ball is dropped and is falling, it will possess kinetic energy because of its motion and it will also have potential energy because it is still above the ground. At the instant the ball strikes the ground, the kinetic energy will be at its maximum while the potential energy will be zero. The change of energy from one form to another is called a transformation of energy. Figure 5-3 gives examples of matter and energy transformation.

While energy can exist in many different forms, matter exists in only three states: solid, liquid, and gas. (See Figure 5-1.)

Matter can be converted from one state to another depending upon conditions of pressure and temperature.

For example, water is a liquid form of matter: however, when subjected to freezing temperatures, water is converted into ice, which is a solid state. Heated to boiling, water becomes a gas in the form of steam. Matter can be in either a state of rest (inertia) or motion (momentum). The physical quantities associated with these states may be mass, volume, or temperature.

Atomic Structure

In 1913, Niels Bohr (1885–1962), a Danish physicist, proposed a model for the atom that is considered the most representative of the structure of matter (Figure 5-4).

Bohr's structural model of an atom appears like a miniature solar system in which electrons orbit around a central nucleus. One distinct difference between

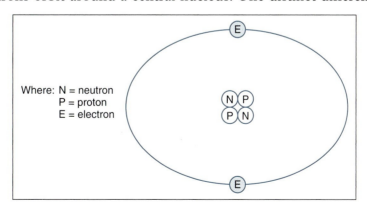

Where: N = neutron
P = proton
E = electron

FIGURE 5-4 A simplified model of a helium atom
Source: Delmar, Cengage Learning.

Bohr's model and an actual atom is that electrons orbit the nucleus of the atom in many planes. Niels Bohr and many of his associates developed a theoretical concept for understanding atomic behavior that has become the foundation of modern physics and is known as quantum or wave mechanics.

All matter is composed of atoms. The atom is the smallest particle into which matter can be divided while still maintaining the unique identity of the matter. The identities of different types of matter are distinguished by how they react chemically. Atoms that have different chemical constituents are considered distinct elements. The atomic and chemical relationship of one element to another follows a regular pattern that is described by the Periodic Table of Elements (Figure 5-2).

The elements are listed in ascending order based on the atomic number, which is noted by a superscript in the upper-left corner (Figure 5-5). The atomic mass of the element is identified by a superscript in the upper-right corner. Each of the elements are also arranged into one of seven horizontal periods and one of eight vertical groups. All elements in the same vertical column (group) will chemically respond in a similar manner. Table 5-6 includes elements important to radiology.

Each of the elements has a specific number of protons in the nucleus. This is a significant characteristic that distinguishes one element from another. The number of protons in an atom is called the atomic number or Z number. The number of protons plus neutrons is the atomic mass number (A).

Atoms of the same or different elements may be chemically combined to form molecules. Molecules, which themselves have distinct physical properties, form the basis for the complex chemical substances called compounds (Figure 5-6).

For example, two atoms of hydrogen associate to form a molecule of hydrogen gas. When two atoms of hydrogen associate, or bond, with one atom of oxygen a molecule of water is formed. It takes many water molecules to form a compound of water. Compounds in general may be described by their physical properties.

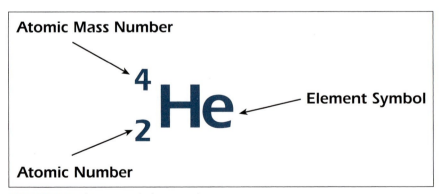

FIGURE 5-5 Atomic symbol nomenclature
Source: Delmar, Cengage Learning.

TABLE 5-6   Elements Important to Radiology

Chemical Symbol	Element	Atomic Number (Z)	Atomic Mass Number (A)
C	Carbon	6	12
O	Oxygen	8	16
Al	Aluminum	13	27
Ca	Calcium	20	40
Fe	Iron	26	56
Cu	Copper	29	63
Mo	Molybdenum	42	98
Ru	Ruthenium	44	102
Ag	Silver	47	107
Sn	Tin	50	120
I	Iodine	53	127
Ba	Barium	56	138
W	Tungsten	74	184
Pb	Lead	82	208

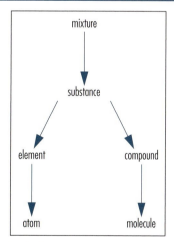

FIGURE 5-6   Structure of matter
Source: Delmar, Cengage Learning.

For example the compound of water may be described by such physical properties as its freezing point (0°, 32°F) and boiling point (100°C, 212°F).

An atom, the fundamental unit of an element, is itself made up of separate particles. All atoms are composed of three particles: proton, neutron, and electron (Figure 5-7).

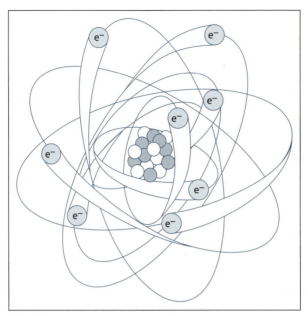

FIGURE 5-7 A three-dimensional diagram of an atom of oxygen, which contains 8 protons, 8 neutrons located within the center nucleus, and 8 electrons within orbital shells moving around the nucleus.
Source: Delmar, Cengage Learning.

Basic Atomic Particles

The atom is best illustrated as having a small dense center, known as the nucleus, which is surrounded by electrons that orbit it at various levels (Figure 5-8).

The nucleus contains two of the three basic particles of the atom, protons, and neutrons, which are responsible for almost all of the mass of an atom. The proton

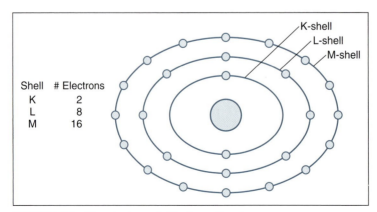

Shell	# Electrons
K	2
L	8
M	16

FIGURE 5-8 The electron shells of a sulfur atom
Source: Delmar, Cengage Learning.

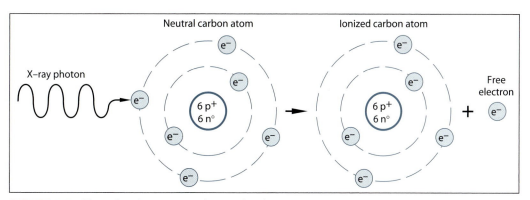

FIGURE 5-9   Neutral carbon atom and ionized carbon atom
Source: Delmar, Cengage Learning.

and neutron are found in the center or nucleus of an atom, and have approximately the same mass (Figure 5-9).

Together, the protons and neutrons may be referred to as **nucleons**. The proton has one positive electrical charge and the neutron is uncharged. For each positively charged proton in the nucleus of an uncharged atom there is one negatively charged (and much less massive) electron outside the nucleus. Since the number of positively charged protons in an atom equals the number of negatively charged electrons, the atom as a whole exists in an uncharged, or electrically neutral state.

Although not a common occurrence in nature, when an atom of a given element loses or gains a proton that atom undergoes structural changes. These structural changes or transitions result in a new element simply due to the change in atomic structure. Atoms of one element evolve to atoms of another element during the natural process of radioactive decay. Radium, with an atomic number of 88, decays (loses protons) over a very long period of time to form the element radon, which has an atomic number of 86. Changes in the number of protons change the identity of the element completely. But this is not the case with changes in the number of neutrons or electrons.

Atoms of the same element may have different numbers of neutrons in the nucleus while maintaining the same chemical identity. If an atom gains or loses neutrons, the result is an atom called an isotope (Figure 5-10).

If an atom gains or loses an electron, the electron is called an ion and the atom is ionized (has a positive charge).

Electrons exist in discrete positions outside the nucleus. These positions are called orbitals and represent the amount of energy individual electrons possess. Just as individual elements are arranged on the periodic table of elements according to their atomic structure, electrons are arranged in a systematic fashion around the nucleus of an atom. The distance of an energy shell from the nucleus determines the binding energy level of the shell. Binding energy is defined as the amount of

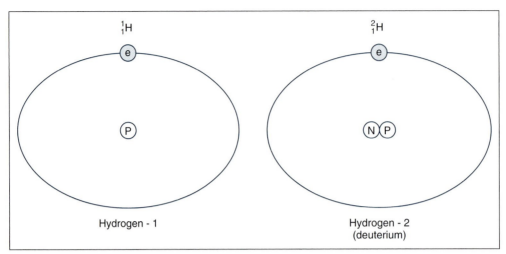

FIGURE 5-10 Two isotopes of hydrogen
Source: Delmar, Cengage Learning.

energy needed to remove an electron from its orbital shell. Electrons are bound to atoms by an amount of their binding energy (Figure 5-11).

Electrons closest to the nucleus have the most binding energy and those farthest away have the least. It takes more energy to knock electrons from the K shell than from the L or M shell.

Each orbital shell is designated by a different letter of the alphabet, beginning with the K-shell, closest to the nucleus, and proceeding through the L-, M-, N-, O-, P, and Q-shells outward from the nucleus (refer to Figures 5-9 and 5-11). Today, scientists no longer use the identifying letters (L, M, N, O, P, and Q) but refer to the orbital shells by the numbers of electrons that can occupy each shell. The occupancy factor is designated according to the formula $2n^2$, where n equals the shell or principle quantum number, starting with the K shell. According to this formula, the maximum number of electrons in each of the shells would be:

K = 2(1) = 2
L = 2(2) = 8
M = 2(3) = 18
N = 2(4) = 32
O = 2(5) = 50
P = 2(6) = 72
Q = 2(7) = 98

Electrons may begin to appear in the next shell before a shell contains its maximum number of electrons. For example, electrons may appear in the N-shell before the M-shell has 18 electrons in it. This is because the number of electrons in the

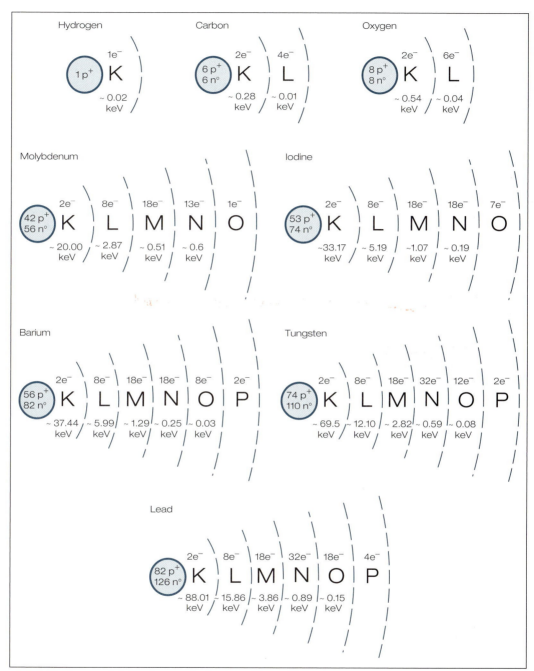

FIGURE 5-11 The closer an electron is to the nucleus, the greater will be the binding energy of the electron
Source: Delmar, Cengage Learning.

outermost shell never exceeds eight as based on the octet rule. The octet rule states that the number of electrons in the outermost shell of an atom can never exceed eight electrons. Atoms containing exactly eight electrons in their outermost shell are inert and chemically stable. This placement of electrons in the orbital shells determines the elements' position within the groups of the periodic table.

The outer-shell electrons also determine the chemical reactivity of an atom. Elements that chemically respond in a similar manner are found in the same vertical column of the periodic table. The number of electrons in the outermost shell of an atom determines the chemical combining characteristic or valence of the element. Elements are commonly shown in an alphabetic abbreviation or a chemical symbol of the element as shown in Figure 5-2.

Hydrogen is the simplest element, with a nucleus of one proton and one orbital electron. A neutron can be added to the nucleus of hydrogen, thus giving an atomic mass number of two (one proton + one neutron). This atom is called deuterium (Figure 5-10). Chemically it is the same as hydrogen because it has one proton and one electron, but atomically it is different (an isotope of hydrogen) because it has one neutron.

Radiation

When energy is emitted and transferred through matter, it is called radiation. Radiation is simply defined as the emission of radiant energy in the form of waves or particles. Radiation may be classified as either non-ionizing or ionizing. If radiation is in the form of matter, it is called particulate radiation. If the radiation is in the form of pure energy that is without mass and charge it is called electromagnetic radiation. There are many types of electromagnetic radiation, such as visible light, radiowaves, or X-rays. Since either type of radiation is capable of ionizing atoms, this radiation is collectively called ionizing radiation (Table 5-7).

Non-ionizing

Non-ionizing radiation does not cause the production of charged particles (**ions**). Examples of non-ionizing radiation are the light from an ordinary light bulb, radio waves, microwaves, and ultraviolet waves.

X-rays are a type of ionizing radiation. Ionizing radiation has the potential to cause harmful effects due to the way it interacts with atoms in living matter. As ionizing radiation passes through living matter, it has the capability to cause atoms to separate into electrically charged positive or negative particles called ions. The ionization of the atoms within cells produces changes that may be harmful. Radiation damage to living tissue results in both short- and long-term effects from the ionization process. The effects of radiation are covered in greater detail in later chapters.

TABLE 5-7   Ionizing Radiation

Particulate
Subatomic particles in motion that originate from the nucleus of radioactive atoms. Radioactive atoms have nuclei that contain excess energy and particles. In an attempt to regain stability, these radioactive atoms emit their excess energy and particles.

Radioactive Decay Process

Alpha Particles	**Beta Particles**
(equivalent to two neutrons)	(equivalent to an electron)
can travel 5 cm	can travel 10–100 cm
Traveling particles of radiation	

Electromagnetic
Electromagnetic radiation differs from particulate in that it consists of bundles of energy (photons) and travels in wavelength form.

Two Types
Gamma radiation, like particulate radiation, originates from nucleus of radioactive atoms; however, it differs in that it exists as wavelengths of energy and is very penetrating to humans.
X-ray is similar to gamma, but originates in orbitals.

Ionizing radiation may be from natural or artificial (man-made) sources. Radioactive materials in the earth (uranium, radium, and thorium), cosmic radiation, and radionuclides in the environment are sources of natural background radiation. X-rays are man-made and are classified as ionizing radiation because they create electrically charged particles (ions) as they pass through living matter. Thus, ionization of living matter by x-rays used in diagnostic radiography creates the need for radiation protection procedures.

Electromagnetic and Particulate Radiation

Matter within the universe exists in a sea of energy. There are many forms of electromagnetic (EM) radiation, such as visible light, radiowaves, and x-rays. Electromagnetic radiation has no mass and no charge and spans a continuum of wide ranges of magnitudes of energy. There are many different types of electromagnetic radiation. Visible light, to which the human eye responds, is intermediate on the electromagnetic spectrum in energy. Just below visible light are infrared radiation, which some insects can see; microwaves, used in cooking and communications; and radiowaves. Just above visible light is ultraviolet radiation, responsible to some extent for human "suntanning." Above ultraviolet, x-rays and gamma rays are found. Gamma rays are identical to x-rays in every respect except in how they are produced. Gamma radiation is a high-energy electromagnetic radiation resulting from a radioactive decay process. X-ray radiation results from the interaction of electrons with the target material of an x-ray tube.

Electromagnetic radiation may be viewed on a scale known as the electromagnetic spectrum. A common property of all EM radiation is velocity. The velocity of EM energy is equal to the speed of light, which is 3 × 10 meters/second (186,4000 miles per second) in a vacuum. EM radiation (energies of approximately 10 eV and higher) is capable of ionizing an atom or a molecule, as may be seen from (Figure 5-12).

Scientists have discovered that under certain circumstances, EM has a dual nature, sometimes behaving as a wave and sometimes as a particle. Electromagnetic radiation is not one continuous waveform but instead consists of separate packets of energy called quanta (singular quantum) or more commonly called a photon. A photon may be thought of as having no mass and being an uncharged bundle of energy that has properties of continuous waves. Therefore, x-rays are commonly referred to as photons or x-ray photons.

The energy and frequency of electromagnetic radiation are directly related—that is, the higher the energy is, the higher the frequency. Energy and frequency are inversely related to wavelength: the higher the energy or frequency is, the shorter the wavelength (Figure 5-13).

If one considers the waveform in Figure 5-14, the distance from the peak of one wave to the next is the wavelength and is measured in meters.

The height of a wave from the lowest valley to the next midpoint is called one cycle. The number of cycles passing through a given point in one second is called the frequency. The frequency is measured in cycles/second, given the name Hertz in SI units, and abbreviated Hz.

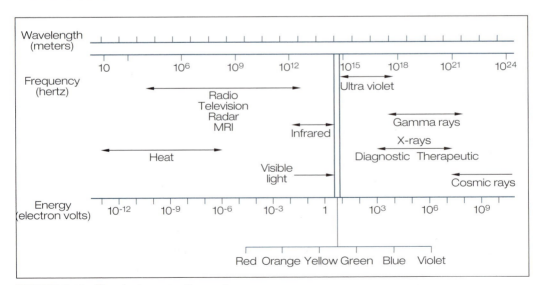

FIGURE 5-12 The electromagnetic spectrum
Source: Delmar, Cengage Learning.

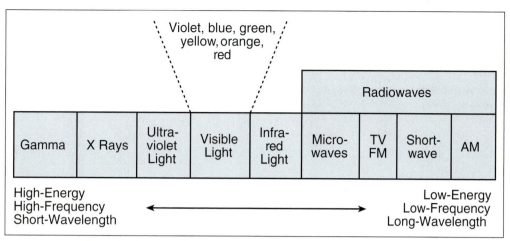

FIGURE 5-13 Example of energy, frequency, and wavelength
Source: Delmar, Cengage Learning.

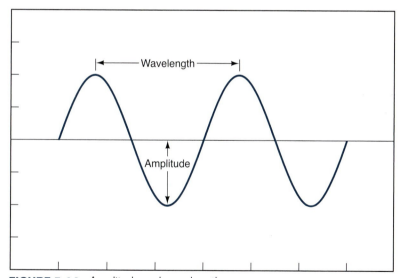

FIGURE 5-14 Amplitude and wavelength
Source: Delmar, Cengage Learning.

Particulate radiation results when any subatomic particle of an atom is released. Two common types of particulate radiation are **alpha particles** and **beta particles** (Table 5-8).

Alpha particles, or alpha rays, are the nuclei of helium atoms, two protons and two neutrons, and have a charge of +2. Beta particles (beta rays) are physically identical to electrons. Both alpha and beta particles have the ability to strike other atoms, causing ionization.

TABLE 5-8   Types of Ionizing Radiation

Particulate Radiation
Source: Originates from the disintegration of the nucleus of radioactive atoms. Particles travel through space as alpha or beta particles.
Electromagnetic Radiation
Source: Gamma rays originate from the disintegration of the nucleus of radioactive atoms. X-rays originate from x-ray tube production.
Gamma rays and x-rays travel through space at the speed of light, and have no mass or charge.

Humans have always been exposed to environmental radiation or naturally occurring background radiation (Table 5-9).

Background radiation originates from the sun, stars, and from naturally occurring radioactive materials in the earth's rocks and water. The actual amount of background radiation humans receive varies with the geographic area.

The soil and rock composition and the elevation above sea level contribute to the amount of environmental or naturally occurring radiation.

Humans receive more radiation exposure at high elevations because there is less atmospheric filtration of the radiation from outer space (cosmic radiation).

TABLE 5-9   Average Annual Radiation Exposure of U.S. Population

Overall average annual exposure is 360 mrem, and all percentages listed are percentages of 360 mrem.

Category	Source	Percentage
295 mrem Natural Background		**82%**
	198 mrem Radon	55%
	97 mrem	27%
	Cosmic, terrestrial, internal	
65 mrem Man-Made		**18%**
	40 mrem Medical X-rays	11%
	14 mrem Nuclear medicine	4%
	11 mrem Consumer products	3%
Other		
	1.1 mrem Occupational	0.3%
	1.1 mrem Fallout	0.3%
	0.4 mrem Nuclear fuel cycle	0.1%
	0.4 mrem Miscellaneous	0.1%

Adapted from data found in National Council on Radiation Protection (NCRP 93).

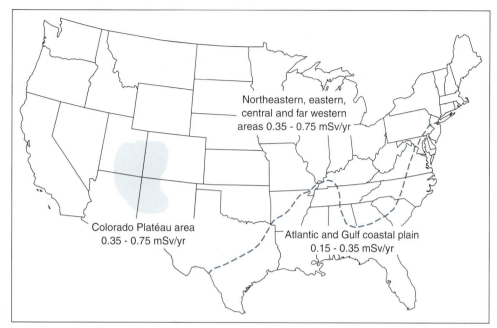

FIGURE 5-15 Natural background radiation variation in the United States
Source: Delmar, Cengage Learning.

For example, humans in Denver, Colorado will receive twice the amount of cosmic radiation as an individual living at sea level (Figure 5-15). The actual amount of radiation a person receives depends on four factors: type of radiation, amount of radiation received, length of time exposed, and the specific body area exposed. These four factors are the important concepts used in developing radiation protection procedures and will be a basis for risk factors discussed in further detail in Chapter 15, Radiation Biology, and Chapter 16, Radiation Protection.

Artificial Sources of Radiation

Since 1895, when Wilhelm Conrad Roentgen named his new discovery x-rays, scientists have been experimenting with its application. Much of the knowledge about the harmful effects of radiation has been gathered as a result of the human health consequences from various applications to humans. From the early uses of ionizing radiation for diagnostic imaging and treatment of disease to application of radium for luminous watch dials, the effects and consequences have led to the current focus on radiation exposure reduction and selective applications. Today, radiation sources may be found in nuclear power plants, atomic weapons, ionization-type smoke detectors, airport luggage screening, and in many industrial and commercial applications. The annual average radiation dose received by humans from medical imaging procedures is much less than the dose received from environmental sources. For example, the average annual radiation exposure of the U.S. population, based on the National Council on Radiation Protection (NCRP) Report NO. 93, is 40 millirems from medical x-rays and 295 millirems from natural background radiation (Table 5-9).

Ionization

Atoms are electrically neutral, their electric charge being zero, because the total number of protons is equal to the number of electrons in the orbital shells. An atom may become ionized if it gains or loses an electron (ionization). Any charged particle is referred to as an ion. The loss of electron results in a net positive charge and the atom is termed a **cation**. The addition of an electron to an atom result in a net negative charge and the atom is called an **anion**. An electron removed from an atom plus the atom from where the electron was ejected is collectively called an ion pair (Figure 5-16).

The effects of radiation on living matter are a result of the ionization (creation of ion pairs) that occurs at the atomic level. During ionization, electrons removed from energy shells result in a positively charged atom. The freed electron (ion) can deposit its energy to surrounding tissue.

As a result of ionization, molecules may be altered causing cellular damage that may result in abnormal cell function or loss of cell function. If enough cells have been damaged, the entire organ or organism may display symptoms of radiation damage.

When an x-ray beam passes through living matter, the x-ray beam undergoes attenuation (Figure 5-16). Attenuation of the x-ray beam refers to any process that prevents x-rays from reaching the patient or the radiographic film. The fact that x-rays are attenuated by the various body structures is the underlying basis for the visible radiographic image (Figure 5-17).

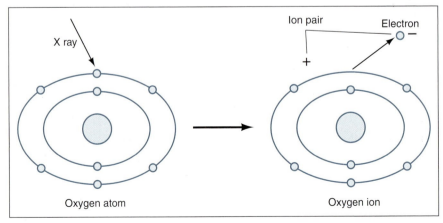

FIGURE 5-16 Ionization of an oxygen atom by x-rays
Source: Delmar, Cengage Learning.

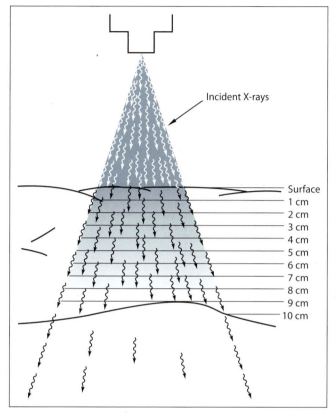

FIGURE 5-17 An x-ray beam undergoes attenuation as it passes through matter
Source: Delmar, Cengage Learning.

For example, x-rays are absorbed preferentially in bone as compared to soft tissue, thus producing the traditional radiographic image (Figure 5-18).

Although the process of attenuation is required for the production of a radiographic image, it also has harmful implications. The greater the absorbed dose of x-rays (radiation), the greater the potential that biologic effects will occur. Both absorption and scatter radiation, or redirection of a x-ray photon after it has interacted with an object, affect attenuation.

X-Ray Interactions with Matter

Using x-rays to produce a diagnostic radiographic image carries both a benefit (diagnostic tool) and potential harm (biologic effects). As an x-ray passes through matter not all of the x-ray photons will interact with the atoms of the matter; some

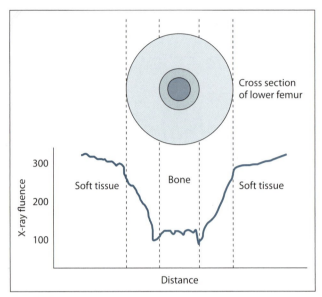

FIGURE 5-18 Absorption characteristics of a body part
Source: Delmar, Cengage Learning.

will pass through. X-rays may also interact with the whole atom, an orbital electron, or directly with the nucleus of an atom; refer to Figures 5-17 and 5-18.

As a result of these various interactions ionization may occur. Because these occurrences are uncontrollable interactions, ionization of atoms is unpredictable. When ionization interactions occur, some alteration in the structure of the atom is anticipated. The type of interaction that occurs will depend on the energy of the incoming x-ray photon. X-ray photons having low energy are most likely to interact with the whole atom. Very high-energy x-ray photons are capable of interacting with the nucleus of the atom. Intermediate-energy x-ray photons generally interact with the orbital electrons.

There are five types of interactions between x-rays and matter: Coherent (Classical or Thompson's) Scattering, Photoelectric Effect, Compton Effect, Photodisintegration, and Pair Production; however only the first three have significance to diagnostic radiography (Table 5-10).

Coherent Scattering

Coherent scattering, also called classical or Thompson's scattering, occurs when a low-energy x-ray photon interacts with an atom (Figure 5-19).

The target atom becomes energized or "excited" and releases this extra energy as a scattered x-ray photon having a wavelength and energy equal to the energy of the original x-ray photon. This released x-ray photon travels in a path

TABLE 5-10   Types of X-ray Interaction with Matter

Type	Characteristics
Coherent Scattering	Also called classical or Thompson's
	Produced by low-energy x-ray photons
	Electrons are not removed but vibrate due to deposit of energy from the photon
	As the electrons vibrate, they emit energy equal to the incoming photon. The energy travels in a path slightly different from the original photon
Photoelectric Absorption	Photon absorption interaction
	Incoming x-ray photon strikes a K-shell electron
	Energy of x-ray photon transferred to electron and x-ray photon ceases to exist
	Vacancy hole in K shell is filled by electrons from outer shells, releasing energy that creates low-energy characteristic photons
	This type of interaction results in increased patient radiation dose
Compton Effect	Also called modified scattering
	Incoming x-ray photon strikes a loosely bound, outer-shell electron
	X-ray photon transfers part of its energy to the electron
	Electron is removed from orbit as a scattered electron
	Ejected electrons may ionize other atoms or recombine with an ion needing an electron
	Photon scatters in another direction, with less energy
Pair Production	Ionization does not occur but the photon has scattered
	Does not occur in diagnostic radiography
	Involves an interaction between the income photon and the nucleus of the atom

different from the direction of the original x-ray photon; thus scattered. In this form of scattering, no energy transfer occurs and therefore no ionization occurs. Coherent scattering generally occurs in low kVp ranges; however, some occurs throughout the diagnostic kVp range, and is responsible for some small amount of radiographic-film fog.

Photoelectric Absorption

Photoelectric absorption occurs when an incoming x-ray photon gives up all of its energy to an inner-shell electron (Figure 5-20).

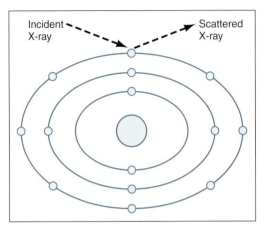

FIGURE 5-19 Coherent scattering
Source: Delmar, Cengage Learning.

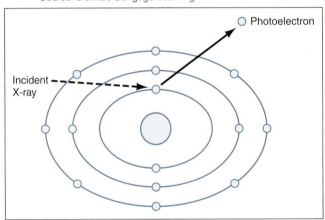

FIGURE 5-20 Photoelectric absorption
Source: Delmar, Cengage Learning.

When this occurs, an electron, called the photoelectron, is ejected from the atom, usually from the inner K or L shell, leaving a vacancy or "hole" to be filled in the shell. When an inner-shell electron is removed from an atom, an electron from an outer shell fills the resulting vacancy. When an outer-shell electron fills an inner-shell vacancy, an x-ray photon may be emitted from the atom and is called characteristic radiation. Therefore, two types of secondary radiation result from a photoelectric interaction: characteristic x-rays and photoelectrons.

Compton Effect

Compton scattering, first described in 1922 by physicist A.H. Compton, is the most common type of x-ray interaction in diagnostic radiology and is responsible for most scattered radiation. Compton scattering occurs when an x-ray photon

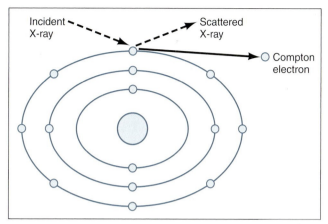

FIGURE 5-21 Compton effect
Source: Delmar, Cengage Learning.

interacts with an electron in the outer orbital shell of an atom. The outer-shell electron, called a Compton electron, is ejected from the atom and results in ionization of the atom (Figure 5-21).

As a result of the interaction, the x-ray photon is redirected with decreased energy and a longer wavelength. The scattered x-ray photon and the Compton electron have the energy to cause additional ionizing interactions with other atoms. Because Compton-scattered x-ray photons may be deflected in any direction, they are of special concern in radiation protection. Those scattering backward in the direction of the incoming x-ray photon are referred to as backscatter radiation. Compton scatter radiation, like most scattered radiation, does not contribute to the diagnostic image. Rather, it causes radiographic-film fog and requires the use of lead shielding for protection of the radiographer and patient.

Photodisintegration

The photodisintegration interaction occurs when a very high-energy x-ray photon (10 MeV or higher) strikes the atomic nucleus, causing a nuclear fragment to be ejected. This process only occurs with very high-energy x-rays and is not likely to occur in diagnostic radiography (Figure 5-22).

Pair Production

Pair production is not likely to occur in the energy ranges used in diagnostic radiology. For pair production to occur a very high-energy incoming x-ray photon, with energy of at least 1.02 MeV, interacts with the nucleus of an atom. The impact of the interaction causes the incoming x-ray photon to disappear, and in its place two electrons appear, one positively charged and one negatively charged (Figure 5-23).

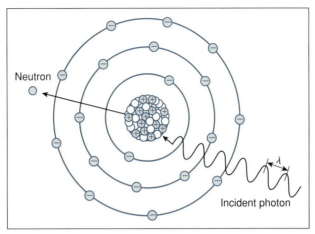

FIGURE 5-22 Photodisintegration
Source: Delmar, Cengage Learning.

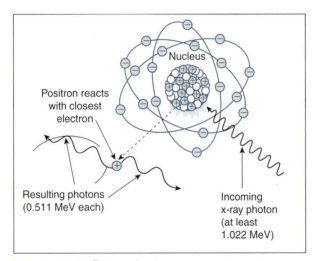

FIGURE 5-23 Pair production
Source: Delmar, Cengage Learning.

Summary

The limited radiographer can best understand the beneficial applications of ionizing radiation as well as its harmful effects by gaining knowledge of radiographic physics. This includes knowledge of the universe and the structure of matter. Also, by being able to conceptualize the ionization process, the limited radiographer can better relate to the daily tasks associated with radiation protection procedures.

REVIEW QUESTIONS

1. In the Système Internationale d' Unités (SI), the measure of electric current is the:
   a. meter
   b. kilogram
   c. ampere
   d. second

2. One sievert (Sv) is equal to _____ radiation equivalent man (REM).
   a. 10
   b. 100
   c. 1,000
   d. 10,000

3. One radiation equivalent man (REM) is equal to _____ milli-sieverts (mSv).
   a. 1
   b. 10
   c. 100
   d. 1,000

4. One gray is equivalent to _____ radiation absorbed dose (RAD).
   a. 1
   b. 10
   c. 100
   d. 1,000

5. A principal characteristic of matter is:
   a. volume
   b. mass
   c. length
   d. flux

6. There are _____ naturally occurring elements identified on the Periodic Table of Elements.
   a. 42
   b. 65
   c. 92
   d. 101

7. The unit of energy is the joule (J).
    a. True
    b. False

8. The number of protons in an atom is called the atomic:
    a. length
    b. number
    c. mass
    d. dimension

9. If an atom gains or loses neutrons, the result is an atom called a/an:
    a. Isotope
    b. nucleon
    c. iatrogenic
    d. none of the above

10. The first energy shell closest to the nucleus contains _____ electrons.
    a. two
    b. four
    c. six
    d. eight

11. As the electromagnetic energy increases, the wavelength gets _____ and _____ penetrating to matter.
    a. shorter, more
    b. shorter, less
    c. longer, more
    d. longer, less

12. When radiation exists in the form of matter, it is referred to as:
    a. super charged
    b. electromagnetic
    c. cantionized
    d. particulate

13. When radiation exists in the form of pure energy, it is referred to as:
    a. super charged
    b. electromagnetic
    c. particulate
    d. cantionized

14. Sources of radiation are:
    1. man-made
    2. terrestrial
    3. cosmic

    Possible Responses
    a. 1 and 2
    b. 1 and 3
    c. 2 and 3
    d. 1, 2, and 3

15. Humans receive the greatest amount of radiation exposure from:
    a. medical x-rays
    b. nuclear fuel
    c. radon
    d. consumer products

16. A non-ionized atom has an electric charge of:
    a. zero
    b. +1
    c. +2
    d. +3

17. After an atom is ionized, its' electric charge status is changed.
    a. True
    b. False

18. Atoms that have been ionized assume a _____ electrical charge:
    a. neutral
    b. positive
    c. zero
    d. minus zero

19. In the photoelectric interaction, the incoming x-ray interacts with a/an:
    a. inner-shell electron
    b. outer-shell electron
    c. nuclear force field
    d. proton in the nucleus

20. The most common type of x-ray interaction in the diagnostic energy range and responsible for most scattered radiation during x-ray examinations is:
a. Compton
b. photoelectric
c. coherent
d. photodisintegration

REFERENCES

Abella, H. A. (April 16, 2007). Report from NCRP: CT-based radiation exposure in U.S. population soars. Diagnostic Imaging Online. CT-based radiation exposure in U.S. population soars. Retrieved from www.diagnosticimaging.com

Abella, H. A. (April 25, 2007). Report from NCRP: Radiation exposure during pregnancy demands well-informed patient management. Diagnostic Imaging.com from http://www.diagnosticimaging.com

American Cancer Society. *Breast cancer facts & figures 2005–2006.* Retrieved from www.cancer.org

American College of Radiology. (2006). *ACR guidelines and standards, ACR practice guideline for general radiography,* 17–20. Retrieved from www.acr.org

American College of Radiology. (2006). *ACR guidelines and standards, ACR practice guideline for performing and interpreting diagnostic computed tomography (CT).* Retrieved from www.acr.org

American College of Radiology. (2006). *ACR practice guideline for radiation oncology.* Retrieved from www.acr.org

American College of Radiology. (2006). *ACR technical standard for diagnostic procedures using radio pharmaceuticals.* Retrieved from http://www.acr.org

American College of Radiology. (2008). *ACR guidelines and standards, ACR practice guideline for the performance of diagnostic mammography.* Retrieved from www.acr.org

American College of Radiology. (2008). *ACR guidelines and standards, ACR practice guideline for the performance of screening mammography.* Retrieved from www.acr.org

Bassett, L., & Butler, D. L. (1991). Mammography and early breast cancer detection. *AmerFamPhys.,* February, Retrieved from findarticles.com

Brusin, J. A. (2007). Radiation protection. *Radiologic Technology, 78*(5), 378–391.

Bushong, S. C. (2008). *Radiologic Science for Technologists: Physics, Biology and Protection.* (9th ed.). St. Louis, MO: Mosby Elsevier.

Campeau, F., & Fleitz, J. (1999). *Limited radiography* (2nd ed.). Clifton Park, NY: Delmar.

Carlton, R. R., & Adler, A. M. (2006). *Principles of radiographic imaging: An art and a science* (3rd ed.). Clifton Park, NY: Delmar Thomson Learning.

Cohen, B. L. (1991). Radiation Standards and hazards. IEEE. *Transformation Education, 34,* 261–265.

Diagnostic Imaging Online (April 24, 2007). *Imaging equipment vendors tout innovations to reduce radiation exposure.* Retrieved from www.diagnosticimaging.com

Feig, S. & Hendrick, R. (1997). Radiation risk from screening mammography of women aged 40–49 years. *National Cancer Institute Monograph*, (22), 119–24. PMID 9709287.

Furlow, B. (2004 May/June). Biological effects of diagnostic imaging. *Radiologic Technology*, 5(5), 355–363.

Gold, R. H., Bassett, L. W., Widoff B. E. (1990). Highlights from the history of mammography, *Radiographics*, Vol 10, 1111–1131. Radiological Society of North America. Retrieved from http://radiographics.rsnajnls.org

Health Physics Society. (2001, February 6). *Answer to question #641 submitted to "ask the experts."* (Category: Radiation workers-pregnant workers). Retrieved from www:hps.org

Idaho State University. (2006). *Radiation and risk. Radiation information networks*. Retrieved from www.physics.isu.edu

International Commission of Radiation on Radiation Protection (ICRP). Amended 21 January 2008. *Pregnancy and medical radiation*. (Report No. 84). Retrieved from www.iscp.org

International Commission of Radiation Units and Measurements: *Radiation quantities and units*. (Report 33). (2007). Retrieved from www.2000.irpa.net

Johns Hopkins Safety Manual. (September 23, 2008). *Personnel monitoring*. Retrieved from www.hopkinsmedicine.org

Lidor, D. (September 16, 2005) *Digital mammography better than x-rays*. Forbes.com (Infoimaging 09.16.05). Retrieved from www.forbes.com

Mathisen, L. (2007). Tragedy times two: Late effects of children who undergo radiation therapy. *RT Image, 20*(16), 17–19.

McClafferty, C. (2001). *The head bone is connected to the neck bone*. New York: Farrar, Straus and Giroux.

McGill University. (2007). *Radiation dose limit*. Retrieved from www.mcgill.ca

Medical Imaging. (May 7, 2007). *How innovations in medical imaging have reduced radiation dosage (executive summary)*. Retrieved from www.medicalimaging.org

Medical Imaging. (May 7, 2007). *How medical imaging has transformed health care in the U.S. (executive summary)*. Retrieved from www.medicalimaging.org

Minigh, J. May/June 2005. Pediatric radiation protection. *Radiologic Technology*, 76(5), 365–375.

Mossman, K. L., Goldman, M., Masse, F., Mills, W. A., Schiager, K. J., Vetter, R. L. (2006, March). *Radiation risk in perspective*. Health Physics Society Position Statement. Retrieved from www.physics.isu.edu

National Cancer Institute. (2005). *Interventional fluoroscopy: Reducing radiation risks for patients and staff*. Retrieved from www.cancer.gov

National Council on Radiation Protection (2004). *Recent application of the NCRP public dose limit recommendations for ionizing radiation*. (NCRP statement No. 10.) Retrieved from www.ncrponline.org

National Council on Radiation Protection and Measurements (NCPR). (1977). *Medical exposure of pregnant and potentially pregnant women*. (Report No. 54). Washington, DC: NCRP.

National Council on Radiation Protection and Measurements. (1981). *Radiation protection in pediatric radiology*. (Report 68). Washington, DC: NCRP.

National Council on Radiation Protection and Measurements (NCRP). (1987). *Ionizing radiation exposure of the population of the United States*. (Report No. 93). Bethesda, MD: NCRP.

National Council on Radiation Protection and Measurements (NCRP). (2007). *Limitations of exposure to ionizing radiation.* (Report 116). Retrieved from www.ncrponline.org

National Research Council, Commission of Life Sciences, Committee on Biological Effects of Ionizing Radiation *(BIERV),* Board of Radiation Effects Research. (1989). *Health effects of exposure to low levels of ionizing radiations.* Washington, DC: National Academy Press.

Norris, T. G. (2002). Radiation safety in fluoroscopy. *Radiologic Technology, 73*(6), 511–533.

North Carolina University Health and Safety, Radiation Safety Division. (2004). *Radiation safety and alara.* Retrieved from www.ncsu.edu

Patton, K. T. (2000). *Structure and Function of the Body.* (11th ed.). St. Louis, MO: Mosby, Inc.

Raussaki, M. T. (2004). *Pediatric Radiation Protection (abstract).* Retrieved from www.springerlink.com

Schleipman, A. R. (2005). Occupational radiation exposure: population studies. *Radiologic Technology, 76*(3), 185–191.

Schueler, B. (2003). *Personnel protection during fluoroscopic procedures.* Mayo Clinic. Rochester, MN. Retrieved from www.aapm.org

Seeram, E. (2001). *Rad techis guide to radiation protection.* Malden, MA: Blackwell Science.

Sherer, M. A., Visconti, P., & Ritenour, E. R. (2006). *Radiation Protection in Medical Radiography.* (5th ed.). St. Louis, MO: Mosby Publishing Company Inc.

Sprawls, P. (2007). *Interaction of radiation with matter.* From: Sprawls Educational Foundation. The Physical Principles of Medical Imaging. Retrieved from http://www.sprawls.org

Thomas, A.M.K., Isherwod, I., & Wells, P.N.T. (Eds.). (1995). *The invisible light: The Röentgen centenary: 100 years of medical radiology.* Oxford: Blackwell Science.

U.S. Department of Labor, Bureau of Labor Statistics, Occupational Outlook Handbook. (2008–2009 Edition). *Nuclear Medicine Technologists.* Retrieved from 222.bls.gov

U.S. Environmental Protection Agency. (2007). *History of radiation protection.* Retrieved from www.epa.gov

U.S. Environmental Protection Agency. (2007). *Ionizing & non-ionizing radiation.* Retrieved from www.epa.gov

U.S. Environmental Protection Agency. (2009). *Estimating risk.* Retrieved from www.epa.gov

U.S. Environmental Protection Agency (2009). *Health effects (understanding radiation).* Retrieved from http://www.epa.gov

United States Environmental Protection Agency. (2007). Ionizing Radiation Factbook, EPA_402-F-06-061. Retrieved from http://www.epa.gov

United States Food and Drug Administration, Centers for Devices and Radiological Health. (September 30, 1994). *FDA public health advisory: Avoidance of serious x-ray induced skin injuries to patients during fluoroscopic-guided procedures.* Rockville, MD: FDA.

Whalen, J. P. & Balter, S. (1984). *Radiation Risks in Medical Imaging.* Chicago: Year Book Medical Publishers, Inc.

Willis, E. & Slavis, T. L. (2005). *Editorials: The alara concept in pediatric CR and DR: Dose reduction in pediatric radiographic exams: A white paper conference executive summary.* Retrieved from www.radiology.rsnajnls.org

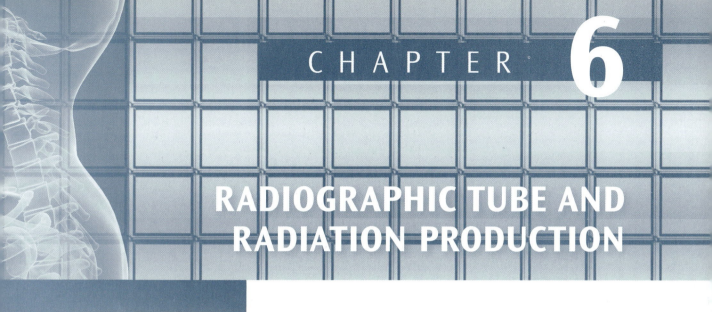

CHAPTER 6

RADIOGRAPHIC TUBE AND RADIATION PRODUCTION

Key Terms

Actual Focal Spot
Alternating Current
Ampere
Anode
Attenuate
Bremsstrahlung Interaction
Cathode
Characteristic Interactions
Conductor
Collimator Shutters
Crest
Current
Effective Focal Spot
Electrification
Electrodynamics
Filament
Filament Circuit
Filtration
Fluoresce
Focusing Cup
Focal Spot
Heel Effect
Insulator
Leakage Radiation
Line Focus Principle
Magnetism
Molybdenum

Chapter Outline

Introduction
Electromagnetic Radiation
Properties of X-Rays
The X-Ray System
X-Ray Production: An Overview
The X-Ray Tube
   The Cathode (–) Assembly
   The Filament
   The Anode Assembly
   The Line Focus Principle
   The Focusing Cup
   Electron Interaction at the Target
   Protective Tube Housing
The Operating Console
Tube Rating Charts
   Tube Heat Capacity

Objectives

Upon completion of this chapter, the student will meet
the following objectives by verifying knowledge of the facts

and principles presented through oral and written communication at a level deemed competent.

⊃ Define terminology related to the radiographic tube and radiation production.

⊃ Recall properties of electromagnetic radiation and x-ray.

⊃ Explain the relationship between energy and x-ray wavelength.

⊃ Recall the major components of a x-ray tube and state their purpose and function.

⊃ Identify important facts and terminology associated with electrification.

⊃ Label the major components of the cathode and anode assembly and recall their purpose and function.

⊃ Explain the advantage(s) of a rotating anode versus a stationary anode.

⊃ Identify correct and incorrect statements regarding the line focus principle and the heel effect.

⊃ Calculate heat units.

Introduction

This chapter introduces the specialized equipment needed to produce the radiographic image and the processes involved in the production of x-rays. Some information presented in this chapter regarding electromagnetic radiation and circuitry will also be covered in other chapters where inclusion is necessary.

The limited radiographer is responsible for producing diagnostic radiographs, and the primary tool to accomplish this task is the x-ray system. The x-ray system consists of the radiographic tube, table, and operating console. Of these, the radiographic tube is the most important component of the x-ray system because it produces the x-rays necessary to obtain a radiographic image, and the radiographer must be familiar with how the system functions.

The processes involved in the production of x-rays are often taken for granted during the busy day-to-day schedule of tending to patients. However, these processes have a way of commanding attention when some phase of the system malfunctions. Generally, the x-ray system can withstand a great deal of usage (and at times, abuse), but knowledge of its operation can prevent many of the causes of system failure.

Electromagnetic Radiation

X-rays are a form of electromagentic radiation or energy. Electromagnetic radiation can travel in a vacuum and differs from sound energy, which requires a medium such as water or tissue to travel. Electromagnetic radiation originates in electric and magnetic disturbances in space. Electromagnetic radiation has the following properties:

- travels at the speed of light (about 186,000 miles per second in a vacuum)
- is quantized; meaning it can exist only in fixed, discrete levels, rather than over a continuous range
- exists in discrete bundles of energy also referred to as quanta

Scientists have found that electromagnetic radiation has a dual nature and the energy is everywhere. Examples of electromagnetic radiation include x-rays, gamma rays, radio waves, and light with the major difference between each being wavelength. The range of electromagnetic energy is portrayed as a spectrum, which is arranged from the shortest wavelength (highest frequency) to longest wavelength (lowest frequency). Refer to Figure 5-12 and Figure 5-13 in Chapter 5, Radiographic Physics.

Properties of X-Rays

X-rays are often referred to as x-ray photons. An x-ray photon is a discrete bundle of energy having no mass, and traveling at the speed of light. X-Rays and electromagnetic radiation may be related to wavelength (the distance from crest to crest). Refer to Figure 5-14 in Chapter 5, Radiographic Physics. Energy and wavelength are inversely proportional, shorter wavelengths correspond to higher energy and longer wavelengths correspond to lower energy.

X-rays and light have many properties in common; however, x-rays have unique properties that make them valuable in diagnostic imaging. Some of the unique properties of x-rays are:

- X-rays can penetrate materials that absorb or reflect visible light.
- X-rays cause certain chemicals to fluoresce (light up). (This property has special application for use in intensifying screen design.)

- X-rays can produce an image on photosensitive film, such as x-ray film, which can then be made visible by chemical development.

Because of their high-energy content, x-rays can produce ions and negative electrons (for additional information, refer to the discussion of ionization in Chapter 5, Radiographic Physics, and Chapter 15, Radiation Biology).

The X-Ray System

X-rays used in medical radiography are electronically produced. Figure 6-1 shows the major components of an x-ray system. The purpose of the x-ray system is to convert electrical energy into x-ray energy.

The x-ray generator converts the electrical power (provided by a utility company) into high-voltage power, which is required by the x-ray tube to produce the x-rays. The generator converts the alternating current (AC) electrical power into

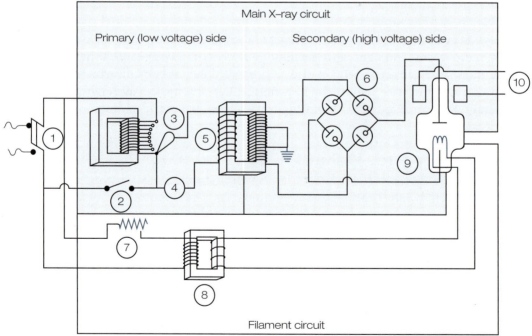

FIGURE 6-1 The complete basic x-ray circuit: (1) main breaker, (2) exposure switch, (3) autotransformer, (4) timer circuit, (5) high-voltage step-up transformer, (6) four-diode rectifiction circuit, (7) filament circuit variable resistance, (8) filament step-down transformer, (9) x-ray tube, and (10) rotor stator
Source: Delmar, Cengage Learning.

a waveform for the production of x-rays. Incoming electrical power also is supplied to the x-ray tube and other components of the x-ray system. The study of moving electrical charges is called electrodynamics.

The movement of electrical charges, or electrons, occurs from one atom to another along the outside of a conductor. A conductor is a material that allows the easy movement of electrons. Most metals, such as copper, are good conductors (Figure 6-2).

Materials, such as rubber or plastic, which resist the flow of electrons, are called insulators. Electrical charges obey certain physical laws, the most important being that like charges repel each other and unlike charges attract each other. A proton (having a positive charge) will be repelled by another proton but will attract an electron (having a negative charge).

When an object has an electrical charge, it is electrified or statically charged. Electrification results from either a deficiency or an excess of electrons and occurs when electrons move from one object to another (Figure 6-3).

Electrical charges possess potential energy because they have the ability to do work by virtue of the repulsion of like charges and the attraction of unlike charges. This potential of electrical charges to do work is called electrical potential. The difference in electrical potential between two points on an electrical conductor is called the potential difference.

If a conductor is connected to a source of electrons, such as one end of a battery and is connected to the other end of the battery to form an electrical circuit, electrons will flow along the conductor and work will be done (Figure 6-4).

The amount of work performed by moving electrical charges is measured in volt (V). Electrons moving through a conductor are referred to as current, which is measured by ampere (A).

If a circuit is modified to resist the flow of electrons, work can be extracted from the circuit in various forms, such as heat or radiant energy. Electrical resistance is measured in ohms (Ω). An ohm is the amount of resistance overcome by one volt to cause one ampere to flow.

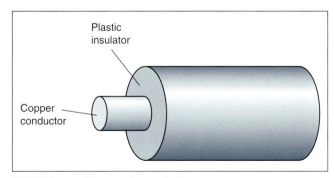

Plastic insulator

Copper conductor

FIGURE 6-2 Typical electrical wire
Source: Delmar, Cengage Learning.

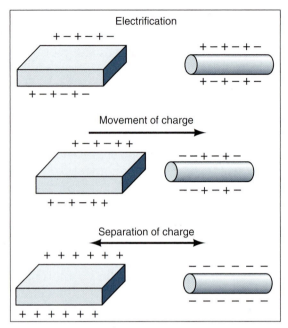

FIGURE 6-3 Electrification
Source: Delmar, Cengage Learning.

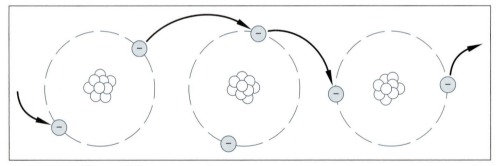

FIGURE 6-4 Electron drift along a conductor
Source: Delmar, Cengage Learning.

The product of current (amperes) and electrical resistance (ohms) is a volt. This equation is expressed as the formula $V = IR$. In this formula the V = voltage in volts, I = current in amperes, and R = resistance in ohms. This is called Ohm's Law and forms the basis for the study of electrical circuits.

The amount of work that electricity does over a given amount of time is called power and is measured in watts (W). Magnetism is the ability of some material to attract iron or iron-like substances. The magnetic property of a substance is defined by the magnetic field it creates. The magnetic field is the zone of influence of the magnetic property and is concentrated at two points called the magnetic poles. The earth itself is a huge magnet, which has its magnetic poles at the geographical north and south. In a similar fashion, the poles of all magnets are called the north and south poles. A basic law of magnetism states that like poles repel each other and unlike poles attract each other. Magnets occur in natural substances or may be created by passing an electrical current through a conductor. This type of electromagnet is important in the operation of x-ray generating equipment.

X-Ray Production: An Overview

X-rays are produced when a very high electrical potential (kilovoltage) is applied across the x-ray tube. To produce x-rays, a system is needed. The x-ray system consists of the x-ray generator, x-ray tube, operating console also called the control panel, and beam modifiers (tube filtration and collimation system). X-ray system circuitry, operating console, and assessories will be discussed in Chapter 7, Imaging Equipment.

The X-Ray Tube

When high-speed electrons collide with matter, electromagnetic photons are produced. Under special conditions, if the electrons collide with matter with a high atomic number and if the electrons have sufficient energy (speed) x-rays are produced. For x-rays to be produced, a set of very special conditions must exist. These include a source of electrons, an appropriate target material (metal), a high voltage, and a vacuum. The x-ray tube is the most efficient means of generating x-rays because it permits these condition to exist.

The x-ray tube converts the electrical energy provided by the generator into an x-ray beam. The x-ray tube consists of a cathode, (−), and an anode, (+), enclosed within a glass envelope which is then encased in a protective housing. The x-ray tube is surrounded by an outer metal housing, which serves to protect the glass tube inserted within (Figure 6-5).

On one side of the x-ray tube is a source of electrons, the cathode. On the other side of the tube is the target (anode), which receives the flow of electrons. The entire cathode and anode assembly, except the stator, is enclosed in a glass envelope from which air has been removed. The x-ray tube must have as much gas or air removed as possible. If the x-ray tube is not highly evacuated of air and other foreign gasses, the electrons will collide with gas molecules, thus reducing tube efficiency. Also an evacuated (vacuum) x-ray tube has a longer life span and will not malfunction as quickly. At the point where the primary x-ray beam exits the glass envelope, a window segment or port is constructed. Some x-ray tubes have a thinner area of the glass envelope to allow less absorption or scatter of the x-ray photons.

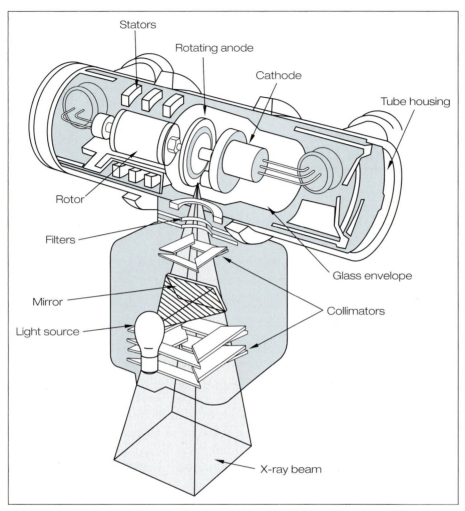

FIGURE 6-5 Schematic drawing of an x-ray tube and collimator (*Courtesy of Siemens Medical Systems, Inc., Iselin, NJ*)

The Cathode (–) Assembly

The cathode assembly consists of the **filament** or filaments, focusing cup, and associated wiring. The production of x-rays is accomplished by providing a high voltage between the negative cathode and the positive anode of the x-ray tube. Whenever electrons are produced at the negatively charged cathode and accelerated toward the anode, they strike the positively charged target area of the anode, and x-ray photons are produced.

The Filament

The filament is mounted in a holder, called the focusing cup, about 2.5 cm (1 inch) or so away from the anode. Modern radiographic tubes have dual (two) filaments; small and large, which are necessary to produce a small and a large focal spot (Figure 6-6).

The filaments are constructed of thin thoriated tungsten wire because tungsten has a high melting point (3,370°C) and because it does not readily vaporize (turn into a gas). Rhenium and molybdenum are also desirable filament materials because of their high melting point. Because a great amount of heat is produced within the x-ray tube, the use of these materials allows the filament to withstand the heat and not melt. Vaporization within the x-ray tube produces particles that deposit on the x-ray tube window and reduce the vacuum within the tube. The purpose of the filament is to provide sufficient resistance to the flow of electrons so that the heat produced will cause thermionic emission to occur. The filament is heated until it glows (incandescence) in the same way as the filament in an ordinary light bulb. Heating the filament provides a source of electrons. The length and diameter of the filament coil, the shape and size of the focusing cup, and their relative positions are factors that affect the shape and size of the spot where the electrons strike the anode. The temperature of the filament controls the quantity of electrons emitted from it. As the temperature of the filament is raised, more electrons are emitted; when kilovoltage is applied between the cathode and anode, the flow of electrical current through the x-ray tube (mA) begins.

Because the filament wire is thin (0.1 to 0.2 mm thick), a major cause of tube failure is the breaking of this wire. Vaporization causes the filament wire to become thin and more susceptible to breaking. Jarring of the x-ray tube can also contribute to filament wire breakage in an older tube.

The radiographic machine is equipped with a double switch on the operating console. One switch, called the **rotor**, is used to heat the filament and to start the anode rotating (to about 3,000 to 10,000 RPM [revolutions per minute]). When

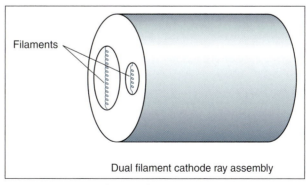

Filaments

Dual filament cathode ray assembly

FIGURE 6-6 Dual filament focusing cup
Source: Delmar, Cengage Learning.

the x-ray machine is first turned on, a low current is sent to the filament wire. When the "prep" or "rotor" button is activated prior to exposure, a higher current is sent to the filament to correspond to the mA selected for the exposure. This boost or increase in current to the filament wire results in an increase in heating of the filament wire and contributes to premature tube failure. The useful life of a diagnostic x-ray tube filament is estimated to be at approximately 10,000 to 20,000 exposures. As a preventative measure, the radiographer should not prolong depressing the "prep" or "rotor" before activating the exposure switch.

The radiographer should have the patient in the final position and be ready to make the exposure so as to avoid holding the rotor switch on for a prolonged time while giving preliminary instructions to the patient. In dual filament x-ray tubes, the small filament (corresponding to the small focal spot) may burn out faster than the larger filament (corresponding to the large focal spot) depending on usage.

The Anode Assembly

The anode assembly consists of the anode, stator, and rotor and serves as the path for the high-voltage flow during exposure. The anode is the positive side of the x-ray tube and has three functions: 1) it serves as a target surface for the high-voltage electrons from the filament (thus the source of x-ray photons); 2) it conducts the high voltage from the cathode back into the x-ray circuitry; and 3) it serves as the primary thermal conductor. The anode target surface is where the high-speed electrons from the cathode side of the tube are stopped suddenly, resulting in the production of x-ray photons. The entire anode is a complex device referred to as the anode assembly. Anodes may be either stationary or rotating (Figure 6-7).

Modern rotating anodes turn very fast, thus allowing a given area on the target to be bombarded by the electron stream for only 7–50 microseconds. Also,

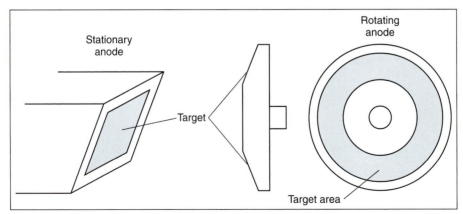

FIGURE 6-7 Stationary anode (*left*) and rotating anode (*right*)
Source: Delmar, Cengage Learning.

the faster the anode rotates, the greater the amount of heat dissipated (given off) from around the target area. The radiographer can help prolong the lifespan of the radiographic equipment by performing an anode warm-up procedure. Details of such procedures are specified by the x-ray tube manufacturers and are designed to bring the anode heat from room temperature to near the range of operation. Such a procedure also assists in maintaining the high vacuum inside the glass envelope.

To help dissipate the large volume of heat, however, the anode may be made to rotate so that the heat is spread over the entire surface of the anode during exposure. Some x-ray tubes may be constructed with a rhenium-tungsten alloy anode. The combination of rhenium ($z = 75$) and tungsten ($z = 74$) further reduces the heat load and subsequent thermal stress and may reduce the potential for surface roughening, cracking, or pitting. Additionally, the combination increases the efficiency of x-ray projection as well as resistance to the heat-related problems previously mentioned.

The portion of the anode where the high-voltage electron stream will impact is referred to by different names such as focal point, focal spot, or the focal track. The target is considered to be the point source of the x-ray photons and it is from this point that the source to image distances (SID) are measured.

The Line Focus Principle

The cathode (negative) side of the x-ray tube has previously been referred to several times but its importance cannot be overemphasized. Electrons flow from negative (cathode) toward the positive (anode) side of the tube. The tungsten wire filament is mounted on the cathode in a cup-shaped depression, called the focusing cup, that serves to focus the stream of fast-moving electrons on the anode target (Figure 6-8).

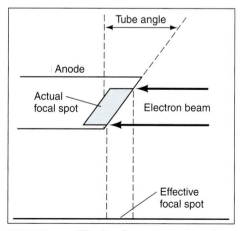

FIGURE 6-8 The line focus principle and the effective focal spot
Source: Delmar, Cengage Learning.

The line focus principle is a result of the electron stream striking an angled target (e.g., 10 degrees, 20 degrees to the central ray). The part of the anode on which the electron stream impacts is called the focal spot. The effect is that of making the resulting x-ray beam smaller than the electron beam. Consequently, when an anode disk having less of an angle is used with a small focal spot, the recorded radiographic image will have greater detail.

The electrons from the filament actually strike the anode in a rectangular shape, such as 1.0 mm × 3.0 mm, but effectively create an image on a film more square, 1.0 mm × 1.0 mm.

Thus, the radiographer must understand the difference between the actual focal spot and the effective focal spot. The size of the effective focal spot is based on 1) the angle of the target and 2) the size of the filament. There is a practical limit to how small the angle of the target can be. Use of too small an angle may cause an unacceptable reduction in x-ray output toward the anode side of the x-ray beam, thereby accentuating what is called the heel effect, which will be discussed in greater detail in Chapter 9, Fundamentals of Radiographic Exposure. Equipment manufacturers use a dimension known as the nominal focal-spot size to designate different sizes of focal spots.

The Focusing Cup

The focusing cup (refer to Figure 6-5) is used to direct the flow of electrons. The electrons flow from negative (cathode) to positive (anode) across the x-ray tube (difference in potential). The focusing cup surrounds the filament and also has a negative potential, as does the filament (cathode). This combination of negatively charged cathode and negatively charged focusing cup allows the electrons to bombard the positively charged anode (target) in a specific focus area (focus spot size) based on the line focus principle. Otherwise, when the electrons impact the target, they would spread heat over the whole target surface. The filament is heated by a high electrical filament current, which is measured in amperes.

When the electrons are released, they collect in a space around the filament and remain there until an electrical force is applied to move them. The force applied to move the electrons is measured in thousands of volts and is called kilovoltage (kV). The kilovoltage is applied through the potential difference across the x-ray tube, creating a net negative charge at the target on the anode side. The kilovoltage force accelerates the electrons at a high velocity across the gap from the cathode to the anode, where they strike the part of the anode known as the target (refer to Figure 6-5).

The electron stream that flows between the cathode (negative) and anode (positive) makes up the x-ray tube current, measured in milliamperes (mA), and is called milliamperage.

The electron stream is focused on one part of the anode, called the target. The anode is made of tungsten and may be either a stationary wedge or a rotating disk.

Tungsten is used because it has a very high melting point—3, 370°C and an atomic number (z) of 74 (z = 74). It can therefore withstand much more heat than other metal materials. There is an enormous amount of heat created by the interaction of electrons in the anode, and tungsten is an excellent material for absorbing high degrees of heat. It should be pointed out that the ability of the target material to withstand heat affects both the quantity (mAs) and the quality (kVp) of the x-ray energy.

By increasing the mAs result there is a direct increase in the quantity of electrons, which in turn causes an increase in blackness on the radiographic film. Increased kVp results in increased x-ray penetration (creates shorter wavelength x-rays), with greater efficiency of the x-ray penetration. Additionally, as kVp increases, scatter radiation increases.

Electron Interaction at the Target

When the electrons are flowing at a high rate of speed and are decelerated or stopped suddenly at the anode and interact with the atoms of the target material, the production of radiant energy (x-rays) occurs. There are two types of target interactions that can produce diagnostic-range x-ray photons: bremsstrahlung interactions and characteristic interactions. The interaction that will occur depends on the electron kinetic energy and the binding energy of the electron shells of the atom. Tungsten and rhenium are materials with high atomic number atoms that facilitate these interactions.

Bremsstrahlung is a German word meaning to break or slow. The term *"brems"* refers to when an electron interacts with the nucleus of an atom in the target material. The strong positive charge of the atom's nucleus displaces the negatively charged electron and causes the electron to "slow down" and to divert the electron's path of travel. The energy that is lost when the electron slows down (bremsstrahlung) is emitted as an x-ray photon. Within the diagnostic x-ray range most photons are produced by bremsstrahlung target interactions (Figure 6-9).

Characteristic interactions occur only when the incoming electron interacts with an inner-shell electron. In this situation, the incoming electron must possess enough energy to knock an inner-shell electron from its orbit, thus ionizing the atom. The incoming electron will usually continue but in a slightly different path. This process releases energy in the form of characteristic radiation also known as secondary radiation. Refer to Chapter 5, Radiographic Physics, for additional information on photoelectric interaction and Figure 5-21.

Protective Tube Housing

When the electrons are flowing at a high rate of speed and are stopped suddenly at the anode where they interact with the anode target material, the production of radiation energy (x-rays) occurs. Unfortunately, the majority of energy used to

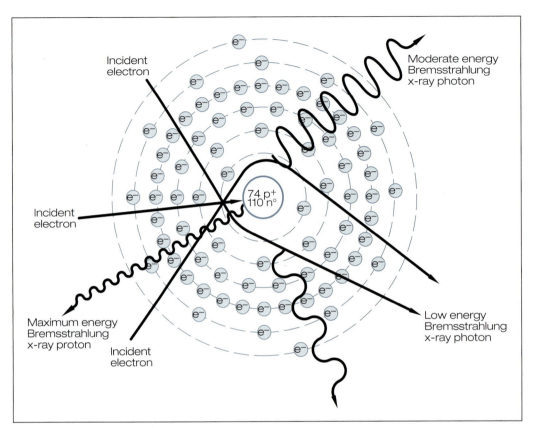

FIGURE 6-9 The bremsstrahlung interaction in a tungsten atom
Source: Delmar, Cengage Learning.

produce x-rays results in heat (98 to 99%) and very little results in useful x-rays (1–2%). The vast amount of heat production at the target may result in excessive x-ray tube heating. X-ray tubes are backed with a good heat-conducting metal to facilitate cooling by conduction. In addition, the tube is enclosed in a metal housing containing oil through which the heat is transferred and dispersed. The special dielectric oil used to fill the space between the glass envelope and the x-ray tube housing also insulates the high-voltage components. This insulation protects the radiographer and the patient from receiving an electric shock. The housing at the cathode end of the tube is usually lined with lead for additional absorption. Construction of the x-ray tube housing also controls leakage and scatter radiation, isolates the high voltages, and provides a means to cool the tube. The housing also serves to cushion the x-ray tube from bumps and jarring that may occur during routine operation.

X-rays produced at the anode are emitted in all directions from the tube window or port (Figure 6-10).

The primary beam consists of all the x-ray photons emitted through the glass window. The remaining photons are unwanted and the x-ray tube housing is designed to absorb them. The x-ray tube housing has a window to permit unrestricted exit for the useful x-ray photons from the glass envelope. Any x-ray photons that escape from the housing except at the window or port are leakage radiation. The amount of leakage radiation produced is generally monitored and enforced by state radiation safety standards and in most states must not exceed 100 mR/hr at 1 meter.

X-ray tube filtration and the collimator shutters alter the quantity and quality of the x-ray beam (Figure 6-11). Filtration serves to absorb many of the low-energy, long wavelength photons. Filtration of the primary beam improves image quality and protects the patient from the low-energy, long wavelength photons. Inherent filtration consists of the x-ray tube and housing. Added filtration is considered any additional filtration material.

The collimator, shown in Figure 6-11, also referred to as a variable collimator, consists of sets of lead shutters mounted at right angles to one another. The shutter pairs move in opposing directions, which allows for a variety of field sizes which limits the area being irradiated. Collimators are equipped with a light source, which represents the primary radiation beam. A crosshair in the light source represents the central ray (CR) or the portion of the primary beam emerging off of the target at a right angle. Additional information about x-ray tube filtration and collimation may also be found in Chapter 9, Fundamentals of Radiographic Exposure, and Chapter 16, Radiation Protection.

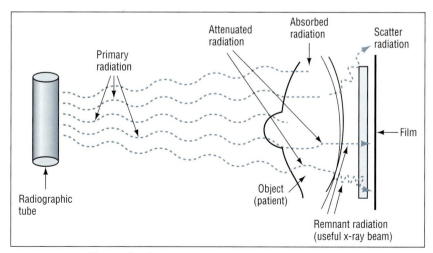

FIGURE 6-10 Types of radiation
Source: Delmar, Cengage Learning.

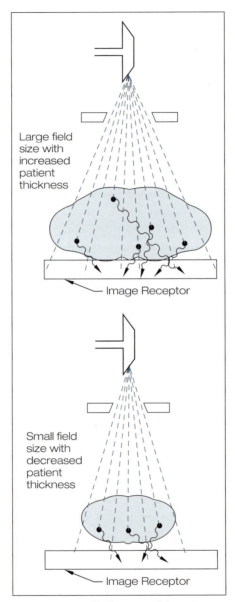

FIGURE 6-11 Collimation of the primary radiation helps reduce the amount of scatter radiation
Source: Delmar, Cengage Learning.

Figure 6-10 shows the terminology used to describe x-rays as they leave the x-ray window or port, travel to, and interact with the anatomic area being examined. The primary (useful) beam consists of the x-ray beam that has passed through the x-ray tube's window, filtration, and collimator shutters. Notice as the x-ray beam passes through the anatomic part being examined, body tissues attenuate (change) the radiation-based interactions with the tissues (Figure 6-10). Scatter radiation occurs when x-rays interact with matter and a change in their direction results. The direction of Scatter radiation is uncontrollable so the radiographer must stand behind a lead barrier during the x-ray examination. The patient's radiosensitive body areas may be protected from scatter radiation by the use of lead shields whenever their application will not obscure necessary diagnostic information. The term remnant radiation is sometimes used to refer to the useful radiation consisting of both primary and secondary radiation.

The Operating Console

The operating console or control panel is located in a control booth, which contains protective, lead shielding. The location of the control booth and the amount of lead used in its construction are dependent on the type of x-ray equipment, its position within the room, the occupancy of adjacent areas, and other factors. Most control booths have a lead glass window so the radiographer can observe the patient.

The types of switches, buttons, and meters on the operating console vary with the type, model, and brand of the equipment (Figure 6-12).

At a minimum, the operating console will allow the operator to select the exposure factors, read indicators of the exposure setting before and during the exposure, and exposure buttons or switches.

Tube Rating Charts

The purpose of a tube-rating chart, shown in Figure 6-13, is to extend the life of a x-ray tube and to ensure that the tube can withstand the heat created by the workload.

Each filament of each x-ray tube has a unique radiographic tube rating chart provided by the manufacturer. There are certain instantaneous ratings that are excessive and can seriously damage or cause a melting point on the anode surface. Such considerations include:

1. Never use high kVp on a cold target. The target must be warmed with several low exposures (low kVp, low mAs; e.g., 50 kVp and 10 mA) before making a single high exposure. A x-ray tube's target will become cold after about an hour of non-use. Always warm the target when beginning the day's work or when the tube has cooled for a long period.
2. Never use an excessive single exposure, even on a warn anode.

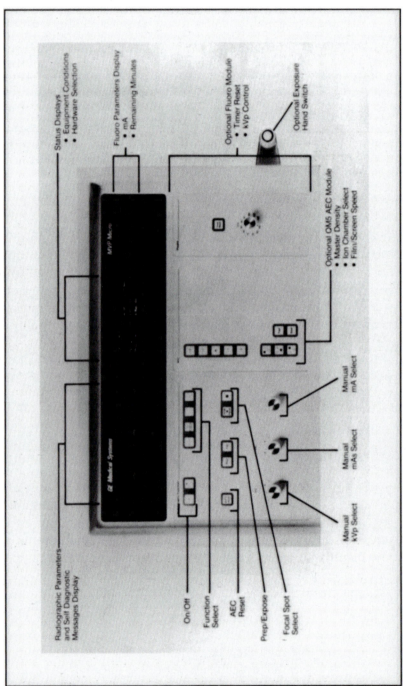

FIGURE 6-12 The control console of a diagnostic x-ray machine *(Courtesy of GEMedical Systems)*

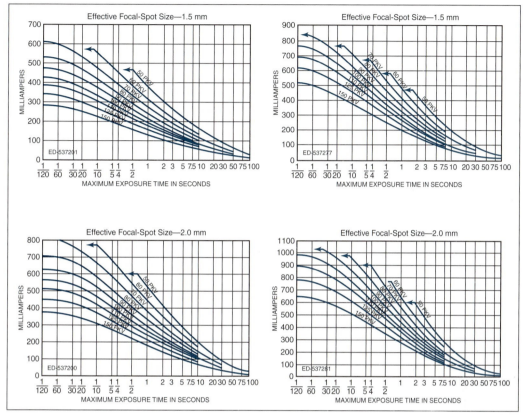

FIGURE 6-13 Representative tube rating charts for a diagnostic x-ray tube
Source: Delmar, Cengage Learning.

3. The number of multiple exposures (e.g., twenty) that may be made at any given time must not exceed the x-ray tube's total heat capacity.

4. A x-ray tube that uses a fixed anode—one that does not rotate—is limited in its heat capacity and thus uses lower kilovoltage (kVp) and milliamperage (mA) levels (e.g., mobile radiography units).

Radiographers generally need only be concerned with warming a cold anode and not exceeding a single exposure rate on the anode. Radiographers should follow the manufacturer's recommendations regarding general maintenance and operation of x-ray systems.

Tube Heat Capacity

Tube heat capacity has been referred to several times because many of the malfunctions associated with x-ray tubes are directly related to heat. X-ray tube heat capacity is measured in heat units (HU). Heat units are simply a mathematical combination of exposure factors, kilovoltage (kVp), seconds (s), and milliamperage (mA) written in formula as kVp × s × mA. For detailed discussion about these exposure factors, refer to the Chapter 9, Fundamentals of Radiographic Exposure.

For now, let's say that the exposure factors 70 kVp × 1.0 seconds × 100-mA equal 7000 HU. The preceding formula may be used to calculate HU for single phase current.

Whether or not the number of HU would be more than the heat capacity of a given x-ray tube would depend on its total capacity and how much heat in HU had already been applied. Depending on the x-ray tube's intended workload, heat units vary from as little as 100,000 HU to 400,000 HU or higher. It is prudent for the radiographer to know and respect the manufacturer's recommended tube capacity.

REVIEW QUESTIONS

1. The cathode beam of an x-ray tube is the:
   a. primary x-ray beam
   b. focused electron beam within the tube
   c. current heating the filament
   d. secondary radiation

2. The target metal used in x-ray tubes should have the following two properties:
   a. high atomic number, high melting point
   b. low atomic number, low melting point
   c. low atomic number, high melting point
   d. high atomic number, low melting point

3. The process of boiling off of electrons from a hot, metallic filament is called:
   a. Compton scatter
   b. pair production
   c. photoelectric effect
   d. thermionic emission

4. The positive terminal of an x-ray tube is the:
   a. cathode
   b. anode
   c. focusing cup
   d. filament

5. The cloud of liberated electrons that remains in the vicinity of the hot filament is called:
   a. tube current
   b. filament current
   c. positrons
   d. space charge

6. The negative terminal of an x-ray tube is the:
   a. cathode
   b. anode
   c. target
   d. rotor

7. X-rays are produced in the:
   1. focal spot
   2. anode
   3. target

   Possible Responses

   a. 1 and 2
   b. 1 and 3
   c. 2 and 3
   d. 1, 2, and 3

8. The effective focal spot:
   1. is smaller than the actual focal spot
   2. is on the anode
   3. determines the resolution

   Possible Responses

   a. 1 and 2
   b. 1 and 3
   c. 2 and 3
   d. 1, 2, and 3

9. A rotating anode:
   1. dissipates heat
   2. has a larger target than a fixed anode
   3. is driven by a motor

Possible Responses

a. 1 and 2
b. 1 and 3
c. 2 and 3
d. 1, 2, and 3

10. The tube housing:
     1. helps contain scattered x-rays
     2. is designed to aid in heat dissipation
     3. contains the glass envelope

Possible Responses

a. 1 and 2
b. 1 and 3
c. 2 and 3
d. 1, 2, and 3

11. The most important component of a radiographic unit with regard to image production is the x-ray tube.
     a. True
     b. False

12. The x-ray tube focusing cup has a _____ charge.
     a. positive
     b. negative

13. Heat units may be determined with the following formula:
     a. $kVp \times s \times mA$
     b. $kVp \times mA$
     c. $kVp \times s \times 1.41$
     d. $kVp \times mA \times 1.35$
     e. none of the above

14. The rotating anode is generally made of an alloy material with a high melting point. The following element(s) represent the most efficient material(s) for x-ray production:
     a. gold
     b. tungsten
     c. rhenium-tungsten
     d. a and b
     e. b and c

15. The amount of electrons generated in the x-ray tube determines the _____.
   a. quality
   b. quantity
   c. mA
   d. a and c
   e. b and c

SUGGESTED READINGS

Bushong, S. C. (2008). *Radiologic science for technologists: Physics, biology and protection* (9th ed.). St. Louis, MO: Mosby Elsevier.

Carlton, R. R. & Adler, A. M. (2006). *Principles of radiographic imaging: An art and a science* (3rd ed.). Albany, NY: Delmar Thomson Learning.

Palakow, N. (2005). All systems go. *RTImage, 18*(5), 27–29.

Quinn, B. C. (2007). *Practical radiographic imaging* (8th ed.). Springfield, IL: Charles C. Thomas.

Shepard, C. T. (2003). *Radiographic image production and manipulation*. New York: McGraw-Hill Companies, Inc.

Key Terms

Automatic Exposure Control (AEC)

Automatic Program Radiography (APR)

Autotransformer

Calipers

Circuit Breaker

Filament Circuit

Fixed Kilovoltage Technique

Full-Wave Rectification

Half-Wave Rectification

High kVp Technique

High-Voltage Cables

High-Voltage Transformer

Kilovolt Peak Meter

Line Voltage Compensator

Milliameter (mA)

Phototimer

Primary Circuit

Radiographic Tube

Rectifiers

Secondary Circuit

Synchronous Timer

Timers

Variable Kilovoltage Technique

Chapter Outline

Introduction
  Equipment Safety
Radiographic Equipment
Primary and Secondary Circuits
  Primary Circuit
  Secondary Circuit
Types of Equipment
Accessory Items
  Calipers
  Exposure Charts (Technique Charts)
  Cassettes

Objectives

Upon completion of the chapter, the student will meet the following objectives by verifying knowledge of the facts and principles presented through oral and written communication at a level deemed competent.

⊃ Explain permanently installed radiographic equipment and its maintenance.
⊃ Identify and discuss the various types and purposes of basic radiographic equipment.

⊃ Discuss the purposes, advantages, and disadvantages of routine and specific radiographic equipment.
⊃ Describe the purpose and disadvantages of mobile equipment and relate complexity of procedures.
⊃ Describe accessory equipment and the usage of different types.
⊃ Develop a basic exposure chart.

Introduction

This chapter deals with the electrical equipment needed to produce the radiographic image. It is important that prospective radiographers possess functional knowledge about the equipment they will use to practice their profession. Knowledge of the basis of the operation of radiographic units provides the radiographer with the background to use the imaging equipment most efficiently.

Equipment Safety

The diagnostic radiology area can pose electrical and mechanical hazard to both patient and radiographer. To prevent injuries, staff must be attentive to maintaining an environment that is safe and equipment that is functioning properly. Palakov (2005) suggests the following strategy for maintaining a safe environment.

- Equipment should provide a high level of electrical isolation between the patient and the ground.
- All equipment operated from electrical outlets should be inspected at regular intervals. The visual inspection should include power plugs and power cords. A qualified inspector should periodically measure resistance and leakage current between the grounding plug and all exposed conducive surfaces of instruments and equipment.
- All staff should be aware of the location of the circuit breaker and it should be visible and unobstructed.
- During the electrical inspection and when collimator lights are replaced, the electricity should be turned off at the circuit breaker.
- All staff should be aware of the location of a fire extinguisher and its proper application. A tri-class type ABC dry chemical extinguisher is recommended for electrically related fires.
- A repair logbook should be kept of all repairs and downtime on equipment.
- A visible "warning" repair tag should be placed on malfunctioning equipment until repairs have been made.

Radiographic Equipment

Radiographic equipment is the instrumentation needed for the performance of the tasks associated with radiographic procedures. Generally, we think of the permanently installed equipment—that which is used for either fluoroscopy or radiography (Figure 7-1). However, many items used as accessories in the production of radiographic images (e.g., grid cassettes, compression bands, etc.) are also considered radiographic equipment.

The most important component of any radiographic unit is the tube. (The tube was discussed in detail in Chapter 6.) The tube is a rotational or fixed part of a unit that also includes an electrical system and controls for circuits, generators, fuses, and switches. According to its purpose, a piece of equipment may be large, with many different components, or small, like a dental unit that hangs on the wall (Figure 7-2). All equipment must be handled with care and have regular maintenance, quality assurance, and testing to provide reliability.

Radiographic units may be divided into two basic parts: the primary circuit (also called the low-voltage circuit), and the secondary or high-voltage circuit.

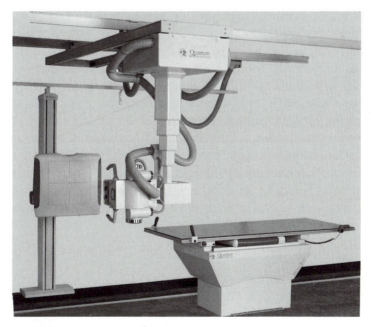

FIGURE 7-1 Permanently installed radiographic equipment
(Quantum Medical Imaging, Ronkonkoma, New York, USA)

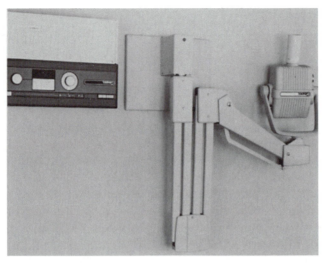

FIGURE 7-2 Dental x-ray machine used for intraoral radiographs (*GENDEX Corporation, Milwaukee, WI*)

Primary Circuit and Secondary Circuit

When a radiographic unit is installed, there must be a current source that comes from an outside source. The local utility company is responsible for the main supply of the incoming 110 or 220 volts of alternating current that will be used for any facility. Lines are brought in from outside and connected to a junction box inside, where the radiographic unit control console is connected.

To produce x-rays, the line voltage must be controlled and changed to a direct current of many thousands of volts. This is done by the high-voltage transformer. A transformer is an electromagnetic device that will increase or decrease the voltage of alternating current. In an x-ray machine, the high-voltage transformer increases the low voltage of the primary circuit to the high voltage needed by the secondary circuit.

Primary Circuit

The primary circuit begins at the main power switch on the control console of the radiographic unit and leads to the primary coil of the high-tension transformer (Figure 7-3). Major components included in the primary section of the circuit are the autotransformer, kilovolt peak meter, line voltage compensator, filament circuit, circuit breaker, and timers.

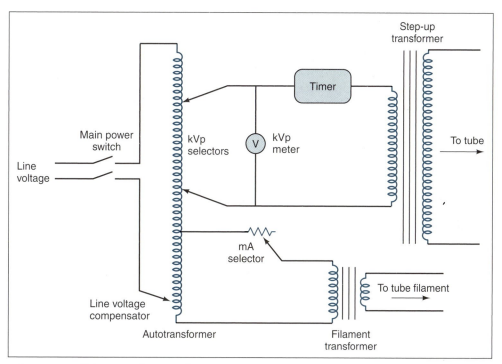

FIGURE 7-3 Schematic diagram of the primary side of an x-ray machine circuit
Source: Delmar, Cengage Learning.

Autotransformer. This special type of transformer is used with the major and minor kVp selectors to provide a means to vary the voltage magnitude, through a step-up transformer and a step-down transformer. A step-up transformer increases voltage and decreases current. A step-down transformer decreases voltage and increases current.

Kilovolt Peak Meter. This meter is connected to the autotransformer. Its function is to display the potential difference in kilovolts going to the high-voltage transformer.

Line Voltage Compensator. This component is connected across or in parallel with the primary circuit to the autotransformer. Its function is to increase or decrease the line voltage if there is a drop or surge in the line voltage. Any change in input voltage will cause a change in output of radiation. Automatic line voltage compensators are included in modern radiographic units.

Filament Circuit. The filament circuit is connected to the autotransformer. Its function is to supply current to the filament of the radiographic tube. The circuit supplies lower voltage and higher current by means of a step-down transformer, which is controlled by a rheostat or variable resistor.

Circuit Breaker.   This is a protective device used to automatically terminate the current in the event that predetermined values are exceeded, i.e., excessive exposure or too much current from the line source. The breaker may be reset mechanically with a switch. If exposure factors cut off the breaker, then lower settings must be selected.

Timers.   Duration of exposure time is controlled by a switch in the timing circuit. The switch, which is built into the electrical circuit, will remain closed for the length of time selected by the radiographer at the control console or panel. Several types of exposure-timing devices are commonly used.

1. *Synchronous timers*: A synchronous timer is controlled and driven by an electrical synchronous motor. It is not generally used because it is not reliable and has limited exposure-time range. Exposure times are not usually accurate for shorter than 1/60 of a second.
2. *Electronic timers*:
   Impulse—A precise timing circuit that operates with an alternating current. The circuit is energized to variable time intervals, from milliseconds to seconds. It is accurate and may be used for rapid film production.
   mAs—A more specific electronic timer is used to control and terminate the time when the correct mAs is reached. This type of mAs timer is protection for tube current.
3. *Automatic timers*: A timing device that automatically terminates the exposure when the correct amount of radiation (density) has reached the film. The accuracy of this device depends on carefully positioning the anatomical part being radiographed correctly to the sensing element of the timing device.
   Automatic exposure-control devices are categorized as phototimer and ionization chamber.
   Phototimers utilizes a light-sensitive photomultiplier tube placed behind a fluorescent screen. The fluorescent screen, placed in front of or behind the film, produces light from radiation transmitted through the film. The light is picked up by the photomultiplier tube which terminates the exposure, after a predetermined charge that corresponds to the density of the film is reached. The amount of screen fluorescence (intensity) is directly proportional to the amount of radiation (intensity) that reaches the film.
   Ionization chambers utilizes a chamber located between the patient and the film. This chamber measures the amount of radiation reaching the film and shuts off the exposure at a predetermined setting.

Timer Tests.   Two types of devices are used for testing the accuracy of timers. One is a simple manual spinning top designed to test single phase current (see Figure 7-4). Single phase units are less common today because most radiology departments or offices have advanced, full-wave rectification radiographic units that utilize three-phase current. This type of current should be tested with an electric meter. The device used for single phase units is placed on top of a film cassette and manually rotated (like a spinning top) not too fast or too slow. The single opening on the disk will show up on the film as dots that represent electrical current flow for 60-cycle current at 120 impulses per second. In order to determine the number of dots to be seen on the film, the exposure timer should be set for a given time and the time divided into 120; e.g., 0.1/120 = 12 dots.

Electric mAs meters used for testing three-phase current are a little more involved because the dots overlap as a result of multiple electrical impulses (see Figure 7-4). This type of device records an arc on the film. The meter is placed on the film cassette and exposed at a given time. The resulting exposure will show an arc of overlapped dots. The degree of the arc must be measured with a protractor provided with the meter. The degree of the arc is divided into the number of impulses; e.g., 90°/360 = 0.4. Instructions for using the mAs meters generally come with the individual device.

Secondary Circuit

The high-voltage, secondary circuit begins with the secondary coil of the step-up transformer (see Figure 7-5). It also includes the **milliameter (mA)**, milliampere second meter (mAs), **rectifiers**, **high-voltage cables**, and **radiographic tube**. All components

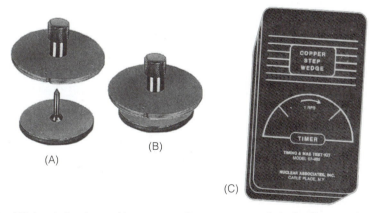

(A)   (B)   (C)

FIGURE 7-4 (A) A spin top is used to measure timer accuracy of single-phase equipment. A brass disc base with a spindle at its center, and the top with a small hole near its edge is exhibited. The spin top, which is easily rotated, is shown in (B). (C) A timer and mAs tester. This device may be used for single-phase, as well as three-phase radiographic equipment. It is a synchronous rotator-slit timer tester, and is used for checking timer accuracy and mAs uniformity. The manufacturer provides directions for appropriate use of the timing and mAs device.

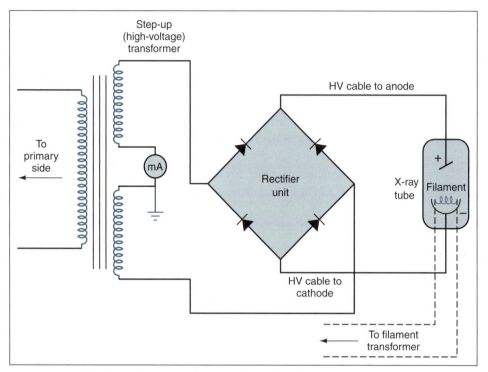

FIGURE 7-5 Schematic diagram of the secondary side of an x-ray machine circuit
Source: Delmar, Cengage Learning.

of the secondary circuit are immersed in oil for purposes of electrical insulation and cooling in a separate section away from the radiographic unit console.

High-Voltage Transformer. The step-up or high-voltage transformer consists of two iron coils wrapped with windings of electrical wire. The coil on the low-voltage side, carrying the current from the primary circuit, is called the primary coil. The coil on the high-voltage side carries the stepped-up, or increased voltage to the secondary circuit and is called the secondary coil.

Milliameter (mA). The mA meter is used to measure the current in milliamperes flowing through the radiographic tube. It is connected in series with the high-voltage circuit.

Rectifiers. Rectifiers are used to change alternating current to direct current, or current flowing in one direction (Figures 7-6A and B). Alternating current is used in the primary circuit for two reasons: 1) it is the type of electricity supplied by the electrical utility, and 2) transformers will only work on alternating current. However, direct current is necessary to operate the radiographic tube so that electrons can be produced and kept flowing in one direction. Any reverse or change in current flow would cease electron production and could damage the tube. Rectification is controlled in modern equipment by devices called *diodes*. Modern radiographic equipment uses solid-state, silicone diode rectifiers to convert alternating current to direct current. Half-wave rectification and Full-wave rectification are the two types of rectification used in modern diagnostic radiology x-ray machines:

1. Half-wave rectification (Figure 7-6A). This type of rectification is used where current is directed by one or two diodes. Negative voltage is suppressed so that the flow of current is only utilized during the positive flow of alternating current. It is also called impulse current because one cycle of alternating current is applied.
2. Full-wave rectification (Figure 7-6B). This type of rectification is used in most radiographic units because it is the most efficient. It uses four diodes so that both the positive and negative impulses are used. There is a constant flow of positive current in one direction.

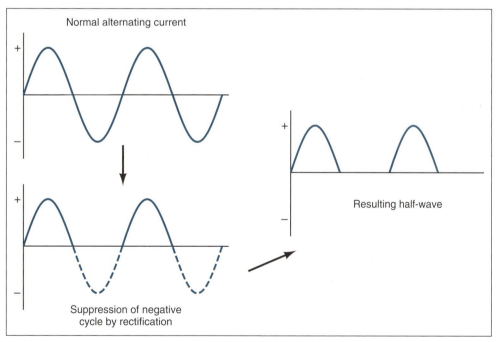

FIGURE 7-6A Half-wave rectification of normal alternating current and the resulting waveform
Source: Delmar, Cengage Learning.

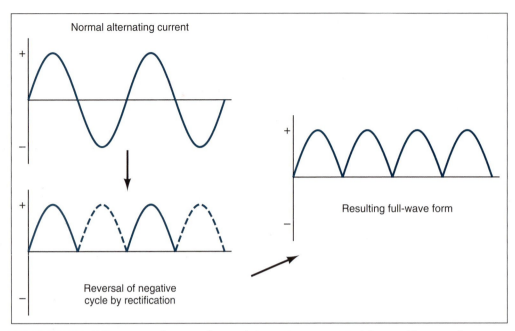

Normal alternating current

Reversal of negative
cycle by rectification

Resulting full-wave form

FIGURE 7-6B Full-wave rectification of normal alternating current and the resulting waveform
Source: Delmar, Cengage Learning.

High-Voltage Cables. Two large cables are used to connect the radiographic tube to the high-voltage generator. One cable is attached to the cathode side of the tube; the other is connected to the anode side of the tube. The cables are designed to prevent any electrical hazard, such as arcing over of current flow from one terminal to the other.

Radiographic Tube. This component is the most important part of the radiographic unit. It is the component that creates the electrons that are used to produce the x-rays that are the basis for radiographic images. Again, the tube is described in detail in Chapter 6.

Types of Equipment

Various types of units, either combined radiographic and fluoroscopic units (RF) or radiographic units only, may be found where radiographic images are produced. They may be installed for general or specific examination purposes, e.g., chest unit or head unit. In addition to installed units, there are portable units, used principally at the bedside. Important items of information to learn and remember about all radiographic units are:

1. *The electrical capacity of the unit in terms of milliamperage and kilovoltage.* Unless a radiographer is working with outdated equipment, a standard unit may have exposure ratings of from 100 to 1200 mA, kVp settings up to 150, and a dual focus tube (large and small focal spots). Other exposure factors include various time settings ranging from milliseconds to several whole seconds, i.e., $\frac{1}{360}$–10 seconds, although radiographs are generally made at fractions of seconds.

2. *The limitation of any unit, especially portables.* In regard to portables, although the radiographer today is so concerned with limitation of exposure, the degree of equipment maneuverability is very important. That is, portable radiography may be complex when the patient's condition is unstable or body position must be maintained, as in orthopedic traction. Extensive orthopedic traction for trauma patients usually requires an experienced radiographer's judgment for making films. Some specific units, such as head units, have limitations that restrict examining the patient who is either sitting or lying on a stretcher and cannot be moved. If the head unit is placed in a tight area or the radiographer does not understand its maneuverability, a head unit may become limited to use with the sitting position only.

3. *The purpose and combinations of exposure factors—the mA, time (s), and kVp selections.* The way in which all exposure factors affect the visible image must be clear to the radiographer. The function of all switches and meters on the control panel must be understood (Figure 7-7).

4. *The purpose and effectiveness of radiographic accessory items.* The way in which accessory items aid in the production or enhancement of the radiographic image is essential knowledge for the radiographer.

Accessory Items

Radiography uses numerous accessory items. Some may be unique to a particular radiographic procedure, such as those used in CT, MRI, or ultrasound. The most common items are cassettes, grid cassettes, calipers, film holders, film markers, film printers, compression bands, tape, and sponges. These items are generally found in any radiographic room. Although most are described and their uses explained in Chapters 8 and 9, calipers and cassettes are discussed in this chapter.

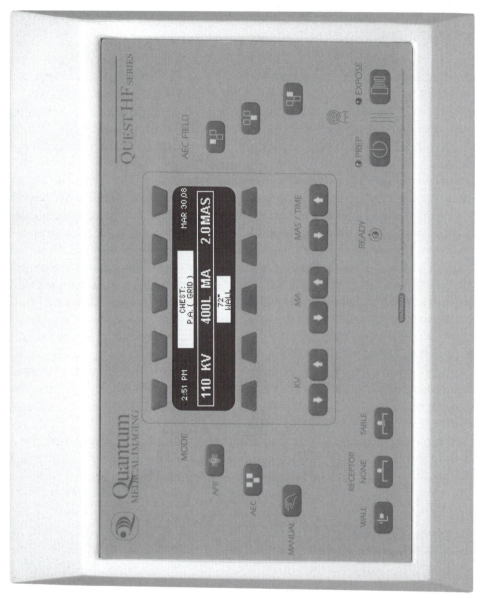

FIGURE 7-7 Modern computerized control console. The exposure factors that have been selected are clearly exhibited. (Quantum Medical Imaging, Ronkonkoma, New York, USA)

Calipers

A caliper is a measuring device, used in radiography to measure the volume of tissue thickness of a body part. Tissue volume is a variable in exposure technique that must be accounted for in image production. It is a mistake to believe that one can simply and accurately visually judge tissue volume. Beyond a certain point, quality begins to suffer when one attempts to "guess" what every set of technical factors will be through visual estimation only. Moreover, it may often be useful for the radiographer measuring tissue volume with the caliper to be aware that tone and texture of tissues may be determined through touch. These discoveries, of course, cannot be made if one never measures tissue. Thus, we can see the deception of assuming exposure latitude. Exposure latitude allows for gradual margin of error in radiographic quality within certain kVp measurement ranges. An important advantage of measuring tissue volume is consistency of exposure techniques. The same patient may be measured at different times by different people, but the result should be the same, thus reflecting equal exposure factors. It does not take into account conditions, such as ascites (abdominal fluid), where exposure must be manipulated to maintain equal radiographic quality in density and contrast. The effect of tissue measurement may become less critical when some exposure factors are standardized and technique charts are developed on the basis of one-centimeter variations of tissue thickness (i.e., 2 kVp per centimeter measurement). The radiographer may be able to visually evaluate tissue thickness by judging the distance between two lines that measure one centimeter.

To place the caliper properly, the (horizontal) sliding part of the device must be parallel to the base of the device and the vertical part must remain perpendicular to the base. The sliding part must not be pushed tightly against the tissue; it should be allowed to rest evenly along the part being measured. Measurement is always taken along the imaginary line where the central ray traverses the body part and at the same angle as the central ray. Extreme differences or variations in the part to be radiographed should be compensated for by determining an average thickness within the total area of the part.

Figure 7-8 is an illustration of a caliper used for determining the amount of tissue volume that will be penetrated by the exposure factors mAs, kVp, and time (sec). Keep in mind that penetration is controlled by kVp (see Chapter 9 for further explanation). Also, think of time as a factor of duration. There should be adequate time for mAs and kVp to produce the image. That is, density (controlled by time $\times$ mA) and penetration (determined by kVp) result in photographic quality. This is discussed in more detail in Chapter 9. Tissue thickness and volume therefore must be taken into account no matter how exposure factors are determined.

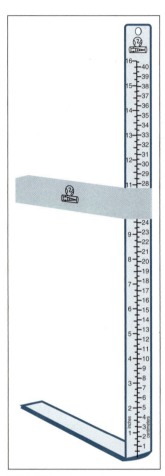

FIGURE 7-8 Type of calipers may be employed for measurement of a body part
Source: Delmar, Cengage Learning.

Exposure Charts (Technique Charts)

Although some facilities may no longer use exposure charts, there remains a need to understand volume of tissue in relationship to exposure factors for penetration and quantity of radiation. Measurement of tissue volume, or thickness of part, is the basis for exposure charts. Thus, these charts serve as a guide for use in producing consistent images of anatomical parts.

Importantly, in addition to consistency, technique factors are determined to protect the patient against overexposure or underexposure. Charts are usually set up for each radiographic room. Various types of charts may exist today, depending on a facility's size and equipment (e.g., small facilities, offices, large facilities). The following types are examples of technique charts: 1) fixed kilovoltage, 2) variable kilovoltage, 3) automatic exposure control (AEC) or phototiming, 4) automatic programmed radiography (APR), and 5) high kVp. There are various other charts that are not mentioned here in the interest of brevity. Brief explanations of the named techniques follow.

1. **Fixed kilovoltage technique** uses an optimum kilovoltage that will penetrate a given part of the body (e.g., hand, knee, chest, abdomen, pelvis, etc.). The mAs is varied based on the centimeter (cm) measurement of the part and the projection. Anatomical parts may be established in groups of small, medium, and large ranges of thickness. Adult measurements are used to establish average techniques. An example with a fixed kVp established at 80 and a varied mAs based on a range of centimeter measurements is provided below.

AP Abdomen	kVp	mAs
14–20 cm = small	80	50
*21–25 cm = medium	80	80
26–32 cm = large	80	110

   *Average: cm = 21–25
      kVp 80
      SID 40″ (100 cm)
      Film speed 200
      Grid 12:1 ratio

This example reflects optimum kVp that produces long scale contrast, which will adequately penetrate a specific anatomical part on the highest percentage of adults. Once kVp is established through exposure of a phantom (e.g., abdomen, chest, knee, skull, etc.) for a region of the body, the only exposure factor changed will be the mAs. Thickness ranges are based on average adult measurements of body regions and are used to establish mAs values. Thickness ranges and percentage frequencies are illustrated in Table 7-1 (Quinn, 1993). The table shows average thickness ranges for various projections and the percentage frequencies for adults. The most practical variable for average groupings is time. That is when the kVp and mAs are sufficient an increase or less likely a decrease in time may suffice for adequate exposure. The patient receives lower radiation dosage and there is greater consistency in image production.

TABLE 7-1 Average Adult Part Thickness By Region

Region	AP	PA	Lat	Percent Frequency
Thumb, Fingers		1.5–4		99
Hand	3–5			99
Hand			7–10	93
Wrist	3–6			99
Wrist			5–8	98
Forearm	6–8			94
Forearm			7–9	92
Elbow	6–8			96
Elbow			7–9	87
Arm	7–10			95
Arm			7–10	94
Shoulder	12–16			79
Clavicle		13–17		82
Foot	6–8			92
Foot			7–9	91
Ankle	8–10			86
Ankle			6–9	96
Leg	10–12			85
Leg			9–11	89
Knee	10–13			92
Knee			9–12	92
Thigh	14–17			77
Thigh			13–16	76
Hip	17–21			76
Cervical Vertebrae C1–3	12–14			77
Cervical Vertebrae C4–7	11–14			98
Cervical Vertebrae C1–7			10–13	90
Thoracic Vertebrae	20–24			76
Thoracic Vertebrae			28–32	81
Lumbar Vertebrae	18–22			69
Lumbar Vertebrae			27–32	77
Pelvis	19–23			78
Skull		18–21		96
Skull			14–17	88
Sinuses Frontal		18–21		97
Sinuses Max.		18–22		88
Sinuses			13–17	96
Mandible			10–12	82
Chest		20–25		82
Chest			27–32	84

Reprinted with permission of the American Society of Radiologic Technologists from Arthur W. Fuchs's Relationship of tissue thickness to kilovoltage. The X-ray Technician [now Radiologic Technology] 19:6, 287–293, 1948.

2. **A variable kilovoltage technique** chart is rarely, if ever, used today with modern equipment and is mentioned only for information and background. In this case, a base kVp must be used and 2 kVp per centimeter added according to measurement of the part being examined. For example, a minimum base of at least 40 kVp may be used. The kVp is determined by using phantom anatomical parts to produce images. Using 40 kVp as a base, measure the part and add 2 kVp per centimeter as illustrated below for a knee (kVp may need to be 50 base).

$$12 \text{ cm} \times 2\text{kVp} = 24$$
$$24 + 40 = 64\text{kVp}$$

Appropriate mAs must be determined through trial and error, again with an anatomical phantom. However, it remains that a sufficient level of kVp must be established to provide consistency in penetration from the lowest to the highest volume of tissue for a given part. Following is a brief chart that provides variable kVp examination of a knee.

AP and Lateral Knee: mAs 15; SID 40″ (100 cm); Grid 12:1 ratio

Part Thickness	kVp
0 cm	$2 \times 10 = 20 + 40 = 60$
11 cm	$2 \times 11 = 22 + 40 = 62$
*12 cm	$2 \times 12 = 24 + 40 = 64$
*13 cm	$2 \times 13 = 26 + 40 = 66$
*14 cm	$2 \times 14 = 28 + 40 = 68$

*May be set as acceptable average ranges. Images produced at lower kVp ranges may be produced without a grid.

Remember kVp controls penetration but produces scatter as it is increased and results in reduced contrast in the recorded image. The primary concern is adequate penetration of the structure with sufficient density. This is discussed in Chapter 9. As mentioned previously, technique charts are developed through trial and error of exposure of anatomical phantoms. Also, manufacturers can provide basic charts to work with following the calibration of equipment after installation.

3. **Automatic exposure control (AEC).** Technique charts are needed with AEC. There must be minimum factors established, that is, kVp, mAs with backup time, or mAs. A photo cell or ionization chamber is used to terminate the exposure when optical density has been reached by the image receptor. This

technique requires accurate patient positioning. The part being examined must be carefully centered in front of the timing device. Measurement of the part is not usually needed for AEC.

Two electronic timing devices have been designed for AEC. One is a photo-timer and the other, an ionization chamber. Both are photocells. The earliest device, the phototimer, is generally placed behind the cassette.

Sufficient radiation must travel through the patient and film and terminates when enough exposure is reached at a predetermined level of kVp, mAs, and backup time. Cassettes are made of radiolucent or a no lead back so that x-rays are not stopped or attenuated. A photomultiplier tube is used to convert x-rays into an electric current, which charges a capacitor continuing through a rheostat that varies resistance.

Ionization chambers are commonly used today in place of the often ineffective and outdated phototimer. Compared to a single field of exposure for phototimers, the ionization chamber uses multiple fields (usually three), as may be seen on the front of a chest machine. The ionization chamber is placed between the patient and cassette. Ionization chambers have two thin parallel radiolucent aluminum or lead electrodes with gas (air) between the electrodes. When struck by radiation the air is ionized, forming charged particles. When voltage is applied across the electrodes the charged particles are attracted to ion pairs, creating current flow. The current flow is directly proportional to the incoming radiation and automatically stops the production of radiation when the correct amount of exposure is transmitted through the structure.

4. **Automatic program radiography (APR)** uses microcomputers to determine kVp and mAs (time). It is only necessary to touch a screen with pictures of a given part of the body and size. The technique is automatically selected and phototimed. These techniques are calibrated and loaded into the machine when it is installed by a service engineer. The radiographer may select from a series of buttons to adjust to differences in patient structure absorption. A switch to manual controls may be available with the equipment.

5. **High kVp technique** charts are designed to utilize high kilovoltage for penetration, usually from 100 kVp and greater. These techniques are used for barium sulfate studies or chest films. The kVp is standardized for all similar procedures with a corresponding lower mAs. Basically, the same approach would be used to establish high kVp charts as for fixed kVp charts.

All radiographic units, regardless of the technique, must be evaluated through quality controls.

Cassettes

A cassette is used to provide mechanical support and protection for the film and contains intensifying screens. Cassettes must be lightweight as well as lightproof (Figure 7-9).

Cassette fronts are made of material that offers almost no filtration to the passage of radiation. Because absorption of moisture may occur and cause expansion and contraction with temperature extremes, warping can result. Materials generally used in construction are: 1) a plastic that will absorb moisture but is radiolucent and 2) a metal alloy such as aluminum or magnesium.

Cassette backs are made of metal, aluminum, or steel. A thin sheet of foil may be attached to the inner side of the back of the cassette to prevent radiation from being scattered back through the cassette to fog film. In the case of photo-timed exposures, unnecessarily long exposures may result unless the photo-tube sensitivity is increased to sufficiently compensate for lead backing in the cassette.

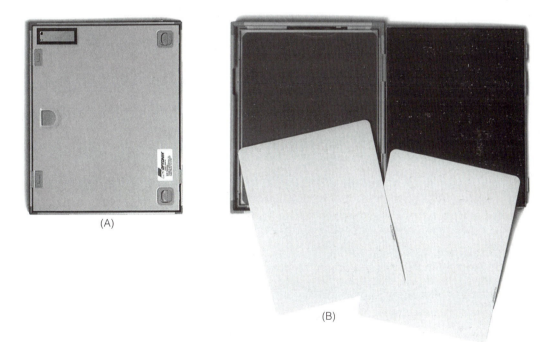

(A)

(B)

FIGURE 7–9 (A) A closed image receptor (x-ray cassette) used to hold the film. (B) The receptor is opened and shows the screens for the receptor. The front and back screens would be mounted inside the receptor where the film would be placed between them when used to record the image. The purpose of screens is to intensify the action of radiation. (*Courtesy of GE Medical Systems*)

REVIEW QUESTIONS

1. Rectification is a process that changes:
   a. direct current to alternating current
   b. alternating current to direct current
   c. high-voltage direct current to low-voltage direct current
   d. high-voltage alternating current to low-voltage alternating current

2. Self-rectification in an x-ray circuit leads to a voltage wave that is the same as:
   a. full-wave
   b. half-wave
   c. direct current
   d. two of the above

3. Which of the following is found in the filament circuit?
   a. step-up transformer
   b. step-down transformer
   c. target
   d. exposure timer

4. Which of the following devices would be located between the secondary coil of the high-voltage transformer and the x-ray tube?
   a. rheostat (milliampere selector)
   b. rectifier
   c. autotransformer
   d. filament transformer

5. The function of the filament circuit is to:
   a. supply low-voltage current to the anode
   b. supply high-voltage current to the filament
   c. supply low-voltage current to the filament
   d. supply high-voltage current to the autotransformer

6. Which of the following devices is found in the primary circuit?
   a. rectifier circuit
   b. x-ray tube
   c. autotransformer
   d. filament

7. Which type of x-ray timer terminates the exposure when a fluorescent screen produces light from the x-rays?
   a. synchronous
   b. impulse
   c. mAs
   d. phototimer

8. Another name for a rectifier is:
   a. autotransformer
   b. diode
   c. filament
   d. voltmeter

9. A device used to measure thickness of a body part is a:
   a. caliper
   b. meter stick
   c. yard stick
   d. tape measure

10. Cassettes:
    1. provide mechanical support for the film
    2. contain intensifying screens
    3. must be light proof

    Possible Responses

    a. 1 and 2
    b. 1 and 3
    c. 2 and 3
    d. 1, 2, and 3

11. The single most significant component of the radiographic unit is:
    a. step-up transformer
    b. half-wave rectifier
    c. tube
    d. none of the above

12. Devices used for testing the accuracy of 3-phase current units are called:
    a. stop watches
    b. manual spinning tops
    c. electric mAs meters
    d. a, b, and c

13. The principle of technique charts is for the radiographer to have a clear understanding of the following factors:
    1. kVp
    2. mAs
    3. time
    4. SID

    Possible Responses

    a. 1 and 2
    b. 1 and 3
    c. 1, 2, and 3
    d. 1, 2, 3, and 4

REFERENCE

Palakov, N. (2005). All systems go: Maintaining safety in the diagnostic radiology suite. *RT Image,* January, 26–29.

SUGGESTED READINGS

Bushong, S. C. (1997). *Radiologic Sciences for Technologists: Physics, Biology and Protection* (6th ed.). St. Louis, MO: C. V. Mosby.

Curry, T. S., Dowdey, J. E., & Murry, R. C. (1990). *Christensen's physics of diagnostic radiology* (4th ed.). Philadelphia: Lea & Febiger.

Papp, J. (2002). *Quality management in the imaging sciences* (2nd ed.). St. Louis, MO: C. V. Mosby.

Quinn, C. B. (1993). *Fuch's radiography exposure, processing and quality control.* (5th ed.). Springfield, IL: Charles C. Thomas.

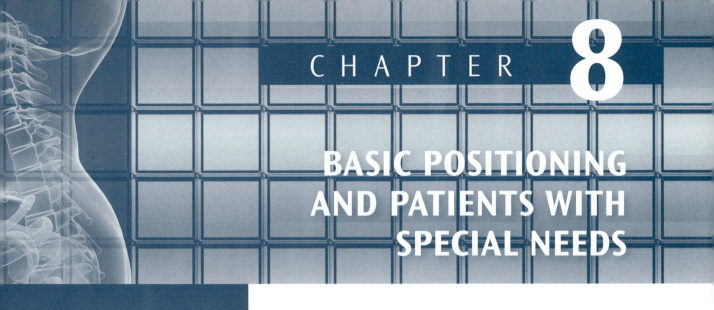

CHAPTER **8**

BASIC POSITIONING AND PATIENTS WITH SPECIAL NEEDS

Key Terms

Anatomic Position
Anterior
Anterior Position
Asthenic
Body Habitus
Body Planes
Coronal
Decubitus
Film Markers
Hypersthenic
Hyposthenic
Oblique Position
Radiographic Position
Radiolucent
Sagittal
Sthenic
Surface Landmarks
Transverse

Chapter Outline

Objectives

Upon completion of the chapter, the student will meet the following objectives by verifying knowledge of the facts and principles presented through oral and written communication at a level deemed competent.

- Explain the basic principles of positioning.
- Differentiate between projection and position.
- Define body planes.
- Discuss four major classifications of body habitus.
- Assess some of the problems associated with special patients needs and approaches to the imaging procedures.
- Describe the true anatomical position.

Introduction

This chapter is not intended to present a comprehensive unit in radiographic positioning—an in-depth study of positioning requires much more space than we are dealing with at this point. However, the information provided should instruct students in the fundamentals of radiographic positioning and familiarize them with positioning terms. Additionally, the chapter addresses positioning with regard to special needs of pediatric and geriatric patients. This information is included because these patients do not always fit into every radiology environment.

The Radiographic Routine

Positioning routines used by one medical facility will not necessarily be the standard for all other medical facilities or physicians offices. Doctors vary in their education and medical radiology experience and this may be reflected in their requests for particular radiography positions or projections. In cases where the radiographer knows that an accessory or special position/projection might better facilitate the diagnosis, she/he should provide this information to the doctor.

There are, however, certain routines for each body part. These routine suggestions are based on the following radiological imaging principles referred to as the routine or basic principles of positioning.

- Proper radiographic positioning may not be effective if practiced without a solid basic knowledge of human anatomy.
- The patient must be made comfortable to avoid the interactive pull of muscle strain that can result in motion.
- The patient's entire body should be in alignment with the part being examined, to avoid a rotated or twisted effect that may obscure information.
- When proper body position has been obtained, appropriate immobilization of the part being examined is essential. Sandbags, tape in some cases, and compression bands are simple and effective immobilization devices. There are also many commercial devices available for immobilizing the patient's position whenever needed.
- Use a size film to adequately place the anatomical part in the film's center but large enough to allow a small margin at the film's edges (1/2 inch to 1 1/2 inches). Place the long axis of the anatomical part being examined parallel to, in the center of, and adjacent to the long axis of the film. It is very important that the anatomy be parallel to the film surface to avoid anatomical distortion.
- Direct the central ray to the center of, and perpendicular to, the long axis of the film.

Further delineation of the above goals is provided in the following concepts.

Projections

Take two projections 90 degrees or at right angles to each other. According to the area being examined, for example long bones, this generally means an anterior-posterior (AP) or a posterior-anterior (PA) and a lateral. In anatomic areas containing a joint such as the lower leg (ankle joint) or the femur (knee joint) an oblique position may also be required.

Always include a joint on radiographs of long bones. In trauma situations, include the entire structure or at a minimum include the joint closest to the injury on the radiograph. In trauma radiography of long bones such as the humerus, forearm, femur, tibia, and fibula, both joints should be included. In some cases, this may require an additional exposure, if the patient's limb is too long for both joints to be included. An oblique position of the part may be required.

Right angle views are necessary to (1) avoid superimposed structures that may obscure pathology; (2) provide alignment of fractured bones or placement of internal structures; and (3) demonstrate foreign body localization. Most medical facilities or doctor offices provide a manual that describes projections required for each radiographic procedure.

Comparison Images

In certain imaging requests of long bones or joints, the request may be to take both sides (right and left) for comparison although only one side is affected. The purpose of comparison radiographs is to provide additional diagnostic information for "comparison" of the affected side with the non-affected side. The patient may question this procedure; however, a simple explanation will often lessen his/her concern. This practice may be more common for children in early growth stages.

Erect/Upright Images

In many cases, a radiographic request will require that the patient be in an erect position for lower limb and pelvic girdle radiographs. When the patient is in the erect position, the lower limb is receiving the weight of the entire body. Erect radiographs also allow for distribution of air and fluid in certain areas of the body. For example, for evaluation of normal chest structures, radiographs should always be taken with the patient in the erect position. Abdominal radiographs also provide information about the status of gas and fluid distribution in the body cavities. When the patient's condition is such that they cannot safely assume an erect or upright position, a decubitus position will provide some information about gas and fluid levels. For additional information refer to the section titled positioning terminology.

Motion Control

Motion control is considered a radiation protection procedure. If the patient moves, motion occurs, resulting in a blurring of the image (loss of definition). Repeat radiographs due to motion result in additional unnecessary radiation exposure to the patient.

A very easy motion control tip is to make sure that patients understand how they can help during the examination. To gain patient cooperation requires that the radiographer explain what is going to happen during the examination and to ask for the patient's help in "holding still" during the examination. Using the fastest exposure time and a comparable speed for screen/film combination is recommended to eliminate image blur resulting from motion.

Use of immobilization aids such as sandbags and sponges may also help the patient to control motion. The use of radiolucent sponge blocks may be placed under the area being examined. This provides support for the injured limb and helps to reduce motion. Proper alignment of the patient may also reduce motion.

Part Placement of the Part on the Film Holder or Image Receptor

Radiography is an art and a science. The artistic side of radiography can often be reflected in the care the radiographer takes in placing the anatomic part on the film holder or image receptor. The anatomic part should be placed on the film holder so the boundaries or borders of the part are included on the finished radiograph. As a general rule, the long axis of the body part should be aligned with the long axis of the film holder or image receptor. In some cases, when two or more projections are needed, the long axis of the anatomic part should be aligned on the film holder or image receptor in the same direction.

Another basic rule of positioning is that the body part should be aligned so that no rotation or twisting occurs. It must be remembered that the anatomic part being imaged is attached to the entire limb or to the trunk of the body and the entire area must be aligned. If any part of the patient's body is twisted or if the trunk or abdominal/pelvic areas are resting in an uncomfortable position, rotation of the actual part may occur, resulting in a poor and obscured image.

Film Markers and Identification

A minimum of three types of **film markers** must be included on each radiograph. The patient's identification, date, and anatomical side markers (R or L) must be included on each radiograph. Additional markers or identification will vary from facility to facility, but may include the radiographer's initials; time indicators; arrow indicators for erect or decubitus; inspiration (INSP) and expiration (EXP) markers; and internal (INT) and external (EXT) makers. The placement of the identification marker should not obscure or superimpose over anatomy of clinical interest.

Cassettes/Image Receptors

Extremity radiographs may be positioned directly on the cassette or image receptor. Whenever a body part measures over 10–12 centimeters, a grid must be used. Smaller anatomic body areas such as the knee, foot, or ankle generally measure less than 10 centimeters. If, however, the part contains excess fluid or blood due to trauma or has a thick cast applied, a grid may be necessary. Refer to Chapter 9, Fundamentals of Radiographic Exposure, for additional information about grids.

Body Habitus

Physical appearance of the body or body build is also referred to as **body habitus**. There are four major body types or classifications; **sthenic, hyposthenic, asthenic,** and **hypersthenic**. These body types are important in understanding the location of internal body structures. The radiographer should become very familiar with these body shapes and their related internal structures.

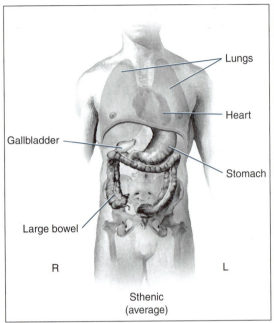

FIGURE 8-1 Sthenic body habitus
Source: Delmar, Cengage Learning.

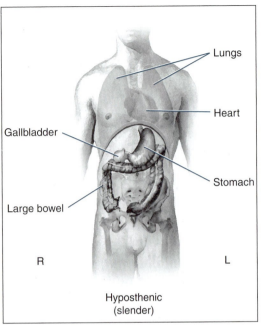

FIGURE 8-2 Hyposthenic body habitus
Source: Delmar, Cengage Learning.

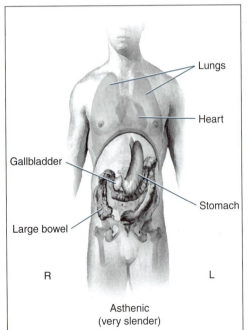

FIGURE 8-3 Asthenic body habitus
Source: Delmar, Cengage Learning.

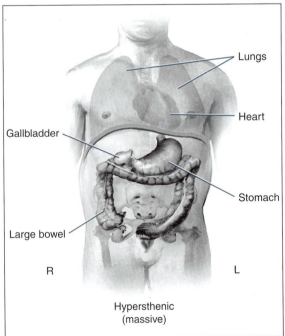

FIGURE 8-4 Hypersthenic body habitus
Source: Delmar, Cengage Learning.

Sthenic refers to the average or normal body shapes and represents about 50% of the population. It means strong, physically fit and this serves as the basis for a guideline to establish radiographic exposure techniques and routine positions. Notice the shape and location of internal structures in Figure 8-1.

Hyposthenic is the body habitus represented by slender or thin people and represents about 35% of the population. Generally, less exposure is required for this body type (Figure 8-2).

Asthenic is the body habitus that is extremely slender and generally frail in appearance and usually weak. It represents about 10% of the population. The body shape appears long and narrow with the abdominal organs lower and vertical in position near the midline (Figure 8-3).

Hypersthenic is the body type that is large and stocky and represents about 5% of the population. The chest and abdomen are broad and deep. The internal organs are higher and lie in a more horizontal position. These persons are often overweight (Figure 8-4).

Body Positions and Planes

Anatomic Position

The true anatomic position is known as the standing (erect) position with the body facing forward, the feet together, and the arms down by each side with the palms of the hands facing forward. The position is used to describe the relationship of body parts to each other. (See Figure 8-5).

Body Planes

Three primary body planes are used to identify the body in different sections: coronal, sagittal, and transverse (Figures 8-6 and 8-7). The coronal plane (also referred to as the frontal plane) divides the body into anterior and posterior portions. It is a vertical plane at right angles to the sagittal plane.

The sagittal plane divides the body into right and left portions. It is a vertical plane parallel to the midsagittal or median plane, which divides the body into right and left portions through the trunk and head.

The transverse plane (horizontal or axial plane) is at right angles to the vertical axis of the body (Figure 8-7).

Surface Landmarks

Table 8-1 provides a list of some commonly used surface landmarks that may be palpated to locate specific vertebral bodies.

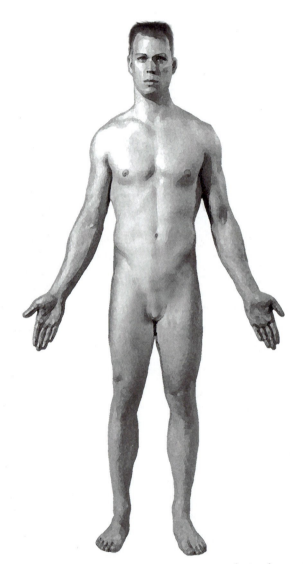

FIGURE 8-5 The anatomic position is erect, facing forward, with arms extended and palms forward, feet together.
Source: Delmar, Cengage Learning.

Table 8-2, Standard Terminology for Positioning and Projection, provides terms identified by the American Registry of Radiologic Technologists. As previously stated, providing comprehensive knowledge of **radiographic positions** is not an intention of this book. However, the basic concepts presented in this chapter should help the student become familiar with the correct way in which to place any part of the

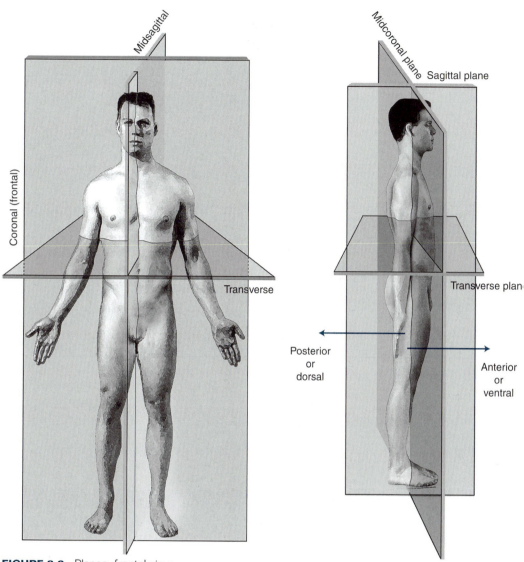

FIGURE 8-6 Planes: frontal view
Source: Delmar, Cengage Learning.

FIGURE 8-7 Planes: side view
Source: Delmar, Cengage Learning.

body for any imaging procedure. Additionally, it is expected that an appropriate and definitive radiographic anatomy and positioning book is available for student review.

The American Registry of Radiologic Technologists provides a listing of radiographic positions and projections in the handbook prepared for certification examinees. This listing and accompanying figure drawings are included in the

TABLE 8-1   Surface Landmarks

Vertebra/Vertebrae	Exterior Landmark
C1	Mastoid tip
C2, C3	Gonion
C5	Thyroid cartilage
C7	Vertebra prominences
T1	Approximately 2 inches superior to sternal notch
T2, T3	Level of sternal notch
	Superior margin of scapula
T4, T5	Level of sternal angle
T7	Level of inferior angle of scapula
T10	Level of xiphoid process
L3	Costal margin
L3, L4	Level of umbilicus
L4,	Level of superior aspect of iliac crest
S1	Level of anterior superior iliac spine
Coccyx	Level of symphysis pubis and greater trochanter

TABLE 8-2   Standard Terminology for Positioning and Projections

Radiographic View: Describes the body part as seen by the x-ray film or other recording medium, such as a fluoroscopic screen. Restricted to the discussion of a *radiograph* or *image*.
Radiographic Position: Refers to a specific body position, such as supine, prone, recumbent, erect, or Trendelenburg. Restricted to the discussion of the *patient's physical position*.
Radiographic Projection: Restricted to the discussion of the *path of the central ray*.

Positioning Terminology	
A. Lying Down	
1. *supine*	lying on the back
2. *prone*	lying face downward
3. *decubitus*	lying down with a horizontal x-ray beam
4. *recumbent*	lying down in any position
B. Erect or Upright	
1. *anterior position*	facing the film
2. *posterior position*	facing the radiographic tube
3. *oblique position*	(erect or lying down)

a. anterior (facing the film)	
i. *left anterior oblique*	body rotated with the left anterior portion closest to the film
ii. *right anterior oblique*	body rotated with the right anterior portion closest to the film
b. posterior (facing the radiographic tube)	
i. *left posterior oblique*	body rotated with the left posterior portion closest to the film
ii. *right posterior oblique*	body rotated with the right posterior portion closest to the film

Note: From *Certification Handbook and Application Materials for Exams Administered in 2006* (p. 44), by The American Registry for Radiologic Technologists, 2006, St. Paul, MN: Author. Used with permission.

appendix to this chapter (Appendix 8-A). These positions and projections may also be found and studied in most comprehensive radiographic positioning and procedures textbooks.

Patients with Special Needs

Pediatric Radiography

This section provides information about the special needs of young children and adolescents and the requirements of the disabled and older adult. Pediatric and geriatric patients as well as disabled patients have the same needs as all patients: a safe, comfortable, and secure environment. The radiography environment may appear cold and imposing and the radiographer may be reluctant or even afraid to undertake routine diagnostic radiography procedures on patients with special needs.

To perform radiography procedures effectively on the pediatric patient, the radiographer must have an understanding that different techniques of communication apply to children depending on their age or developmental stage. Also, gaining cooperation from a child may depend on their previous experiences and on the severity of their illness. It is unreasonable to expect seriously ill children to cooperate. Children often need the emotional support that only parents can provide. Gaining a child's trust is also an important component to successful pediatric radiology. Trust requires that the radiographer be sensitive to the age-appropriate needs of children. Some of these age-appropriate needs and communication techniques are addressed as follows.

Infants (Birth to 1 year). Infants respond to external stimuli and internal needs of hunger, pain, and the need to feel secure. A light, gentle touch and a soothing voice can be used to calm a crying infant. Infants relate to faces and like eye contact, but they cannot focus very far away, so remain in their visual field when talking. They like to be held firmly and gently and many respond to being rocked while the holder walks around with them. Infants should never be left alone or unattended, even if properly immobilized. Security objects such as a blanket rattle, pacifier, or stuffed animal should never be taken from children unless absolutely necessary (Peart, 2001).

Toddlers (1 to 3 years).   Toddlers can present the greatest challenge to the radiographer. They know what they like and may loudly voice their opinion when asked to do things they do not like. The word "NO" is a part of their vocabulary for which they may not even understand its full meaning. Toddler's can relate to simple requests but since their attention span is short, they may need lots of reminders and calming reassurance. Toddlers may carry with them vivid memories of prior discomforts experienced with people in health care settings and may begin crying the minute you appear on the scene. Toddlers are more likely than infants to have a strong attachment to a security object, and this item may be used to communication with the toddler. When talking with a toddler, either raise the child up to eye contact height or stoop down to their level to communicate (Peart, 2001; Spieler, 2005).

Preschoolers or Children between 3 to 5 years of age.   Children in this age group are in constant motion, exploring the world and all the objects therein. These children like to exert their independence and can often be heard giving their opinion of any situation. Ask for their help and give them a task to do. Positioning a doll next to preschoolers and letting them repeat your instructions to the doll may divert their attention and gain their cooperation. Sandbags and similar devices can be purchased or made in the shape of familiar animals; like a frog sandbag. Immobilization of the preschooler should be a last resort (Peart, 2001).

School-Aged Children (6 to 10 years).   School-aged children can think logically and communicate with the radiographer. Engaging the school-aged child in activities related to the procedure creates a diversionary distraction. Providing opportunities for school-aged children to make choices engages them in the task at hand. Answering questions about the procedure and providing simple, direct, and honest answers is important for gaining cooperation from the school-aged child. Creating a child-friendly imaging environment with strategically placed pictures and toys provides an important non-verbal message of welcome (Peart, 2001).

Adolescents (more than 10 years).   One of the most important characteristics of this age group is their modesty and self-awareness of the changes occurring to their bodies as a result of puberty. Special attention should be given to respecting their concern for "taking their clothes off." Pregnancy in this age group may also be a concern. Questions about pregnancy or possible pregnancy should be asked away from parents or guardians. Do not presume that adolescents do not have any say in their treatment. Many older teenagers are emancipated minors who are financially independent and are in charge of their medical care and treatment decisions (Peart, 2001).

Parents in the X-Ray Room.   The decision to permit a parent or legal guardian to accompany the child into the x-ray room is often incorporated in facility policy. If no such facility policy exists, the radiographer must make the decision. With infants, toddlers, and even preschoolers, the presence of a familiar face can be very reassuring and make the diagnostic imaging procedure a success (Peart, 2001). Also, many young children will behave more age appropriate for a stranger than they will for a parent. Whatever decision is made by the radiographer, it is important to remember decisions are not necessarily final. If the presence of a parent is making it more difficult to complete the examination, the parent can always be asked to leave the room. In cases where the child cannot cooperate and must be immobilized, the parent is likely to be upset and not be of value in calming the child.

Immobilization

Diagnostic imaging of the pediatric patient or adolescent generally requires that the radiographer modify not only the technical factors but also the entire approach to patient care and positioning. Infants and small children can be immobilized for most imaging examinations without the need for someone to hold them. Commercially available pediatric immobilization devices should be used whenever possible.

If circumstances require that someone hold a child during a x-ray exposure, the person selected should be someone who does not receive occupationally related radiation. Generally, this is the child's parent, provided that the parent is not pregnant. If the parent is not available, the radiographer should recruit a person who does not receive occupational radiation exposure and is not pregnant. The person recruited should be provided a leaded apron and lead gloves, if the hands will be in the radiation field. The radiographer should demonstrate exactly how the child should be held and how to sit or stand to minimize exposure to primary radiation. Having the person position their body at arm length from the child will reduce some of exposure to scatter radiation. Figure 8-8 demonstrates how to hold a child appropriately for a chest radiograph and how the person holding the child should be dressed.

Commercial Immobilization Devices.   Immobilization of children poses many challenges for the radiographer. The most common is the reaction of parents or caregivers when they see their child restrained. Traditionally, immobilization of children

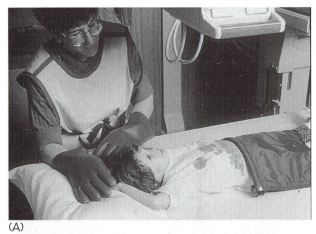

(A)

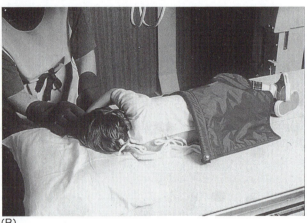

(B)

FIGURE 8-8 (A) AP and (B) lateral chest—child.
Appropriate method of protection and holding a child during
radiographic exposure
Source: Delmar, Cengage Learning.

has been managed with simple pieces of cloth, often referred to as arm bands, to hold the child's arms and feet in place. One device that is commonly known is called a Pigg-O-Stat® (see Figure 8-9). One type of band, which may be called a support or compression band, consists of a single piece of cloth (usually duck cloth or similar sturdy cloth) that is secured to rails on both sides of the radiographic table. Any radiology facility that provides pediatric imaging will have the appropriate equipment available for working with children. If a children's hospital is available, it would be of great benefit for students to have a short rotation there or at least a guided instructional tour.

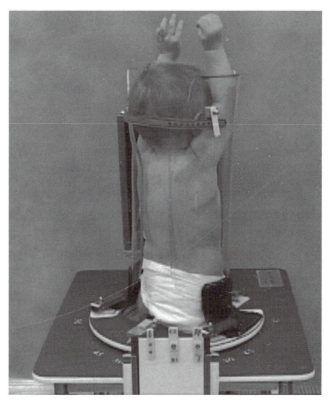

FIGURE 8-9 Pigg-o-Stat used as suitable method for pediatric chest radiography *(Reprinted with permission of Modern Way Immobilizers, Inc.)*

Tips for gaining cooperation from the pediatric patient include the following (adapted from *Creative Tips for Radiographing Kids*, Spieler, 2005, p. 15):

- Use a demonstration doll or animal to show what will happen and how the exam will take place.
- Have an arsenal of funny items to wear when taking radiographs of children. Floppy hats and colorful jackets may help to avoid a child's "white coat" fear.
- Toys that are appropriate and can withstand regular cleaning also help to distract the child's attention.

Also, singing a familiar song and talking in a low, calm voice can help to assure the child.

The radiographer should always be prepared to deal with the pediatric patient. Preparation helps in making the examination go more smoothly with successful outcomes.

Child Abuse

Child abuse knows no bias of gender, race, or socioeconomic background. Unfortunately, the abuser is usually not a stranger but often the child's caregiver, parent, sibling, or a family friend or relative. Child abuse in most states is chargeable under general felony and misdemeanor criminal statutes such as murder, mayhem or assault with intent to maim, assault and battery by means of a dangerous weapon, and assault and battery.

Most medical facilities have developed policies and procedures related to reporting suspected child abuse. Child abuse, also referred to as battered child syndrome (BCS), is currently called nonaccidental trauma (NAT). Radiographers should be aware of their responsibilities concerning NAT in the state in which they are working. For purposes of the following discussion, the term *child abuse* will be used to encompass all forms of abuse and neglect.

The radiologist, referring physician, radiographer, and all medical staff members are critical watchdogs for the signs and symptoms of child abuse. The importance radiological professionals play in diagnosing child abuse cannot be overstated. Unfortunately, not all states have mandated abuse reporting laws. Such laws have as their primary purpose the identification of child abuse and neglect and, secondarily, the protection of children through state monitoring of families and the provision of services. Many medical facilities have operating guidelines for handling suspected abuse regardless of whether it is a child or adult.

The role of the radiologist and radiographer in cases of suspected abuse is usually that of a consultant acting with limited clinical and laboratory information. When radiological findings indicate the possibility of abuse, the radiologist or film-reading physician has the responsibility to indicate the suspicion in the imaging report and in direct verbal communication in accordance with facility policy.

Radiographers are also accountable to report suspected or confirmed child abuse. In this situation, the radiographer should consult with the supervisor or facility administrator as to the proper procedure to follow.

Signs of Abuse. A few of the warning signs of physical abuse are fairly easy to recognize and include but are not limited to unexplained bruising, burns, black eyes, and fractures. The radiographer should observe injuries that seem unusual for the child to have suffered under normal circumstances. The radiographer should be alert to parent or guardian explanations, especially those that seem unrealistic.

Diagnosis of sexual abuse is generally based on history and physical examination with supporting laboratory studies. Those involved with diagnostic radiography studies should be aware that sexual abuse is frequently associated with physical abuse.

When clinical or imaging findings are suspicious for potential abuse, a radiographic skeletal survey is obtained. The purpose of the skeletal survey is to document the presence of findings of abuse for legal reasons so that the child may be removed from the environment of abuse.

A skeletal survey for suspected abuse generally includes some or all of the following radiographs: chest, skull, upper arms, forearms, hands, pelvis, upper legs, lower legs, ankles, and feet areas. In some cases, skeletal surveys and CT scans are also recommended for severe injuries or in the event of death. Each medical facility will have its own policy for these types of routines.

Geriatrics

Geriatrics, also gerontology, is the branch of medicine concerned with the problems of aging. Included are all aspects of aging, including physiological, pathological, psychological, economic, and sociological problems. The importance of geriatrics is emphasized by the fact the expected lifespan is increasing. An estimated 25,000 persons in the United States are 100 years old or older, and by the year 2080 this number will increase to more than 100,000 (*Taber's Cyclopedic Medical Dictionary*, 1997, p. 790).

Radiographers should be aware of biological changes that accompany aging and use the knowledge to adapt the radiographic routine. Elderly patients have special needs that require different care than younger patients. Although there are individual variations in aging processes, there are predictable chronic and acute medical conditions that require radiography examinations. In the elderly population, the radiographer should be aware that the chief complaint or primary diagnosis indicates only one of many potential medical complications.

It is the radiographer's responsibility to assess each patient's cognitive and physical ability prior to beginning an imaging procedure. Some of the biologic changes that can accompany aging include the following (adapted from *Radiologic Technologists' Responses to Elderly Patients*, Rarey, 1998, pp. 566–572):

- Decreased depth perception may result in a loss of judgment when stepping up onto and down off the examination or radiographic table.
- Visual loss may impair the older patient's ability to navigate between the examination room and the dressing room or bathroom. Visual loss may also interfere with the older patient's ability to read examination instructions and to complete medical information questionnaires.
- Hearing loss may interfere with the older patient's ability to hear instructions. This is particularly evident when the older person is unable to follow breathing instructions during chest radiography.

- A decrease in muscle mass results in poor mobility and poor balance. Older patients are also more likely to suffer from osteopenia and osteoporosis, making them more susceptible to bone fractures.
- A decrease in fat pads can make it more painful for older patients to lie on examination tables. Also, the older patient may have fragile skin, which is more susceptible to cuts and scraps during the procedure. Care should be taken when moving or assisting the older patient to avoid skin injuries.

One of the most important aspects of dealing with the older patient is the communication factor. Calling the patient by name, smiling, and having a brief conversation helps to create a welcoming environment and also allows the radiographer to determine the patient's ability to hear and comprehend information about the radiographic procedure. The elderly often exhibit reduced strength and endurance, which results in increased risk of injury. To accommodate the needs of the older patient, the radiography staff should walk through the facility and evaluate each area including the waiting or reception area, dressing room, bathroom, and radiography suite. In performing the evaluation, the staff should consider each area from the older patient's perspective. For example, are there signs that direct the patient in case they should become disoriented? Is the signage legible, accessible, consistent, bilingual, and in Braille? Is the facility well-lit and free of clutter that may cause an accident? Are there places for patients to stop and rest, or to call for help in long stretches of hallways?

The older patient often requires accommodations during radiographic positioning. The radiographer should keep in mind the anatomy that should appear on the image, while considering the restraints of the older patient's body habitus. In extreme cases, the radiograph may be obtained by assisting patients onto the table and positioning them comfortably on their side. The image receptor (IR) would be supported and the x-ray beam directed horizontally to obtain the AP or PA projections.

Radiographic findings that are consistent with aging, chronic pathologies, and the lifestyle choices of many elderly patients include those listed in Table 8-3.

Imaging Patients with Dementia or Alzheimer's Disease

Dementia is a broad term that refers to cognitive deficit, including memory impairment. There are many causes. The current classifications include dementia of Alzheimer's disease; vascular dementia; AIDS dementia; dementia due to head trauma; dementia due to Parkinson's, Huntington's, or Creutzfeldt-Jakob disease; and dementia induced by substance abuse (*Taber's Cyclopedic Medical Dictionary*, 1997, p. 73).

TABLE 8-3   Common Radiographic Findings for Elderly Patients

Examination	Findings
Chest	Calcifications of great vessels
	Cardiomegaly
	Chronic obstructive pulmonary disease (COPD)
	Pacemaker or other evidence of previous cardiac surgery
Plain abdomen	Aneurysm
	Calcifications in organs and vessels and the biliary tract
Spine and Pelvis	Compression fractures
	Osteoporosis
	Osteoarthritis
	Paget's disease
Extremities	Fractures
	Gout
	Osteoporosis
	Paget's disease
	Rheumatoid arthritis
	Degenerative joint disease

Note: From "Improving the Geriatric Radiography Experience" by D. L. Wright, 1998, Copyright *Seminars in Radiologic Technology*, Adapted with permission.

Specifically, Alzheimer's is a "chronic progressive disorder that accounts for more than 50% of all dementia. The most common form occurs in people older than 65, but the presenile form can begin between the ages of 40 to 60" (*Taber's Cyclopedic Medical Dictionary*, 1997, p. 303).

Some appropriate procedures may help the radiographer to obtain quality radiographs on patients with memory impairment. Respect is common to all patient interactions in diagnostic imaging procedures and appropriate courtesy titles such as Mr. or Mrs. or a professional title should be used. When providing services to the patient with dementia, the radiographer may find it necessary to repeat directions. The radiographer can create a non-threatening environment by using a calm and easygoing manner when having to repeat directions or questions. The radiographer should expect to have to reintroduce him or herself and remind the patient what is happening. Short sentences that convey one thought at a time and waiting for an answer before asking the next question is essential. The communication skills used with the dementia patient are similar to those used when imaging the young child.

REVIEW QUESTIONS

1. The concept of body habitus is based on the physical appearance of the body. Of the four major types of classification, _____ is the most common.
   a. sthenic
   b. hyposthenic
   c. asthenic
   d. hypersthenic

2. The following refers to the path of the central ray:
   a. radiographic view
   b. radiographic positions
   c. radiographic projection
   d. Trendelenburg

3. Radiographic positioning is most effective when applied with a solid basic knowledge of:
   a. human anatomy
   b. physiology
   c. film size
   d. patients' history

4. Generally, there should always be two projections taken of each area being examined.
   a. True
   b. False

5. The most effective control of motion that would blur the image is to:
   a. talk to the patient
   b. use the fastest exposure time
   c. always immobilize the patient
   d. align the body appropriately

6. Proper identification of a radiograph or image usually includes:
   1. anatomical marker R or L
   2. patient's name
   3. date

   Possible Responses
   a. 1 and 2
   b. 1 and 3

c. 2 and 3
d. 1, 2, and 3

7. The true anatomical position is described to refer to the body:
   1. in the erect position
   2. facing forward
   3. with the arms down along the sides
   4. with the palms forward

   Possible Responses

   a. 1 and 2
   b. 1 and 3
   c. 1, 2, and 3
   d. 1, 2, 3, and 4

8. There are three primary planes used to identify the body in different sections.
   a. True
   b. False

REFERENCES

Peart, O. (2001). Pediatric imaging: Talking to tots. *RT Image, 14*(21), 20–23.
Rarey, L. (1998). Radiologic technologists, responses to elderly patients. *Radiologic Technology, 69*(6), 566–572.
Spieler, G. (2005). Creative tips for radiographing kids. *ASRT Scanner. 38*(1), p. 15.
Taber's Cyclopedic Medical Dictionary. (15th ed.). (1997). Philadelphia: F.A. Davis Company.
Wright, D. L. (1998). Improving the geriatric radiography experience. *Seminars in Radiologic Technology, 6*(2) 46–52.

SUGGESTED READING

Viggiano, T. (2005). Keeping kids still. *Advance Extra!-Diagnostic Radiography Supplement. Advance for Imaging and Radiation Therapy,* Special Supplement, November 28.

RADIOGRAPHIC POSITIONS AND PROJECTIONS

I. **Thorax**
    A. Chest
        1. PA upright
        2. lateral upright
        3. AP Lordotic
        4. AP supine
        5. lateral decubitus
        6. posterior oblique
        7. anterior oblique
    B. Ribs
        1. AP and PA, above and below diaphragm
        2. anterior and posterior oblique
    C. Sternum
        1. lateral
        2. RAO breathing technique
        3. RAO expiration
        4. LAO
        5. PA sternoclavicular joints
        6. anterior oblique sternoclavicular joints
        7. PA axial sternoclavicular joints
    D. Soft Tissue Neck
        1. AP upper airway
        2. lateral upper airway

II. **Abdomen and GI studies**
    A. Abdomen
        1. AP supine
        2. AP upright
        3. lateral decubitus
        4. dorsal decubitus
    B. Esophagus
        1. RAO
        2. left lateral
        3. AP
        4. PA
        5. LAO
    C. Swallowing Dysfunction Study
    D. Upper GI series★
        1. AP scout
        2. RAO
        3. PA
        4. right lateral
        5. LPO
        6. AP
    E. Small Bowel Series
        1. PA scout
        2. PA (follow through)
        3. ileocecal spots
        4. enteroclysis procedure
    F. Barium Enema★
        1. left lateral rectum
        2. left lateral decubitus

★ single or double contrast

3. right lateral decubitus
4. LPO and RPO
5. PA
6. RAO and LAO
7. AP axial (butterfly)
8. PA axial (butterfly)
9. PA post-evacuation
G. Surgical Cholangiography
1. AP
H. ERCP
1. AP

III. **Urological Studies**
A. Cystography
1. AP
2. LPO and RPO 60°
3. lateral
4. AP 10–15° caudad
B. Cystourethrography
1. AP voiding cystourethrogram female
2. RPO 30°, voiding cystogram male
C. Intravenous Urography
1. AP, scout and series
2. RPO and LPO 30°
3. PA post-void
4. AP post-void, upright
5. nephrotomography
6. AP ureteric compression
D. Retrograde Pyelography
1. AP scout
2. AP pyelogram
3. AP ureterogram

IV. **Spine and Pelvis**
A. Cervical Spine
1. AP angle cephalad
2. AP open mouth
3. lateral

4. cross table lateral
5. anterior oblique
6. posterior oblique
7. lateral swimmers
8. lateral flexion and extension
9. AP dens (Fuchs)
10. PA dens (Judd)
B. Thoracic Spine
1. AP
2. lateral, breathing
3. lateral, expiration
C. Scoliosis Series
1. AP/PA scoliosis series (Ferguson)
D. Lumbar Spine
1. AP
2. PA
3. lateral
4. L5-S1 lateral spot
5. posterior oblique 45°
6. anterior oblique 45°
7. AP L5-S1, 30–35° cephalad
8. AP right and left bending
9. lateral flexion and extension
E. Sacrum and Coccyx
1. AP sacrum, 15–25° cephalad
2. AP coccyx, 10–20° caudad
3. lateral sacrum and coccyx, combined
4. lateral sacrum or coccyx, separate
F. Sacroiliac Joints
1. AP
2. posterior oblique
3. anterior oblique
G. Pelvis and Hip
1. AP hip only
2. cross-table lateral hip
3. unilateral frog-leg, non-trauma

4. axiolateral inferosuperior, trauma (Clements-Nakayama)
5. AP pelvis
6. AP pelvis, bilateral frog-leg
7. AP pelvis, axial anterior pelvic bones (inlet, outlet)
8. anterior oblique pelvis, acetabulum (Judet)

V. **Cranium**
  A. Skull
    1. AP axial (Towne)
    2. lateral
    3. PA (Caldwell)
    4. PA no angle
    5. submentovertical (full basal)
    6. PA 25–30° angle (Haas)
    7. trauma cross table lateral
    8. trauma AP, 15° cephalad
    9. trauma AP, no angle
    10. trauma AP, axial (Towne)
  B. Facial Bones
    1. lateral
    2. parietoacanthial (Waters)
    3. PA (Caldwell)
    4. PA (modified Waters)
  C. Mandible
    1. axiolateral oblique
    2. PA no angle
    3. AP axial (Towne)
    4. PA semi-axial, 20–25° cephalad
    5. PA (modified Waters)
    6. submentovertical (full basal)
  D. Zygomatic Arch
    1. submentovertical (full basal)
    2. parietoacanthial (Waters)
    3. AP axial (Towne)

4. axial oblique
5. lateral
  E. Temporomandibular Joints
    1. lateral (Law)
    2. lateral (Schuller)
    3. AP axial (Towne)
  F. Nasal Bones
    1. parietoacanthial (Waters)
    2. lateral
    3. PA (Caldwell)
  G. Orbits
    1. parietoacanthial (Waters)
    2. lateral
    3. PA (Caldwell)
  H. Paranasal Sinuses
    1. lateral
    2. PA (Caldwell)
    3. parietoacanthial (Waters)
    4. submentovertical (full basal)
    5. open mouth parietoacanthial (Waters)

VI. **Extremities**
  A. Toes
    1. AP, entire foot
    2. oblique toe
    3. lateral toe
  B. Foot
    1. AP angle toward heel
    2. medial oblique
    3. lateral oblique
    4. mediolateral
    5. lateromedial
    6. sesamoids, tangential
    7. AP weight bearing
    8. lateral weight bearing
  C. Calcaneus (Os Calcis)
    1. lateral
    2. plantodorsal, axial
    3. dorsoplantar, axial

D. Ankle
1. AP
2. AP mortise
3. mediolateral
4. oblique, 45° internal
5. lateromedial
6. AP stress views

E. Tibia, Fibula
1. AP
2. lateral
3. oblique

F. Knee
1. AP
2. lateral
3. AP weight bearing
4. lateral oblique 45°
5. medial oblique 45°
6. PA
7. PA axial – intercondylar fossa (tunnel)

G. Patella
1. lateral
2. supine flexion 45° (Merchant)
3. PA
4. prone flexion 90° (Settegast)
5. prone flexion 55° (Hughston)

H. Femur
1. AP
2. mediolateral

I. Fingers
1. PA entire hand
2. PA finger only
3. lateral
4. oblique
5. AP thumb
6. oblique thumb
7. lateral thumb

J. Hand
1. PA
2. lateral
3. oblique

K. Wrist
1. PA
2. oblique 45°
3. lateral
4. PA for scaphoid
5. scaphoid (Stecher)
6. carpal canal

L. Forearm
1. AP
2. lateral

M. Elbow
1. AP
2. lateral
3. external oblique
4. internal oblique
5. AP partial flexion
6. axial trauma (Coyle)

N. Humerus
1. AP non-trauma
2. lateral non-trauma
3. AP neutral trauma
4. scapular Y trauma
5. transthoracic lateral trauma
6. lateral, mid and distal, trauma

O. Shoulder
1. AP internal and external rotation
2. inferosuperior axial, non-trauma
3. posterior oblique (Grashey)
4. tangential non-trauma
5. AP neutral trauma
6. transthoracic lateral trauma
7. scapular Y trauma

P. Scapula
   1. AP
   2. lateral, anterior oblique
   3. lateral, posterior oblique
Q. Clavicle
   1. AP
   2. AP angle 15–30° cephalad
   3. PA angle 15–30° caudad
R. Acromioclavicular joints
   1. AP bilateral with and
      without weights

S. Bone Survey
T. Long Bone Measurement
U. Bone Age
V. Soft Tissue/Foreign Body

VII. Other Procedures
A. Arthrography
B. Myelography
C. Venography

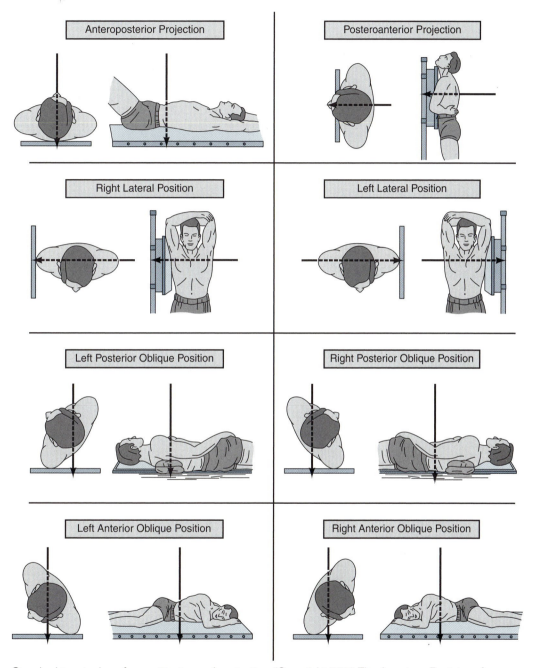

Standard terminology for positioning and projection *(Copyright 2006 The American Registry of Radiologic Technologists)*

CHAPTER 9

FUNDAMENTALS OF RADIOGRAPHIC EXPOSURE

Key Terms

Beam Filtration
Beam Restriction
Central Ray
Compression of Tissue
Contrast
Density
Distance
Distortion
Exposure Factors
Film Contrast
Film Fog
Film Resolution
Filtration
Geometric Properties
Grids
Heat Unit (HU)
Heel Effect
Intensifying Screens
Inverse Square Law
Kilovoltage
Kilovoltage Peak (kVp)
Large Focal Spot
Magnification
Milliamperage (ma)
Milliamperage Seconds (mAs)
Motion

Chapter Outline

Objectives

Upon completion of the chapter, the student will meet the following objectives by verifying knowledge of the facts

Object-to-Image Receptor Distance (OID)

Photographic Properties

Processing

Recorded Detail

Screen-Film Contact

Small Focal Spot

Source-to-Image Receptor Distance (SID)

Subject Contrast

Time

and principles presented through oral and written communication at a level deemed competent.

◯ Differentiate between the photographic and geometric properties related to the radiographic image.

◯ Define and explain radiographic density as it relates to photographic properties of the radiographic image.

◯ Define and explain radiographic contrast as it relates to photographic properties of the radiographic image.

◯ Define other types of contrast: subject contrast, film contrast.

◯ Define exposure latitude and kilovoltage ranges.

◯ Explain what recorded detail means in the visible image.

◯ Describe how mA, kVp, time, SID, and heel effect control and affect density and contrast in the radiographic image.

◯ Explain the effect of motion on the formation of the radiographic image.

◯ Explain the effect of magnification on the formation of the radiographic image.

◯ Explain the effect of distortion on the formation of the radiographic image.

◯ Given appropriate information, explain how to calculate exposure factors mA, time, kVp, and SID and their collective photographic effect.

◯ Explain the difference between object-to-image receptor distance (OID) and source-to-image receptor distance (SID).

Introduction

In this chapter, the student will learn how to manipulate exposure factors according to their interactive effect on the radiographic image. Standardization of radiographic exposure factors, although theoretically based, must be understood in the application of day-to-day radiography. More importantly, the student must understand exposure latitude and how it provides a margin of error which varies depending on mathematical ranges of exposure factors (mA, time, kVp, SID). The quality of the visible radiographic image depends largely on the perception of the viewer. However, with a solid background in the knowledge of human anatomy and an understanding of the technical factors that create a radiographic image, the health professional is able to evaluate the image in discipline-specific terms.

This chapter is intended for instruction of film/screen technology because there are still facilities that utilize this type of imaging. Digital technology is discussed in Chapter 10.

Image Production

A radiograph is produced from x-rays passing through a patient's body and interacting with the emulsion (surface) of a radiographic film. The finished radiograph is expected to provide a quality diagnostic image of the body part adjacent to the film. The image comprises the outlines and densities of the body part it represents (e.g., stomach, lungs). When processed with appropriate chemicals, the film emulsion yields a radiograph that, when placed on an illuminated light source (viewbox), provides visual information from which the physician can make a radiographic diagnosis.

A diagnostic quality radiograph should have adequate density (blackness), good contrast (range of gray shades), clear recorded detail (definition and resolution), and no visual distortion or magnification (size and shape) of the anatomy being examined. A physician interprets the anatomy in a radiograph based on visual properties. These properties can be categorized into two areas: density and contrast (categorized as photographic properties) and the recorded detail and absence of distortion and magnification (categorized as geometric properties). Table 9-1 summarizes the general parameters for interpreting radiographs. Each of the properties will be discussed further in the chapter.

TABLE 9-1   Image Interpretation Areas

Photographic Properties	Geometric Properties
Density	Recorded Detail
Contrast	Distortion
	Magnification

Exposure Factors

Production of the visible radiographic image is controlled by the following **exposure factors: milliamperage (mA), time, kilovoltage peak (kVp),** and **source-to-image receptor distance (SID).** However, other factors—heel effect, tube alignment to the film and body part, object-film distance, tissue thickness/pathology, screen selection, collimation and beam filters, fog, and film processing—also influence image production.

Exposure factors and other technical considerations will be discussed in relation to their effect on the image by photographic or geometric consequence. For the sake of simplicity, henceforth mA, time, kVp, and SID will be referred to as factors.

Photographic Factors

The two major photographic factors of the image are 1) *density* and 2) *contrast.*

Density

Density is seen as the overall blackness of the total image. Density is controlled by **milliamperage-seconds (mAs)**—it represents the quantity of radiation being produced for a certain length of time in an energized radiographic tube. The mAs to be used during any given radiographic exposure, e.g., 100 mA, 200 mA, 300 mA, are set by the radiographer at the control console of the radiographic unit (Figures 9-1A and B).

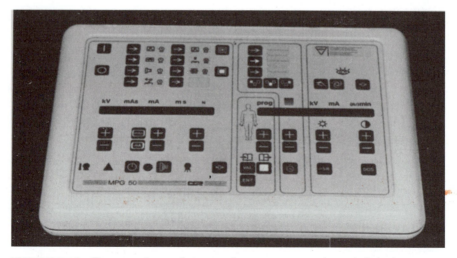

FIGURE 9-1A The control console is a modern, computerized panel. Only the exposure factors that have been selected are shown on the panel. Older machines may still show individual mA stations and the time (seconds) dial selector. (*Reprinted courtesy of Eastman Kodak Company*)

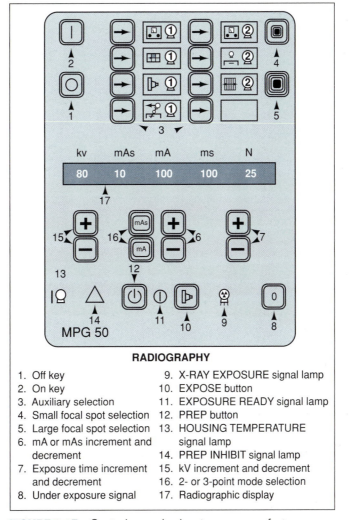

FIGURE 9-1B Control console showing exposure factors selected for a specific exposure. Controls are defined in the key.
Source: Delmar, Cengage Learning.

The density of the radiograph is directly proportional to the amount of mA used for exposure and length of time the exposure is delivered (referred to as mAs setting). A good principle to remember is that, proportionally, 200 mA at 1.0 seconds will produce twice as much density on a film as will 100 mA at 1.0 second. Higher mA selections will increase the production of electrons inside the tube (hence, quantity of radiation). Therefore, as more electrons are produced, more radiation reaches the film and more blackness or density will be seen on the film. Density is directly proportional to mA and time. If the mA is doubled, the quantity of radiation will double. If the time is doubled, the quantity of radiation will double. Both mA and time (mAs) have a direct effect on the degree of film darkening (density).

Time and Density. Time is a factor of duration. It expresses the length of time that electrons (mA) are produced in the tube. As previously indicated, mA and time together are known as milliampere-seconds or mAs. Actually, time indicates how long a given amount of mA will last. In other words, milliamperes × time (seconds) = milliampere second (mAs). For example:

$$300 \, mA \times 0.1 \, sec = 30 \, mAs.$$

The quantity of radiation, therefore, must be stated as mAs for four reasons: 1) mAs indicates quantity of radiation and how long the exposure lasted; 2) dosage is a product of mAs (e.g., a 300 mA selection and a time of 1 second would produce 300 mAs); 3) doubling the time has the same effect as doubling the mA (300 mA × 2 sec = 600 mAs; the quantity of radiation doubles and density or visible blackness in the recorded image doubles); and 4) the relationship between mA × T should remain constant during repeated exposures as long as the radiation output is consistent and the generating equipment has been properly calibrated by a company service representative.

The fourth factor above is related to the *Reciprocity Law*. This law means that any combination of mA × T factors that are equivalent mAs should produce the same amount of density. See the following example for further elaboration.

mA	TIME (s)	CALCULATION	mAs
50	$\frac{1}{5}$ sec.	$50 \times \frac{1}{5}$ sec. =	10 mAs
100	$\frac{1}{10}$ sec.	$100 \times \frac{1}{10}$ sec. =	10 mAs
200	$\frac{1}{20}$ sec.	$200 \times \frac{1}{20}$ sec. =	10 mAs
300	$\frac{1}{30}$ sec.	$300 \times \frac{1}{30}$ sec. =	10 mAs

All of the above combinations should produce the same amount of density in the image (overall blackness). Thus, if a faster time is needed to avoid motion, mA and time may be changed according to the equation in the example.

Because time is a factor of duration, it is important to always identify the fastest exposure time compatible with other exposure factors (mA, kVp, SID) to avoid capturing any patient or organ motion in the recorded image.

Factors that control the mAs selection are: 1) the size of the focal spot to be used and 2) the amount of exposure time needed. Focal spots are the primary factor controlling recorded detail (a geometric property). However, their ability to withstand heat units inside the tube is critical to how much mAs may be applied for a given technique. Other factors will be discussed in this chapter in topics related to recorded detail (subtopic of Geometric Factors) and to motion (subtopic of Distortion and Magnification). Smaller focal-spot (filament) size in the tube results in sharper recorded detail of the anatomy seen in a radiographic image. For this reason, whenever practical, a smaller focal-spot size should be used. However, if the anatomy being radiographed is thick (large tissue volume, above 12 cm), a larger focal-spot size must be used due to the increased production of internal tube heat. Thus, a disadvantage of the smaller focal-spot size is that it cannot tolerate the heat generated with the long or increased exposure time that may be required for thick body parts. The lower mA stations (e.g., 100 mA, 200 mA, and 300 mA) reflect a smaller focal spot. Larger focal-spot sizes are automatically switched on in the generator circuitry with larger mA selections (400 mA, 500 mA, 800 mA, and higher). Combinations of the formula mA $\times$ T = mAs follow.

SMALL FOCAL SPOT	LARGE FOCAL SPOT
300 mA $\times$ 0.10 T = 30 mAs	600 mA $\times$ 0.05 T = 30 mAs
300 mA $\times$ 0.5 T = 150 mAs	600 mA $\times$ 0.25 T = 150 mAs

The examples show that mA $\times$ T may be used to achieve the same density on the recorded image using different focal-spot sizes. This factor is also related to the Reciprocity Law referred to on page 238 (see related examples).

The mA stations and their related focal-spot sizes vary with equipment and the particular **heat unit (HU)** capacity of the specific manufacturer's radiographic tube (Table 9-2).

The formula for determining HU capacity is:

$$mA \times T \times kVp$$

For example:

$$300 \, mA \times 1 \, sec \times 80 \, kVp = 2400 \, HU$$

For 3-phase units (6 pulse and 12 pulse), the formulas are:

6 pulse:	$1.35 \times 300 \, mA \times 1.0 \, sec \times 80 \, kVp = 32,400$
12 pulse:	$1.41 \times 300 \, mA \times 1.0 \, sec \times 80 \, kVp = 33,840$

If the total tube capacity is 300,000 HU, then the exposure cited in the first example would use only a small portion (0.08%) of the total capacity. The tube therefore could still withstand much more heat, which would allow several more exposures within the same range.

TABLE 9-2   Advantages/Disadvantages of Small and Large Focal Spots

Focal-Spot Size (FSS)	Advantages	Disadvantages
Small Focal Spot (100, 200, 300 mA stations)	Results in greater recorded detail of image.	Longer (slower) exposure time may result in patient motion. Focal spot cannot tolerate heat generated by a long exposure time.
Large Focal Spot (400, 500, 800 mA stations)	Shorter (faster) exposure time minimizes risk of patient motion. Focal spot can tolerate increased heat generated by longer exposure times.	Results in loss of recorded detail of image.

Other factors that interact to change the direct effect of density are kVp, SID, **heel effect,** *film processing,* and **film fog.**

Quantity of radiation for technique charts may be determined by trial and error using various combinations of mA × T on a phantom or device that represents the equivalency of human body structure. *Never use real human subjects* to establish technique factors. Once the average adult quantity of radiation has been established for a given part of the body, (e.g., head or chest), it is seldom necessary to adjust the mA. Only the time factor and sometimes the **kilovoltage** will need to be adjusted for various thickness ranges of anatomical structures. Table 9-3 shows examples of time variations.

kVp and Density.   kVp controls contrast. It does, however, affect density in two ways. As kVp is increased, the stream of electrons in the tube moves more efficiently across the tube and results in increased part penetration (discussed later with kVp). A second effect is that as kVp is increased, more radiation energy is produced, resulting in more scattered radiation, which increases density to the film (recorded image). This can be controlled by use of a grid (discussed under Accessories).

TABLE 9-3   Examples of Time Variations for Average Adult Chest

Chest	mA	cm Measurement	T	mAs
	300	Small 15–18	$1/30$	10
	300	Medium 19–22	$1/15$	20
	300	Large 25–32	$1/10$	30

Note: The chart shows how the time can be adjusted to accommodate various chest-size ranges without changing the mA. However, these calculations may not be appropriate for a given radiographic unit.

Distance and Density. Distance, or SID, has a significant influence on density. SID obeys the **inverse square law** (Figure 9-2). Understanding the concept of the inverse square law is necessary because it relates to density, radiation intensity, and radiation dosage. These three factors collectively work in concert with the inverse square law, but the most visible to the radiographer is density because it results from a standard SID set by the radiographer. The inverse square law states: *The intensity of radiation is inversely proportional to the square of the distance.* The inverse square law is expressed in the following formula:

$$\frac{I_1}{I_2} = \frac{D_2^2}{D_1^2}$$

Where: I_1 = original intensity
I_2 = new intensity
D_2 = new distance
D_1 = original distance

Intensity is related to the amount of radiation produced in the tube through mA as it is combined with time. Thus, mA $\times$ T = mAs. Since the radiographer sets these factors along with kVp, s/he determines exposure factors to work together as mA $\times$ T $\times$ kVp. The fourth factor SID is usually set at 40 inches standard distance. Occasionally the SID must be changed to produce a specific image. When this is necessary, the radiographer must make changes in technique factors to compensate for an increase or decrease in exposure or essentially the number of photons reaching the film.

The inverse square law formula can be applied to compensate for percentage of change in distance decreased by half, from 40 inches to 20 inches. See the following example.

$$\frac{I_1}{I_2} = \frac{80_2^2}{40_1^2}$$

$$\frac{I_1}{x} = \frac{6400}{1600}$$

$$6400x = 1600$$
$$x = 6400/1600$$
$$x = 25\%$$

In this case, 25% less radiation would be needed to avoid overexposure of the image. Whereas, if 40 inches SID is increased to 80 inches SID, or doubled, the radiation beam would be attenuated or spread over an area four times greater than at 40 inches. Thus, intensity of the beam is attenuated at the increased SID. This would result in an underexposed image on the finished radiograph due to the loss in overall density.

Because intensity reflects the number of photons that may reach the film in terms of radiation interaction, it is most practical to use mAs to compensate for SID changes.

To obtain the same amount of density from 40 inches to an increase of 80 inches, an increase in radiation exposure (photons) is required as indicated by a square law relationship. The following mAs-Distance (SID) formula may be applied to compensate for distance changes.

$$\frac{mAs_1}{mAs_2} = \frac{D_2^2}{D_1^2}$$

Where: mAs_1 = original mAs
   mAs_2 = new mAs
   D_1 = original distance
   D_2 = new distance

This formula expresses a square law change in the distance (SID). The relationship may be changed as a proportional mAs factor. Increasing the distance by twice as much requires four times more radiation exposure using the above formula.

The following example reflects a 25% change in exposure, which was expressed in the previous inverse square law formula.

$$\frac{mAs_1}{mAs_2} = \frac{40_1^2}{80_2^2}$$

$$\frac{30mAs}{x} = \frac{40^2}{80^2}$$

$$\frac{30mAs}{x} = \frac{1600}{6400}$$

$$6400x = 48,000$$

$$x = 7.5$$

The new distance of 80 inches attenuates (spreads) the intensity of the beam of radiation over an area 4 times greater than at the old distance of 40 inches. As is evidenced by either formula, inverse square law or square law, a change in SID must be compensated for by a change in mAs. See Figure 9-2.

Simply put, the radiation beam diverges and proceeds in a straight path (lines). The area covered becomes increasingly larger with lessened intensity as the beam of radiation travels a greater distance from the source. To produce a given density at a different distance, it is necessary to vary the exposure inversely with the square of the distance. The exposure area in Figure 9-2 has increased four times from 40 inches to 80 inches.

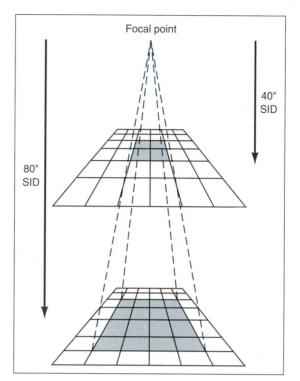

FIGURE 9-2 At 40 inches, a 4-square area represents the SID spread. At 80 inches, twice the distance, a 16-square area represents the SID and shows increased spread for the same quantity of radiation.
Source: Delmar, Cengage Learning.

Heel Effect and Density. Heel effect is a phenomenon related to the structure of the radiographic tube's target (anode) angle. Figure 9-3A shows the long axis of the tube and how the radiation beam is emitted from the focal spot. The radiation intensity diminishes along a line parallel with the long axis of the tube, and is called the heel effect. As shown in Figure 9-3A, the intensity of the exposure increases toward the cathode (filament) side of the tube while it decreases toward the anode (target) side of the tube as a result of the target angle. Because the heel effect causes more radiation to be emitted toward the cathode side of the tube, the heel effect is more pronounced in tubes with steeper target angles (10 degrees) than in tubes with greater target angles (20 degrees) (Figure 9-3B).

The rule should be to align the long axis of the tube parallel with the longer or broader portion of the anatomical structure being examined so that the cathode side of the tube is directed over the thicker part of the structure. One example for

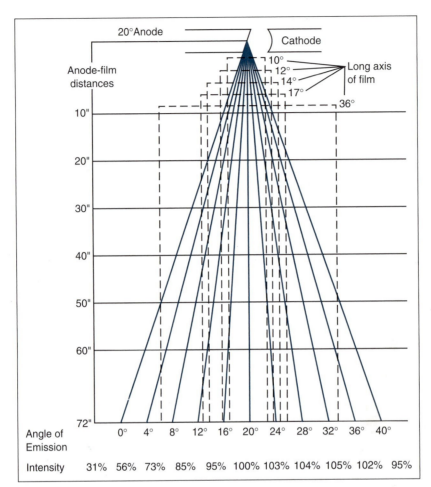

FIGURE 9-3A Representation of the heel effect, where radiation intensity increases toward the cathode end of the tube
Source: Delmar, Cengage Learning.

proper tube alignment is radiographic examination of the femur. The cathode side of the tube should be directed toward the hip region and the anode side over the knee region so that the more intense radiation will pass through the adjacent thicker upper femoral area. Another example is the examination of the lower leg. The cathode side should be directed toward the knee thickness or proximal leg to balance radiation distribution. A final example is a lateral lumbar spine. The cathode side of the tube should be directed over the upper pelvic region.

Film Fog and Density. Density may also be affected by film fog, which is unwanted density that makes it difficult to visualize structures on the radiograph. Film fog

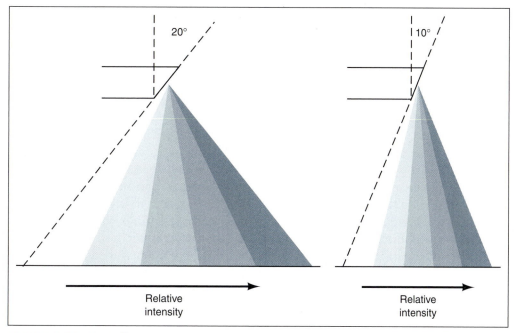

FIGURE 9-3B   Heel effect
Source: Delmar, Cengage Learning.

may be caused by age (old film), light (result is total blackening of film emulsion), scattered radiation exposure, or improper film development. In order to prevent or reduce film fog, the darkroom must be lightproof. The darkroom safelight should be well-positioned and maintained. Film must be used according to its expiration date. Radiographic film must be processed properly, and unused film should be stored in a lead-lined room or container. Any change in processing time or temperature will quickly affect density in a radiograph. Chapter 10 discusses in more detail why time and temperature must remain constant.

Artifacts are foreign or unwanted marks that show up on a radiograph because of improper film handling, improper processing, or faulty equipment. Artifacts can result in a change (either an increase or a decrease) in film density, usually in a particular area of the image.

Contrast

Contrast is the second major photographic factor. There are three types of contrast: radiographic, subject, and film. Each will be discussed as to its role in a diagnostic quality radiograph.

Radiographic contrast results from the distribution of black metallic silver in the film emulsion and is directly controlled by the penetrating effects of kilovoltage.

Radiographic contrast is visualized in the image as gray tones or degrees of gray that reveal the differences between body organs or tissues. Contrast enhances information. If no contrast can be seen between organs, then very little information may be visible in the radiographic image. An excellent example of this phenomena in human anatomy is an obese abdomen where the internal organs appear as equal in tissue thickness and therefore density because of fat content. It is like looking for a white goose in a snow storm. Contrast is controlled by the kilovoltage or, more technically, the quality of energy or wavelength (short or long). You may want to refer to the chapter on physics, Chapter 5.

A variety of long and short wavelengths (low and high energies) will demonstrate a range of shades from black to gray to white (gray tones) and their density differences. The differences are easily seen in the structures visible in the radiographic image. In the blacker portion of a radiograph, the visible structures will have absorbed *less* radiation, and the whiter portion of the visible structures will have absorbed *more* radiation. This means that the whiter structures have greater tissue density.

Radiographic contrast is generally referred to as the overall contrast seen in the image. It includes long-scale (more gray tones) contrast and short-scale (more black and white tones) contrast. Radiation of higher energy (shorter wave-length), 70 kVp or more, will produce long-scale contrast with many gray tones (Figure 9-4A). Additionally,

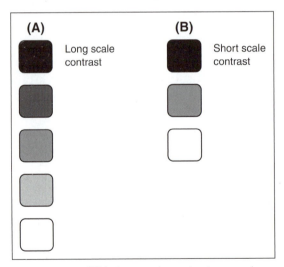

FIGURE 9-4 (A) In long-scale contrast, several degrees of gray to black tones will be produced in the image with higher kVp ranges, i.e., above 70 kVp; (B) In short-scale contrast, the range of gray tones is more abrupt from white to black. Fewer gray tones will be seen in the image. Short-scale contrast is produced at lower kVp ranges, i.e., below 70 kVp. Source: Delmar, Cengage Learning.

tissues having little difference in thickness or density will appear as images with flat gray tones. If there are large differences in the thickness of body structures, e.g., bone versus soft tissue, or if 70 kilovoltage and lower is used, short-scale contrast with more pronounced black and white tones will be produced (Figure 9-4B). Much of the radiographic image contrast is influenced by subject contrast and film contrast.

Subject contrast depends on how much the radiation beam is attenuated or spreads out as it enters, passes through, and exits the various structures within the body. This is what is known as an *aerial image*, which is created by the absorption of radiation in various percentages by different tissue thicknesses (Figure 9-5). Bone will absorb more radiation than soft tissue, but this may vary greatly depending on tissue density, age, disease, or other conditions where structure may change or be complex.

Film contrast is inherent in the type of filming system being used, including 1) the type of film (low-contrast or high-contrast), 2) the processing conditions (the time-temperature method of developing films should be adhered to for visualization of optimal contrast—see Chapter 12), and 3) the use of screens versus no screens. That is, because intensifying screens convert radiant energy to visible light, contrast is increased with screens; whereas without screens (direct exposure), contrast is affected mostly by the natural difference in tissue thickness.

As previously stated, contrast enhances information by making the detail of structures appropriately visible in the image. Without appropriate levels of subject

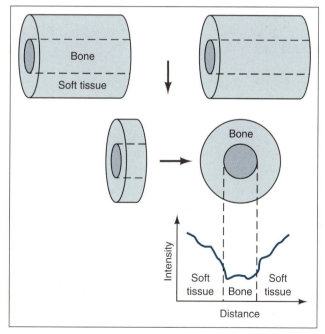

FIGURE 9-5 Aerial image
Source: Delmar, Cengage Learning.

contrast being visualized in the radiographic image, it would be difficult to differentiate human structures and diseases with discernible accuracy.

It was stated earlier, under the discussion on mAs, that the overall amount of density or blackness seen in the radiographic image is controlled by the quantity of mAs used and that the degree of density is proportionate to the mAs (double the mAs, double the density). By comparison, contrast is controlled by kVp and has an approximate effect on the image according to the 15% rule. This rule means that if you are using 80 kVp in your technique factors (i.e., 300 mA, 0.30 seconds, 80 kVp) and you add 15% (12 kVp) more to the original 80, kVp is increased to 92. Such a change would double the kVp penetration effectiveness, but contrast would visibly decrease.

Increasing or decreasing the kVp by 15% has an effect equivalent to increasing or decreasing the mAs by 50%. It should be noted that although kVp and mAs have an interactive effect in increasing or decreasing contrast and density respectively, they may not be interchanged to compensate for the lack of one or the other. As further explanation, note that if structures are underpenetrated due to a lack of kVp, no amount of mAs increase will improve the penetration; added mAs will only add density. Penetration of structure can best be achieved by using the appropriate amount of kVp. Conversely, if an image is underexposed and lacks density, mAs must be added; kVp would add only scattered radiation and thus cause the image to look gray and flat without clarity.

In summary, the two factors of mAs (density) and kVp (contrast) must be used so that the interactive effects are complementary to each other and not compensatory for the lack of one or the other.

Milliamperage-Seconds (mAs) and Contrast. Milliamperage-seconds (mAs) fundamentally controls the quantity of radiation; kVp fundamentally controls contrast. The two factors must not be interchanged. Too much mAs will result in increased density or blackness with an accompanying loss of visible radiographic contrast. It is equally important to note that increasing mAs generally will not improve structure penetration, which is also controlled by kVp.

Distance and Contrast (kVp). The intensity of primary and secondary radiation changes inversely proportional to the square of the distance. Any change in distance will result in a proportionate change in the amount of scattered radiation. Thus, image contrast will not be affected. The degree of density in nearby structures may be lighter or darker, but the level of contrast will be fundamentally unchanged. Additionally, the degree of structure penetration will not, for all practical purposes, be affected. Levels of kVp penetration are equally effective at any distance (e.g., 70 kVp, 80 kVp).

Other Factors. Other factors that influence both density and contrast are beam restriction, beam filtration, and compression of tissue. Although these areas are discussed later in the chapter, they are mentioned here to facilitate easy reference.

Beam restriction or *limitation* reduces the amount of scattered radiation interacting with the body and thereby prevents excessive scatter from fogging the film with increased density and decreased contrast of the visible image.

Beam filtration (filters) is added to the radiation beam to eliminate nonuseful, soft, low-energy (long wavelengths) radiation. This filtration results in hardening of the beam by allowing mostly higher energy (shorter wavelengths) to pass through unchanged. Contrast may be improved then with a decreased amount of lower-energy wavelengths.

Compression of tissue has the effect of reducing tissue thickness. In the area where tissue is compressed, therefore, contrast may be visibly reduced due to increased penetration by kVp. Density will be increased in the same area due to less absorption of radiation.

Geometric Factors

Density and contrast are photographic factors that refer to the properties of the visible radiographic image. Geometric factors deal with the recorded detail of the image and the accuracy with which the true edges of the anatomy may be seen. Recorded detail, distortion, and magnification are the geometric factors of interest.

Recorded Detail

Recorded detail is the degree of information or definition that may be seen in the anatomy or the resolution or sharpness of lines that separates one structure from another. Although motion is rarely seen in a radiographic image because of very rapid exposure-time settings on today's equipment, motion completely destroys information by blurring the visibility of the radiographic (or recorded) image. It does not require a great deal of experience or knowledge to recognize blurring in a radiographic image. It may be compared to the blurring seen in an ordinary photograph when the subject has moved. The fastest possible exposure time therefore is the best recourse against motion and should always be used in accordance with all other factors when making any radiographic exposure.

Focal-spot size (FSS), SID, OFD, and intensifying screens are factors that influence the geometry of the image, and each must be designed to reduce or minimize the geometric blur. "Geometric blur," or *penumbra* (Figure 9-6) is the term used to describe the gradient unsharpness or edge enhancement of an image.

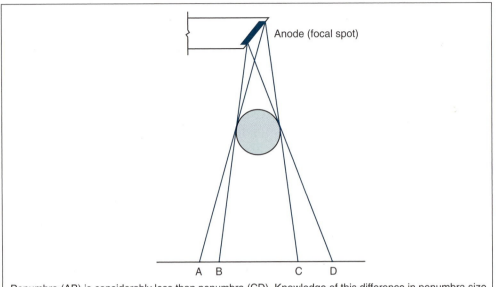

Anode (focal spot)

A B   C D

Penumbra (AB) is considerably less than penumbra (CD). Knowledge of this difference in penumbra size can be used to minimize unsharpness effects by proper positioning of the patient. In essence what is happening is that the film is seeing a smaller focal spot on the anode side as compared with the cathode side. Generally, the area of primary interest is pointed towards the anode side of the x-ray tube.

FIGURE 9-6 Focal spot and its relationship to subject placement (*Reprinted courtesy of Eastman Kodak Company*)

Focal-Spot Size. The effective focal-spot size was discussed in Chapter 6. The relationship of the focal spot to geometric blur is that it is the single most important factor in recording the detail of the anatomy in the radiographic image. The **small focal spot** (produced by the smaller filament) in a dual focus tube will produce better recorded detail than the **large focal spot** (filament) (Figure 9-7). The rule to follow in utilizing focal-spot size is to use the smaller one whenever the exposure factors (mA, T, kVp, and SID) are set low enough to allow its use.

Source-to-Image Receptor Distance (SID). For all practical purposes, SID has no effect on the penetrating power of the kVp. Changes in the SID will not affect contrast as long as the kVp remains unchanged. The rule concerning the relationship between SID and recorded detail is that a greater (increased) SID will reduce geometric blur and thus improve recorded detail. (See the penumbra reduction in Figure 9-8.) Most radiographic images are produced at a standardized 40-inch SID. (See section on distance and density, this chapter.)

Object-to-Image Receptor Distance (OID). The term **object-to-image receptor distance (OID)** refers to the practice/rule of placing the object (anatomy) as close to the

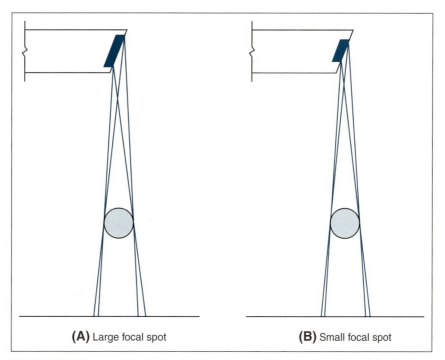

FIGURE 9-7 Penumbral shadow or edge unsharpness occurs because the focal spot on the anode is not a point source. It is comprised of many point sources, each of which projects its own object image onto the film. (A) Large focal spot and its resulting penumbra; (B) Small focal spot and a reduced amount of penumbra. (*Reprinted courtesy of Eastman Kodak Company*)

image receptor (the cassette) as possible. This is a cardinal rule to observe because magnification occurs when the part is not close to the film or image receptor. The result is an overall enlarged and fuzzy image. Although we recognize that placing the anatomy adjacent to the image receptor surface is not always possible, minimizing the gap is important to reducing geometric blur (Figure 9-9). The rule should be to always place the part (object) adjacent to or as close as possible to the receptor surface. Magnification or size distortion may be reduced by decreasing the OID or by increasing the SID. Most radiographs are taken at a standard SID of 40 inches (100 cm), which usually results in a magnification factor of approximately 1.1.

For radiographs taken at 72 inches (180 cm) the magnification factor is approximately 1.05. Several formulas may be used to determine the amount of image magnification. The most practical formula applies the ratio of SID to SOD (the distance from the source of the x-rays to the object being examined; SOD is also referred to as FOD for focal-object distance).

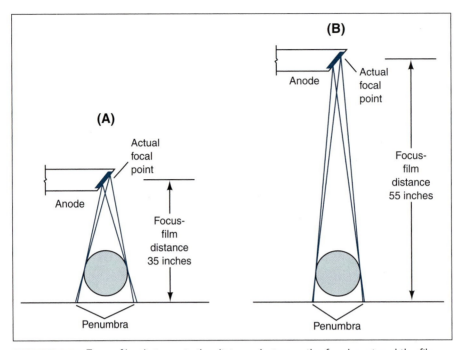

FIGURE 9-8 Focus-film distance is the distance between the focal spot and the film. Generally speaking, focus-film distance directly affects the degree of penumbral shadow and geometric unsharpness. Note that A has a 35-inch focus-film distance and a greater degree of penumbral shadow than B, which has a 55-inch focus-film distance. The radiographic illustrations provided graphically illustrate the difference in penumbral shadow as one goes from a short focus-film distance to a long focus-film distance. (*Reprinted courtesy of Eastman Kodak Company*)

$$MF = \frac{SID}{SOD}$$
$$= \frac{40}{32}$$
$$= 1.25 \text{ times}$$

These same results, however, may be arrived at in a different, but more involved, way. Determining the percentage of magnification requires certain information—that is, the size of the image width (IW) and object width (OW) must be established. While the image width may be measured from the radiograph, the object width must be determined. For example, suppose you are using a 40 inch SID, an 8 inch OFD, and a 10 centimeter (cm) image size. The following formulas may be used to determine object width and amount of magnification.

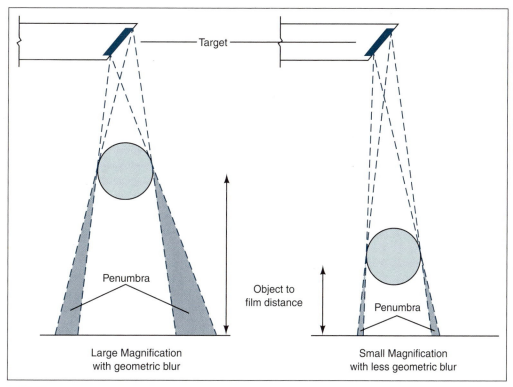

FIGURE 9-9 Improvement in radiographic image due to shorter object-to-film distance (*Reprinted courtesy of Eastman Kodak Company*)

(1) $\quad \text{OW} = \dfrac{\text{SID}}{\text{SID} - \text{OFD}}$

$\qquad = \dfrac{40}{40 - 8} = \dfrac{40}{32}$

$\dfrac{40}{32} = \dfrac{10 \text{ cm}}{x}$

$\dfrac{40}{32} = \dfrac{10 \times 32}{40x}$

$\dfrac{320}{40} = 8 \text{ cm (OW)}$

Once the object width has been determined, the following formula may be used to calculate the magnification factor.

(2) $MF = \dfrac{IW}{OW}$

$= \dfrac{10}{8}$

$= 1.25$

The percentage of magnification may then be calculated according to the following formula.

(3) $\%MF = \dfrac{IW - OW}{OW} \times 100$

$= \dfrac{10 - 8}{8} \times 100$

$= \dfrac{2}{8} \times 100$

$= 00.25 \times 100$

$= 25\%$

Intensifying Screens. Intensifying screens affect recorded detail according to the size of the phosphor crystal (see Chapter 9). Smaller crystal size will create less

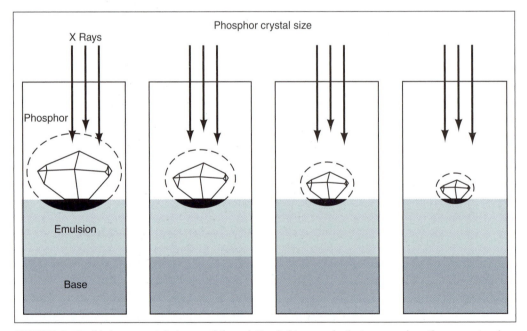

FIGURE 9-10 Various crystal sizes and the relative light spreads that occur when they are struck by incident radiation. Smaller crystal size creates less light diffusion in the radiographic image. (*Reprinted courtesy of Eastman Kodak Company*)

blurring of the image because there is less diffusion of light created by the smaller crystal (Figure 9-10), thus, improved or better recorded detail. Screens are discussed in greater detail under Accessories.

Screen-Film Contact. The loss of **screen-film contact** is infrequent with automatic systems where no one ever touches or opens cassettes. Generally, screen-film contact is lost only in cassettes that are larger in size (14 × 17 in/35 × 43 cm) and when cassettes are constantly opened for loading, unloading, and cleaning. What visually appears with incomplete screen-film contact is a blurring of the image, usually in the center of the film (Figure 9-11A).

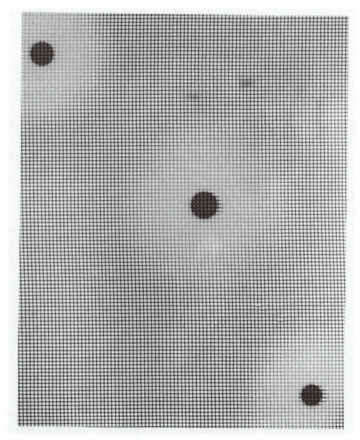

FIGURE 9-11A Poor screen-film contact. These films demonstrate blurring around the areas where the coins have been placed. Poor screen-film contact appears in the area of the screens where there may be poor contact. This is more common with large 14 × 17 in. size screens than with any other size screens. (*Reprinted courtesy of Eastman Kodak Company*)

Film Resolution.   Film resolution is the ability of the crystals within the film emulsion to efficiently record information. This ability is dependent on crystal size. Generally, smaller crystal size will be able to resolve and record more image information with less geometric blur than larger crystal size.

Distortion and Magnification

Distortion of the radiographic image refers to changes in size or shape of the anatomic part. Magnification (Figure 9-11B), foreshortening, and elongation (Figure 9-12) of

FIGURE 9-11B   Notice the size of the coins as a result of magnification compared to the image size of the coins in Figure 9-11A. (*Reprinted courtesy of Eastman Kodak Company*)

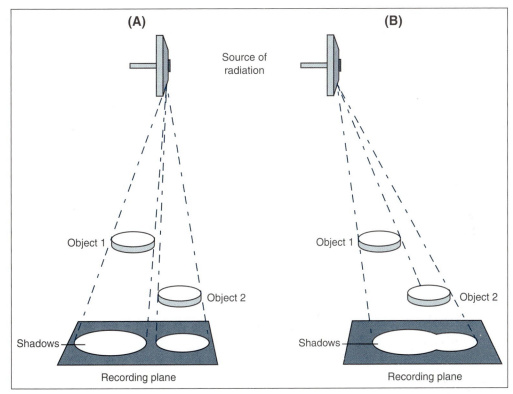

FIGURE 9-12 Some magnification in the radiographic image may be useful (e.g., for a finger). Distortion, however, is rarely helpful. (A) No distortion in the circular objects on the recording plane (film); (B) With a change in the direction (angle) of the radiation, the circular objects elongate and overlap—they appear as one object. The radiation must pass through the object perpendicularly as the object is placed parallel to the recording plane.
Source: Delmar, Cengage Learning.

the actual image size or shape are forms of distortion. A number of factors—OID, SID, motion, focal-spot size (FSS), and tube-to-part alignment—influence geometric image (Figure 9-12).

Motion. Motion is a major factor in reducing image clarity and increasing distortion. A radiograph containing motion is referred to as a "blurred image." A blurred image appears fuzzy with unclear edges. There is one major and best recourse against the loss of information caused by motion and that is to use fast exposure time. However, using as fast an exposure time as is practical and patient immobilization when appropriate will help reduce image distortion caused by motion. If available, fast film/screen may also be used.

There are two types of motion, voluntary and involuntary. The patient primarily controls voluntary motion, whereas the patient cannot control involuntary motion as this type of motion relates to normal body functions (e.g., heartbeat).

It is important to remember to give patients clear instructions to avoid motion or even to practice with them what they are expected to do. Children must be managed in more selective ways. Most facilities will have appropriate techniques for children, especially those designed for children only.

Tube-Part Alignment. Improper alignment of the tube or **central ray** to the body part or the film results in distortion. This distortion may cause the image to appear longer or shorter than its actual length. The physical shape of the anatomic part can also influence the amount of distortion. Whenever possible, to avoid shape distortion, the radiographic tube (central ray) should be perpendicular to the long axis of the part (Figure 9-13).

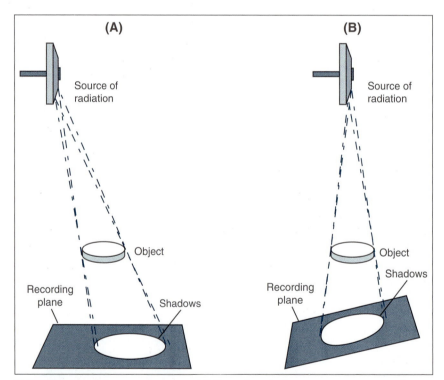

FIGURE 9-13 Tube-part alignment. (A) Even though the source is not vertically above the circular object, it casts a circular shadow, provided the object and the recording plane are parallel; (B) Distortion results when object and image-receptor plane are not parallel.
Source: Delmar, Cengage Learning.

Image-Production Accessories

There are several accessory items that are very important to image production. These accessory items are generally standardized and few changes need ever be made regarding their use and application. It is important, however, to understand the purpose of and effect of these items on the image. These accessory items are: intensifying screens, grids, beam restrictors, filtration, and processing.

Intensifying Screens

Intensifying screens have phosphors that intensify the action of radiation. Although screens are addressed in Chapter 12, some review is appropriate here to help understand the effect of exposure with screens. Two important elements of screens are: 1) the size of the crystal and 2) thickness of the layer of the phosphor. The effect that screens have on density is related to both the crystal size and thickness of the emulsion, which determines the screen speed (response time) or amount of light produced (intensification). There are several categories of screens: detail or slow-speed screens, general purpose or medium-speed screens, and fast or high-speed screens. For convenience and ease of recognition, screen speeds have been given specific numbers by manufacturers.

Screen-speed factor or intensification of screens is determined as a ratio of the amount of exposure necessary without screens to the amount necessary with screens:

$$\text{Intensification factor (speed factor)} = \frac{\text{exposure without screens}}{\text{exposure with screens}}$$

The comparisons are not intended to be more than a simple illustration of the differences in the two types of blue and green screens.

Information regarding intensifying screen phosphors used in various types of screens may be obtained from manufacturers. Green sensitive screens are faster than blue sensitive screens. Some examples of different phosphors follow.

Calcium tungstate (old) $CaWO_4$	Blue
Lanthanum oxybromide	Blue
Gadolinium oxysulfide	Green
Yttrium tantalate	Blue-green

Because we are concerned with the amount of density produced in the combination of screens and film, it is more effective and efficient to think in terms of speed. That is, if one is in the process of changing screens, it is necessary to know what change in exposure factors, if any, will be required. For example, a speed factor of 100 would require 50% more exposure than a speed factor of 200.

Screen speed affects density by the required exposure necessary to produce a given amount of blackness in the radiographic image. Again, using the above factors, if a general purpose screen with a rating of 200 is used and it is then decided that a detail screen with a rating of 100 is needed, an increase of 50% more exposure will be needed to maintain the same density with the slower detail screen. For practical purposes, however, the daily use of screens is standardized, so that exposure factors are determined according to the way in which radiographic procedures are conducted on a routine basis. Procedures may vary from extremities, chest, abdomen, pelvis, spine, and skull examinations in large radiography departments to extremities, chest, abdomen, and pelvis in smaller departments or a doctor's office.

Grids

Grids are precision instruments designed for the single purpose of absorbing scattered radiation, although some primary radiation is absorbed as well. A grid is designed to be used where density of the image is affected by the amount of scattered radiation reaching the film. This is because a greater exposure is needed for producing images of structures that measure above 12 cm in thickness, where more than 70 kVp is required. When kVp settings are increased, more scattered radiation is created. Basically, changing from no grid to the use of a grid requires four times more exposure because of scattered and primary beam absorption by lead strips in the grid (Figure 9-14). The grid works in this way: when a grid is added, it is placed under the table, between the patient and the film. The lead strips in the grid absorb divergent radiation beams scattered away from the direction of the more perpendicular primary beam. The gaps between the lead strips allow the primary beam to reach and interact with the film emulsion whereas the scattered radiation is absorbed by the lead strips. The amount of scattered radiation that is absorbed by the grid is related to *grid ratio*. Grid ratio is defined as the ratio of the height of the lead strips to the distance between the lead strips, as seen in the following diagram (Figure 9-15).

As seen in the diagram, the effect of the grid lines, or its efficiency (cleanup ability), depends on the height of the lead strips and the distance between the strips (wide or narrow). The less the distance between them and greater the height, as in the 16:1 ratio, the more efficient the grid will be in pickup or removal of scattered radiation.

Approximately four times more mAs must be added when a grid is used than when a grid is not used because of absorption by the lead strips. Otherwise, there would be a loss of density that would cause the radiographic image to appear greatly

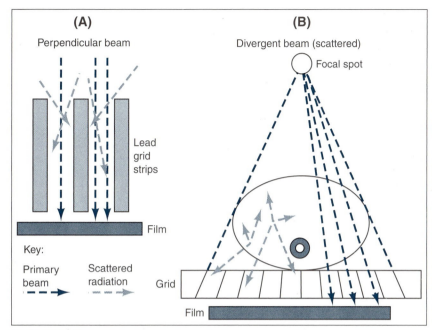

FIGURE 9-14 Grid cross section. (A) An enlarged small portion of a grid shows how scattered radiation is absorbed by the lead strips. It also shows how perpendicular radiation from the primary beam passes between the lead strips to reach the film emulsion. (B) The radiation of the radiation beam, the part being examined, the grid, and the image-recording receptor
Source: Delmar, Cengage Learning.

underexposed. For example, if 5 mAs is used without a grid, 20 mAs must be used with a grid. (See grid conversion chart, Table 9-4).

Beam Restriction and Filtration

These areas are discussed in Chapters 15 and 16. Their effect on density, however, can be stated relatively simply. Primary beam restriction is achieved by the use of collimators, diaphragms, and occasionally cones (Figure 9-16). The purpose of these devices is to minimize the amount of scattered radiation that reaches the film. An increase in scattered radiation reaching the film results in fog, which causes an increase in density and a resultant decrease in contrast. The primary beam should be limited or confined to the area of the structure being radiographed, leaving only a narrow border within the edges of the film. The beam must at least be confined to the size of the film itself. Unnecessarily exposing large areas beyond the film edges results in added density in the radiographic image and increased dosage to the patient.

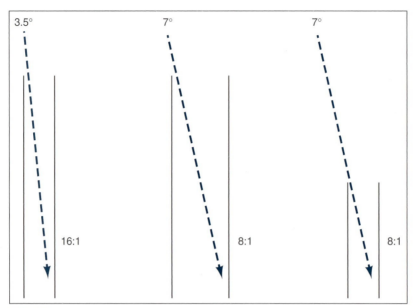

FIGURE 9-15 Effect of grid ratio on scatter angle
Source: Delmar, Cengage Learning.

TABLE 9-4 Basic Grid Conversion Ratios for Changing from Non-Grid to Grid Technique

Non-Grid to Grid*	When mAs Use is Increased	When kVp Use is Increased	Maximum kVp for Grid Ratio
5:1	2 × original mAs	+ 8 kVp	80
8:1	4 × original mAs	+ 20 kVp	90–100
12:1	5 × original mAs	+ 25 kVp	110–120
16:1	6 × original mAs	+ 30 kVp	150

*Note: That kVp increases may be preferable to mAs increases when technique is changed from non-grid exposure to grid exposure. An increase in mAs reduces contrast as well as increases exposure time, whereas an increase in kVp does not increase radiation dosage. Also, unless the kVp is excessive, decreasing mAs permits the penetration value of the total exposure to be retained.

Filtration

Filtration is the process of filtering the beam of radiation through some type of material that will remove lower-energy radiation from the beam and prevent it from reaching the patient. The filter should be a type of material that will allow the more useful higher-energy radiation to pass through unchanged, but will absorb nonuseful lower-energy radiation. Aluminum is a material of choice for filters because it

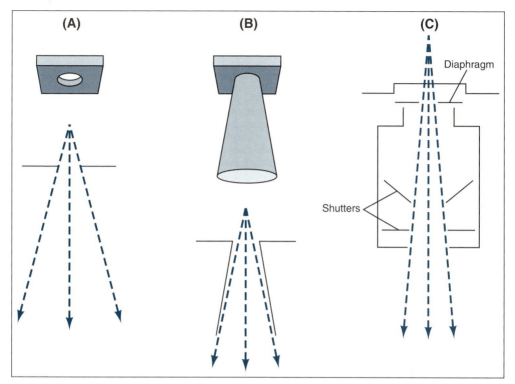

FIGURE 9-16 (A) A sheet of lead with a hole in the center (aperture diaphragm). (B) A sheet of metal or lead (diaphragm) with a cylinder cone attached. The lead is placed close to the radiation source with the cone extending down. The length and diameter of the cone determine the size of the field exposed. (C) A collimator with multiple shutters. The shutters are variable by external controls, but generally are set on automatic field size. Near the tube window is a diaphragm designed to minimize off-focus radiation. The collimator is used for positive beam limitation (PBL) as required by law. A and B are obsolete on modern standard equipment.
Source: Delmar, Cengage Learning.

is less expensive than other materials and it absorbs lower-energy radiation well while allowing passage of higher-energy radiation. The aluminum is placed within the beam, either at the tube-window aperture or at the collimator opening. This is called added filtration and may measure 2.0 mm of aluminum or its equivalent. There is usually 0.5 mm of filtration within the tube itself, made up by the glass tube and its surrounding insulating oil. This is called inherent (built-in) filtration. The total minimal amount of beam filtration should be about 2.5 mm (inherent and added) of aluminum equivalent. If there were no added filtration to the radiation beam and lower-energy radiation were permitted to reach the film, the radiographic image density and patient dosage would increase. For medical radiography, patient dosage is therefore most effectively reduced with 2.5 mm of total filtration.

Processing

Three film processing-related elements can adversely affect film density if they are not appropriately managed. These are *safelights*, *film age*, and *chemicals*. Although these are discussed in detail in Chapter 12, a brief introduction is needed here. The following three requirements may be properly set by following the recommendations of the film manufacturer: 1) the safelight must have the correct color of filter for the type(s) of film used; 2) it must have the correct size (wattage) bulb; and 3) it must be placed at the correct distance from the film-loading area and processor.

Age of film is important. Film comes from the manufacturer with an expiration date. Film boxes should be stored so that the oldest film is always used prior to that more recently dated.

Processor chemicals are precisely controlled by a time-temperature processing method. Any increase in the temperature is likely to add density to the film. Also, if the chemicals are not properly replenished and become exhausted or contaminated for any reason, added chemical density will occur on the film. All of the above, if not controlled, will create fog on the film that will result in increased density.

Summary

A summary of photographic factors and geometric factors appears in Table 9-5.

TABLE 9-5   Summary of Photographic and Geometric Factors

Factors	Controlled by Photographic Factors	Influenced/Affected by
Density	mAs	SID
		Heel effect
		kVp
		Fog processing
Contrast	Kilovoltage	Filters
		Fog (all forms)
		Film processing
		Subject contrast
		Type of film
		Pathology

Secondary Radiation Fog	Size of area exposed
	Compression
	Cones
	Diaphragms
	Grids
	kVp
Geometric Factors	
Recorded Detail	Focal-spot size
	Object-to-image receptor distance
	Motion
	Screen-crystal size
	Film-screen contact
Image Size (Magnification)	Source-to-image receptor distance
	Object-to-image receptor distance
Image Size (Distortion)	Alignment of tube to film
	Alignment of part to film
	Object-to-image receptor distance

REVIEW QUESTIONS

1. Radiographic density is best defined as the:
   a. sharpness of the radiographic image
   b. distortion of the image shape and size
   c. degree of blackness in the radiograph
   d. degree of difference between the light and dark areas

2. Radiographic contrast is best defined as the:
   a. sharpness of the radiographic image
   b. distortion of the image shape and size
   c. degree of blackness in the radiograph
   d. degree of difference between the light and dark areas

3. Select the exposure setting that will result in the greatest density:

	mA	TIME	SID
a.	100	½ second	36"
b.	200	¼ second	30"
c.	300	⅙ second	40"
d.	400	⅛ second	46"

4. To apply heel effect when radiographing a femur, position the thicker anatomic part beneath the:
   a. cathode
   b. anode
   c. cathode or anode
   d. there is little difference

5. A sharp difference between the light and dark areas of a radiographic image is termed:
   a. subject contrast
   b. long-scale contrast
   c. short-scale contrast
   d. inherent contrast

6. To change from a short-scale contrast to a long-scale contrast:
   a. decrease mAs and increase kVp
   b. decrease mAs and decrease kVp
   c. increase mAs and decrease kVp
   d. increase mAs and increase kVp

7. A grid should be used when the body part being radiographed is:
   a. likely to produce motion
   b. thicker than 12 centimeters
   c. subject to variations in size
   d. radiolucent

8. Which of the following technical factor sets is likely to result in the greatest amount of magnification?

	mAs	OID	SID
a.	30	6"	36"
b.	50	5"	50"
c.	75	4"	60"
d.	100	3"	72"

9. The photographic properties of a radiograph consist of the following elements:
   a. recorded detail
   b. density and contrast
   c. magnification and distortion
   d. a and b
   e. a and c

10. The primary purpose of a grid is to reduce the effects of _____ on the image.
    a. density
    b. contrast
    c. scattered radiation
    d. all of the above

11. When any of several combinations of mA and T will produce an equivalent amount of mAs, the result is called:
    a. Ohm's Law
    b. reciprocity law
    c. inverse square law
    d. none of the above

12. Heat unit (HU) capacity is determined by the following formula:
    a. $mA \times T$
    b. $mA \times kVp$
    c. $mA \times T \times kVp$
    d. $mA \times T \times kVp^2$

13. *The intensity of radiation is inversely proportional to the square of the distance* expresses the relationship between:
    a. distance and density
    b. distance and contrast
    c. distance and focal-spot size
    d. distance and radiation intensity

14. A change in SID from an original position of 40 inches to an increased position of 60 inches will change the following effect of _____.
    a. density (mA)
    b. intensity (SID)
    c. penetration (kVp)
    d. all of the above

15. The term "geometric blur" or penumbra is associated with the effects of the following factor(s):
    a. FSS
    b. SID
    c. OID
    d. a and c
    e. a, b, and c

16. When a standard 40 inches SID is used, the approximate amount of magnification of most radiographic images would be:
    a. 1.5
    b. 1.75
    c. 1.1
    d. 2.0

17. Primary beam filtration may be achieved by the use of a device (or devices) known as a:
    a. diaphragm
    b. cone
    c. collimator
    d. all of the above

18. The total amount of minimal beam filtration is:
    a. 2.0 mm
    b. 2.5 mm
    c. 0.5 mm
    d. none of the above

19. Which one of the grid ratios listed below is more efficient than the others?
    a. 5:1
    b. 8:1
    c. 16:1
    d. no one is more efficient than the others

20. The magnification factor may be represented by the following formula:
    a. $\dfrac{SID}{SOD}$
    b. $\dfrac{SID}{SID - OID}$
    c. $\dfrac{Image\,Width}{Object\,Width}$
    d. a and c

REFERENCES

Carlton, R. R., & Adler, A. M. (2006). *Principles of radiographic imaging: An art and a science* (4th ed.). Clifton Park, NY: Thomson Delmar Learning.

Quinn, R. A., & Sigi, C. C. (Eds.). (1980). *Radiography in modern industry*. Rochester, NY: Eastman Kodak Company.

SUGGESTED READINGS

Bushong, S. C. (1997). *Radiologic science for technologists: Physics, biology and protection.* (6th ed.). St. Louis, MO: Mosby, Inc.

Curry, T. S., Dowdey, J. E., & Murry, R. C. (1984). *Christensen's introduction to the physics of diagnostic radiology* (3rd ed.). Philadelphia: Lea & Febiger.

Papp, J. (2006). *Quality management in the imaging sciences.* (3rd ed.). St. Louis, MO: Mosby, Inc.

Quinn, C. B. (2003). *Fuch's radiography exposure, processing and quality control* (6th ed.). Springfield, IL: Charles C. Thomas.

Thompson, M. A., Hallaway, M. P., Hall, J. D., & David, S. B. (1999). *Principles of imaging science and protection*. Philadelphia: W. B. Saunders Company.

CHAPTER 10

DIGITAL RADIOGRAPHY AND PICTURE ARCHIVING AND COMMUNICATION SYSTEMS (PACS)

Key Terms

Analog-to-Digital Converter (ADC)

Bit Depth

Computed Radiography (CR)

Digital to Analog Converter (DAC)

Digital Imaging

Digital Imaging and Communications in Medicine (DICOM)

Digital Imaging Processing

Digital Image Production

Digital Radiography (DR)

Direct Capture

Exposure Index Number

Exposure Index Value

Hospital Information System (HIS)

Matrix

Photostimulable Phosphor (PSP)

Picture Archiving and Communication System (PACS)

Pixel

Radiology Information System (RIS)

Teleradiology

Voxel

Chapter Outline

Introduction
Digital Imaging
Image Method
Digital Image Production
Look-Up Tables (LUT)
PACS, HIS, RIS, and DICOM
Quality Control in CR

Objectives

Upon completion of the chapter, the student will meet the following objectives by verifying knowledge of the facts and principles presented through oral and written communication at a level deemed competent.

❍ Compare digital radiography to screen/film radiography.
❍ Define computed radiography.
❍ Explain direct capture radiography.
❍ Explain digital image production.
❍ Describe Picture Archiving and Communications Systems (PACS).

⊃ Define photostimulable phosphor (PSP).
⊃ Explain digital image processing.
⊃ Identify the purpose of Digital Imaging and Communication in Medicine (DICOM).

Introduction

Computerized radiography has advanced imaging technology in ways that provide increased image quality as well as quality control. Every element of capturing, storing, and reproducing an image has become more efficient. Equally important in imaging is information or data. This too may be achieved through a computed system. Activities related to handling, maintaining, and storing medical imaging records are performed through picture archiving and communication systems or PACS (Figure 10-1). It is therefore very important for the student to have an understanding of computer fundamentals as they relate to advanced imaging techniques.

Digital Imaging

Using computers as opposed to conventional analog film/screen methods produces digital radiographic images. That is, digital images look like conventional film/screen images but are acquired through computerized devices. This type of radiography, however, provides much wider exposure latitudes than film/screen methods. **Digital imaging** has other advantages over film/screen (analog) radiography. First, darkrooms and film are not needed, and electronic storage makes no film storage area necessary. Second, hard copies may be obtained any time, thus, original images are always accessible. Third, images may be electronically transmitted over distances to other health care facilities; this is called **teleradiology**. Fourth, one of the best features of digital processing is that images may be enhanced. Contrast and detail may be electronically manipulated through software programs; this is referred to as image postprocessing.

Image Method

Digital imaging processing is computer generated. It is based on several concepts including a number related to physics, mathematics, engineering, and computer science. Also, digital image processing dates back to early programs of the National Aeronautics and Space Administration (NASA). Computed radiographic images

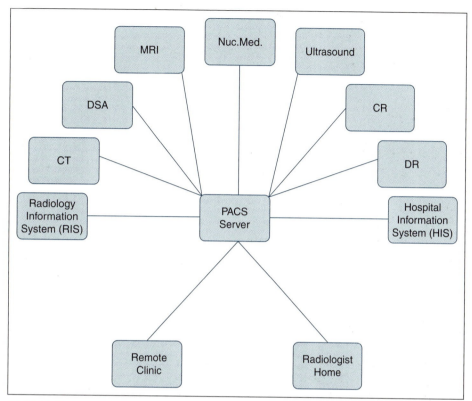

FIGURE 10-1 The Picture Archieving and Communication System (PACS) is a systematic method of connecting all digital information for the purpose of communication and storage within the hospital. The heart of the PACS system is the mainframe server. Additional information systems communicating with the PACS server include the Radiology Information System (RIS) and the Hospital Information System (HIS).
Source: Delmar, Cengage Learning.

may be acquired through different processes. Elements of a computed digital image consist of a **matrix, pixels** (picture elements), **voxels** (volume of tissue), and **bit depth**. A matrix is the basic formation of a two-dimensional image that consists of columns (M) and rows (N). The columns and rows make up small areas called squares. The square elements are called pixels.

The relationship between M and N is square when $M = N$. The size of the image is shown in the relationship $M \times N \times k$ bits. The radiographer or operator determines matrix size, also referred to as the field of view (FOV). When produced with digital imaging processing, digital images of human anatomy are rectangular. Image detail or spatial resolution is produced by the size of the matrix (Figures 10-2A and 10-2B). An increase in the matrix size within the same FOV produces a better image.

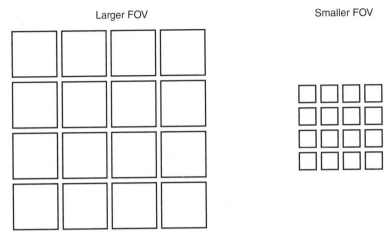

FIGURE 10-2A With the same matrix (5 × 5), a larger field-of-view (FOV) will result in an image with less resolution and a smaller FOV will result in an image with more resolution.
Source: Delmar, Cengage Learning.

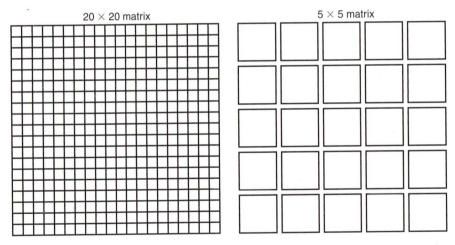

FIGURE10-2B With the same FOV, a 20 × 20 matrix will produce more image resolution and a 5 × 5 matrix will produce an image with less resolution.
Source: Delmar, Cengage Learning.

Relatedly, a decrease in the FOV without a decrease in the matrix size will result in a decrease in pixel size and greater image detail.

As stated previously, pixel means picture element and is the smallest piece of a two-dimensional, rectangular image array of square pixels that make up the matrix. Smaller pixels result in better spatial resolution. According to Seeram, "Each pixel contains a number (discrete value) that represents a brightness level. The numbers correspond to the tissue characteristics being imaged" (2004). In radiography and CT, these numbers are related to the atomic number and mass density of the anatomical tissues. Further, pixel size may be determined using pixel size = FOV/matrix, that is, spatial resolution is better, the larger the matrix and the smaller the pixel size with the same FOV (Figures 10-2A and 10-2B).

Voxel represents volume of pixels. The pixels in the digital image represent the information contained in a volume of tissue. This volume of information is converted into numerical values contained in the pixels, the numbers are assigned brightness levels. In the previously mentioned relationship M × N × k bits, k bits means that each pixel in the digital image matrix M × N represents k binary digits. The number of bits per pixel is the bit depth, which determines the number of shades of gray that affects the density resolution of the image. Simply explained, each pixel has 2^k gray levels; the binary system uses base 2 k bits = 2^k. A bit depth of 8 would be 2^8 (256) shades of gray (Figure 10-3).

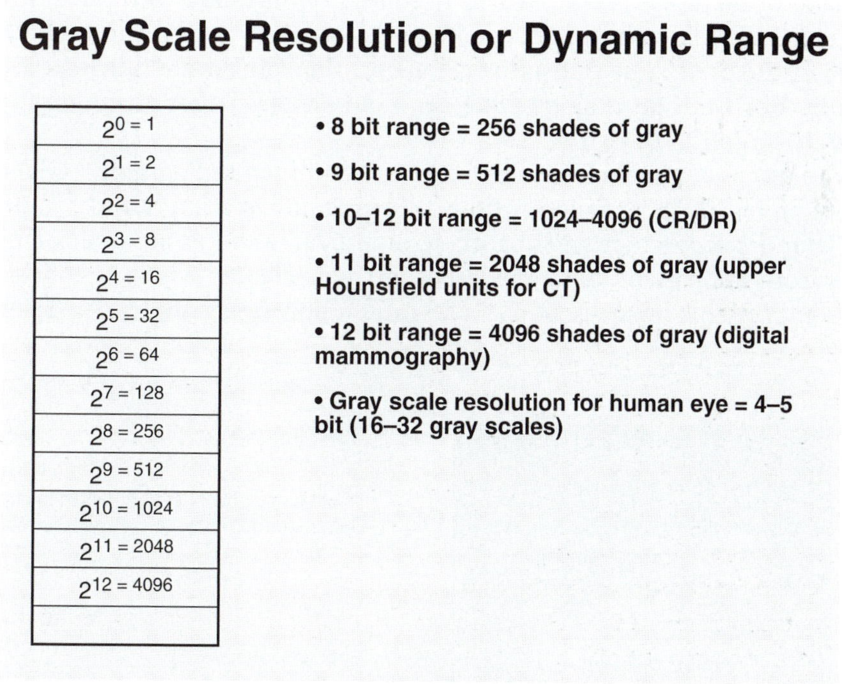

Gray Scale Resolution or Dynamic Range

$2^0 = 1$
$2^1 = 2$
$2^2 = 4$
$2^3 = 8$
$2^4 = 16$
$2^5 = 32$
$2^6 = 64$
$2^7 = 128$
$2^8 = 256$
$2^9 = 512$
$2^{10} = 1024$
$2^{11} = 2048$
$2^{12} = 4096$

- 8 bit range = 256 shades of gray
- 9 bit range = 512 shades of gray
- 10–12 bit range = 1024–4096 (CR/DR)
- 11 bit range = 2048 shades of gray (upper Hounsfield units for CT)
- 12 bit range = 4096 shades of gray (digital mammography)
- Gray scale resolution for human eye = 4–5 bit (16–32 gray scales)

FIGURE 10-3 With a bit system ranging from 2^0 to 2^{12}, any given pixel within the digital image can display from 1 to 4096 different shades of gray.
Source: Delmar, Cengage Learning.

Digital Image Production

In film-screen radiography, the radiographer places the patient into a position on the radiographic table or in a standing position in front of a cassette holder on the wall. The patient is then exposed as the appropriate amount of radiation traverses the anatomy being examined, which creates a latent image on the film. The film is then chemically processed to make the image visible. The finished radiograph is then passed along to the radiologist for interpretation. Many things can happen during this entire process to cause a film to be of poor quality.

By contrast, both **computed radiography (CR)** and **digital radiography (DR)** offer more advantages for image accuracy and enhancement. **Digital image production** components include data acquisition; image processing; image display, storage, and archiving; and image communication.

Data acquisition refers to recording patient information through electron density receptors. This process involves the x-ray tube and digital image receptors rather than intensifying screen/film. The CR image receptor consists of an imaging plate made of metal on plastic, which is coated on one side with photostimulable phosphors (PSP). The phosphor is coated in a layer less than 1 mm in thickness on one side of the plate. The phosphor is barium fluorobromide lubricated with europium Ba Fbr Eu. The imaging plate can hold a static latent image up to 6 hours (Figures 10-4A and 10-4B).

Before discussing the differences between computed radiography (CR) and digital radiography (DR), let us look at the following information outline on processes. Both CR and DR interact and absorb remnant radiation as an analog image that emerges from the patient; thus, the latent image is created which is converted into a digital image. This image is converted in the following examples. As described by

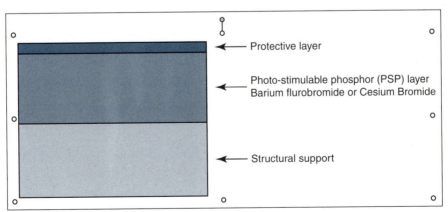

FIGURE 10-4A Cross-sectional area of the computed radiography PSP screen comprised of the protective layer, PSP layer, and structural support
Source: Delmar, Cengage Learning.

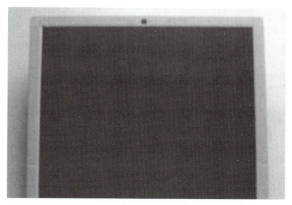

FIGURE 10-4B The inside of the CR cassette contains a phosphor screen that absorbs the radiation signal and stores it as a latent image. The phosphor screen holds the static latent image up to 6 hours before diminishing.
Source: Delmar, Cengage Learning.

Seeram (2004), a digital imaging system works as an analog-digital-analog process (Figure 10-5). Explanations of the system components in Figure 10-5 follow.

- Data acquisition is analog and includes the x-ray tube and image detectors (output signals).
- **Analog to digital converter (ADC)**, changes analog signal to digital image of patient part being examined.
- Computer processing involves producing an output digital image through the binary number system. It is here that the input image can be changed by reducing image noise or by enhancing contrast and sharpness.

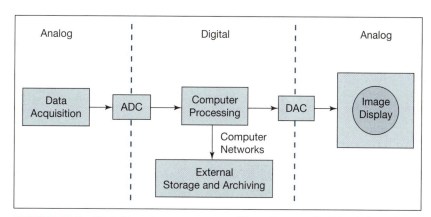

FIGURE 10-5 Digital imaging components *(From Seeram, E. (2004). Digital image processing.* Radiologic Technology, 75(6), 435–452.)

- **Digital to analog converter (DAC),** is a process in which the digital image is converted into an analog signal that can be displayed on a monitor. It is at this point where images are preserved in storage and archived on magnetic tapes, disks, or laser optical disks. Images may be communicated electronically through computer networks to remote sites. Picture archiving communication systems (PACS) are generally used in updated radiology departments.
- Image display takes place when the digital signal that has been converted to an analog image is displayed on a monitor.

Figure 10-6 provides a visual expression of the film/screen system. The system is analog and depends on the transmission of radiation distribution through the patient (image) on film and screen coated with crystals, which cause a continuous light intensity in each specific location on the part being imaged. The digital imaging system in Figure 10-7 reflects a more involved system (see also Figure 10-5).

CR requires processing of the phosphor imaging cassette. DR (also called **direct capture,** direct-to-digital [DDR]) involves no cassette; therefore, no processing is needed as seen in Figure 10-7. This figure shows a digital image that is a numerical representation production of the digital image.

The terms computed radiography (CR) and digital radiography (DR) are used interchangeably. However there are distinct differences between the two imaging systems.

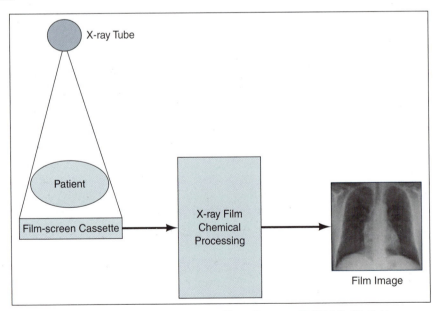

FIGURE 10-6 Film-based imaging steps *(From Seeram, E. (2004). Digital image processing. Radiologic Technology, 75(6), 435–452.)*

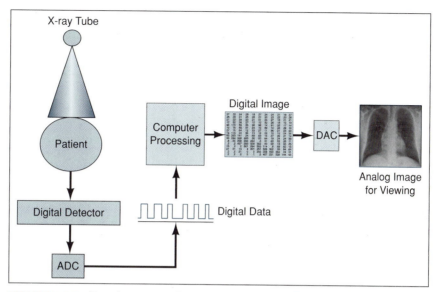

FIGURE 10-7 Digital image production *(From Seeram, E. (2004). Digital image processing.* Radiologic Technology, 75*(6), 435–452.)*

In CR (also known as a cassette-based system), the image receptor or cassette is placed in a special processor known as the CR reader. Once inside the CR reader, the cassette is opened and a **photostimulable phosphor (PSP)** screen is exposed to a laser beam. As the laser beam scans over the PSP, the screen glows and emits visible light. The amount of visible light emitted by the PSP is converted into an analog signal representing the anatomy being radiographed. From here, the analog-to-digital converter (ADC) changes the analog image signal into a digital image signal. Before the CR cassette is removed from the reader unit, the PSP screen is exposed to a bright sodium vapor lamp. The intense exposure erases any residual image on the PSP screen. The digital data are further processed with special proprietary software and the resultant anatomical image is displayed on a visual monitor. Figure 10-8 illustrates the steps and sequence in CR image formation.

While performing CR, the technologist must observe the **exposure index number** (also known as the sensitivity or S-number or Lgm Log Median exposure). An improper exposure index indicates that the image values **exposure index value** will vary among manufacturers and the proprietary software used for reconstructing the CR image.

With DR (also known as direct capture or a cassetteless-based system), no separate image reader unit is required to process the radiographic image. As with all new technologies, these systems are very expensive. Typically, the DR image

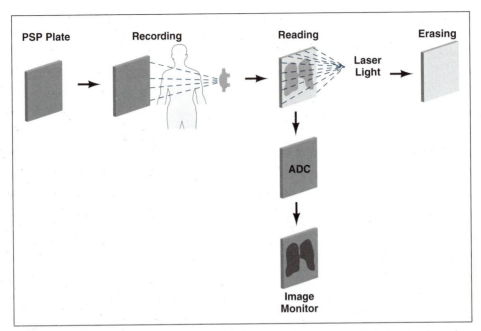

FIGURE 10-8 The steps in the computed radiography (CR) process include a traditional x-ray exposure of the anatomical part using a cassette containing a PSP plate. The PSP plate holds the latent image. After exposure, the cassette is placed in the CR reader where the PSP plate is removed and scanned with a laser light. The laser light interacts with the PSP plate causing the phosphor crystals to emit a visible light signal representing the latent image. This light signal is digitized via the analog-to-digital (ADC) converter. The computer processes this digital information with special mathematical formulas. When an optimal level of density and contrast is obtained, the image is displayed on the image monitor. The final step in this process is to erase any residual latent image left on the PSP screen. Once erased, the PSP plate can be reused to take another image. *(Courtesy of Carestream Health, Inc.)*

receptor is constructed inside the wall or table Bucky and consists of an active matrix array (AMA) of detector elements (DELs) and thin-film transistors (TFTs). The array of DELs captures the remnant radiation or analog signal representing an anatomical image. The TFTs assist the DELs in releasing the analog signal from the AMA. From here, the analog signal is routed through the ADC. The digital data representing the anatomical image are further processed with special proprietary software, and the resultant anatomical image is displayed on a visual monitor. After the DR exposure has been made and the image is processed, the AMA discharges and releases any residual image remaining behind the image receptor. At this point, the cassetteless-based system is ready to use again (Figures 10-9A and 10-9B).

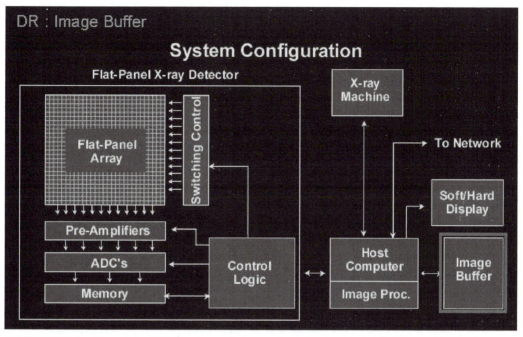

FIGURE 10-9A Overview of the components in the direct capture or digital radiography system *(Courtesy of Carestream Health, Inc.)*

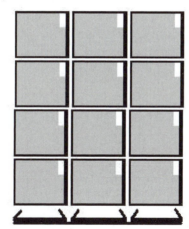

FIGURE 10-9B The DR imaging system contains an flat panel array of detector elements (also known as an active matrix array). Each detector element contains a thin-film-transistor (TFT) that aids in the production of a direct-captured digital image.
Source: Delmar, Cengage Learning.

Look-Up Tables (LUT)

CR and DR imaging systems are highly automated. All digital systems have greater latitude; thus, a wider range of radiation exposures produces an optimal radiograph. Radiographers should remain cautious and continue to use their technique guides or charts for setting proper radiation settings. Additionally, they should not adopt the philosophy that one large amount of radiation exposure can be used on all patient examinations regardless of body habitus and size. Such a practice, which is unethical, leads to an increase in radiation exposure to the patient population as well as to the occupational worker.

When a CR or DR image receptor receives an optimum radiation exposure, the look-up table (LUT) menu sets the proper density and contrast scale for each anatomical part being radiographed. With CR, the PSP plate is exposed first. The correct LUT is selected prior to placing the PSP plate into the CR reader. In DR, the LUT is selected on the control panel prior to making the anatomical exposure. Figure 10-10 illustrates a LUT for spine imaging.

PACS, HIS, RIS, and DICOM

Throughout the radiology department, digital information and data are obtained from all imaging modalities. Large amounts of digital data must be systemically connected for archiving and communication purposes. The **picture archiving and**

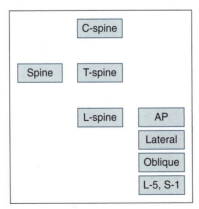

FIGURE 10-10 The look-up table (LUT) is used in both CR and DR imaging. After the analog signal is converted into a digital signal, the LUT sets the proper density and contrast scale for the image.
Source: Delmar, Cengage Learning.

communication system (PACS) provides a systematic network for sending, receiving, and storing all digital images within the medical imaging department. The heart of any PACS system is the mainframe computer server containing proprietary software. Numerous PACS workstations may be distributed all over the imaging department to facilitate workflow (see Figure 10-1). Compared to film/screen radiography, PACS increases efficiency within the department. Multiple users within or outside the imaging facility can view images simultaneously.

PACS can easily interface with the hospital information system (HIS) and the radiology information system (RIS). HIS enables electronic communication and workflow for many areas within the hospital. An example of the HIS includes networking databases for medical records, billing, and electronic charting. The RIS included databases for all imaging procedures. Typically, personnel access the RIS to generate a request to perform a specific medical imaging procedure. Another important software link to the PACS and the RIS is known as digital imaging and communication in medicine (DICOM). DICOM transfers images and other medical information between computers. Essentially, DICOM enables standardization between diagnostic and therapeutic equipment and systems from various manufacturers.

Quality Control in CR

As with film screen radiography, quality control procedures must be performed on digital x-ray equipment and other peripheral devices. Quality control can be defined as a procedure or test used to determine if the unit is performing at optimal levels. Optimal performance means that the equipment is performing according to a set standard or benchmark. The quality control procedures in CR and DR can be categorized into hardware artifacts, software artifacts, and patient positioning artifacts.

Hardware artifacts can occur in the PSP plate, the CR reader, and the hard copy laser printer. The most common causes of CR imaging artifacts are dust, dirt, and scratches on the PSP plate. If the CR plate is not sufficiently erased, a phantom or residual image left over from the previous imaging procedure may contaminate the image of a future imaging procedure. A phantom or residual image will take on the appearance of a double exposed image (i.e., two images on one plate). At times, the CR reader can malfunction causing skipped scan lines leading to a distorted image. As the CR reader ages, the red laser light used to extract the latent image from the PSP screen weakens over time, thus degrading the CR image.

Software artifacts may result from the improper selection of various CR processing parameters resulting in an incorrect histogram analysis, improper dynamic range scaling, and incorrect optical densities and pixel values. Excessive scatter radiation contacting the PSP plate has major consequences on image quality. Too much scatter results in an incorrect histogram analysis of the latent image read from the PSP plate.

Technologist error resulting from improper positioning may cause digital imaging artifacts. Positioning error artifacts include random drop-off of optical density throughout the image, the appearance of a "halo" around the edges of the anatomy, and an incorrect histogram analysis due to too much scatter. If the technologist underexposes a specific procedure, insufficient signal stored in the image receptor could possibly lead to poor image quality.

A common QC tool used in digital radiography is the Society of Motion Picture and Television Engineers (SMPTE) test pattern (Figure 10-11). The SMPTE test pattern consists of a series of horizontal and vertical lines used for measuring spatial resolution. Additional box patterns consisting of shades of black, gray, and white are used to measure levels of contrast resolution. The SMPTE test pattern is

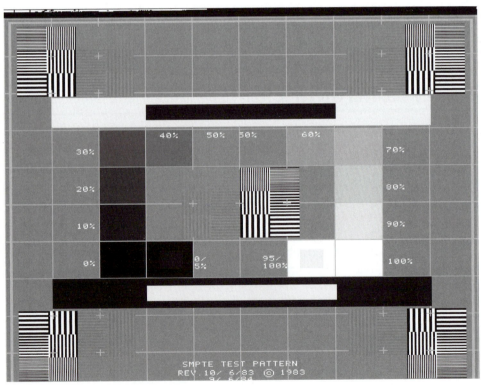

FIGURE 10-11 The SMPTE test pattern is used to evaluate the imaging monitors and laser printers. The SMPTE test pattern measures the spatial and contrast resolution within the digital imaging system. *(Courtesy of Society of Motion Picture and Television Engineers [SMPTE])*

performed quarterly to evaluate consistency among the numerous image monitors and laser printers within the department.

Prior to the start of the workday, the technologist should erase all CR plates to minimize the possibility of a double-exposed image. This is a good practice since a previously exposed PSP plate may retain a residual image. Erasing all CR cassettes will minimize accidental double exposures and minimize patient exposure due to unnecessary repeats.

REVIEW QUESTIONS

1. A major feature of digital processing is:
    1. image production
    2. contrast and detail enhancement
    3. electronic manipulation of the image

    Possible Responses

    a. 1 and 2
    b. 1 and 3
    c. 2 and 3
    d. 1, 2, and 3

2. Gray scale resolution may be referred to as:
    a. archiving
    b. dynamic range
    c. image plate
    d. data acquisition

3. The photostimulable phosphors which are image receptors and are coated on metal or plastic plate in a layer are:
    a. less than 1 mm thick
    b. 2 mm thick
    c. 1.5 mm thick
    d. less than 0.5 mm thick

4. Manipulating contrast and detail through software programs is referred to as:
    a. digital imaging processing
    b. picture elements
    c. postprocessing
    d. matrix formation

5. Technologists may cause digital imaging artifacts by positioning patients improperly, which results in:
   1. a halo around the edges of the anatomy.
   2. drop-off of optical density
   3. an incorrect histogram analysis because of too much scatter

   Possible Responses

   a. 1 and 3
   b. 1 and 2
   c. 1, 2, and 3

REFERENCE

Seeram, E. (2004). Digital image processing. *Radiologic Technology, 75*(6), 435–452.

SUGGESTED READINGS

Carlton, R. R. & Adler, A. M. (2006). *Principles of radiographic imaging: An art and a science* (4th ed.). Clifton Park, NY: Thomson Delmar Learning.

Papp, J. (2002). *Quality management in the imaging sciences* (2nd ed.). St. Louis, MO: C. V. Mosby.

Quinn, C. B. (1993). *Fuch's radiography exposure, processing and quality control* (5th ed.). Springfield, IL: Charles C. Thomas.

Seeram, E. (2005). Digital image compression. *Radiologic Technology, 76*(6), 449–459.

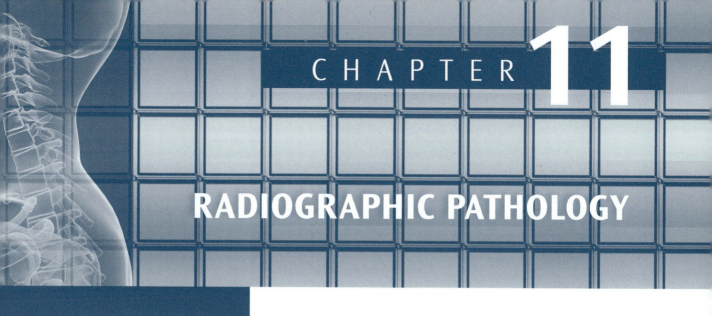

CHAPTER 11

RADIOGRAPHIC PATHOLOGY

Key Terms

Acromegaly
Acute Disease
Air bronchograms
Anasarca
Aplasia
Ascites
Atrophy
Attenuation
Avulsion
Barton's Fracture
Benign
Bennett's Fracture/Dislocation
Boxer's Fracture
Bursitis
Carpal Tunnel Syndrome
Chauffeur's Fracture
Chondrosarcoma
Chronic Disease
Clay Shoveler's Fracture
Colles' Fracture
Congenital
Contusion
Degenerative Diseases
Diagnosis
Dislocation
Dysplasia

Chapter Outline

Overview
Introduction to Pathology
  Additive and Destructive Pathology
  Etiology
Chest and Bony Thorax Pathology and Imaging
Considerations
  Anatomy Overview of the Bony Thorax and Chest
  Plain Chest X-Ray Examination
  Radiographic Pathology of the Chest
  Occupational Lung Diseases
  Lesser-Known Lung Diseases
  Lung Cancer
  Respiratory and Cardiovascular Diseases and Conditions
  The Bony Thorax
Extremities: Pathology and Imaging Considerations
  Introduction
  Trauma Radiography
  Osteoarthritis
The Upper Extremity
  The Hand and Fingers

Objectives

Upon completion of the chapter, the student will meet the following objectives by verifying knowledge of the facts and principles presented through oral and written communication at a level deemed competent.

⊃ Define key terminology related to pathology and related imaging considerations.

⊃ Identify additive and destructive diseases that have an impact on the selection of the x-ray exposure factors.

⊃ Select the appropriate change in the exposure factors when additive and destructive diseases are present.

⊃ Recognize common diseases and conditions of the chest, bony thorax, extremities, vertebral spine, and abdomen and recall facts about each that may impact the standard positioning routine and selection of the technical x-ray exposure factors.

⊃ Discuss the limited radiographer's role in imaging abuse.

Overview

Radiography has a significant role in the diagnosis and monitoring of diseases and injuries. The limited radiographer's role is to consistently produce high-quality radiographs so that physicians have the necessary information they need to make an accurate diagnosis. To accomplish this task, limited radiographers should be familiar with the radiographic appearance and etiology (origin) of the most significant diseases and injuries, as well as a prognosis (likely outcome) and current treatment protocols. Also of importance to the limited radiographer is the knowledge that certain diseases or injuries may require changes in the radiographic routine. Examples of such changes include:

- Alteration in the selection of technical x-ray exposure factors.
- Adaptation of routine positioning to accommodate the patient's condition.
- Additional care and attention to the patient prior to, during, and after the x-ray examination.

This chapter provides an introduction to the vast and complex subject of radiographic pathology. In an attempt to provide adequate and practical information, the authors selected topics that the limited radiographer is likely to encounter. The selections were dictated by the premise that the scope of practice for limited radiography is generally confined to imaging examinations that do not require the use of contrast agents. Whenever possible, the authors have attempted to provide a link between pathology, selection, and alteration of technical x-ray exposure factors, and modification of standard patient positioning.

Radiographers are encouraged to seek additional information as needed in textbooks and resources dedicated to human pathology, radiographic anatomy, and positioning.

Introduction to Pathology

The term *pathology* originates from the Greek term *pathos* which means suffering. Pathology, a branch of the medical sciences, attempts to discover the nature of disease and its causes, processes, development, and consequences. A disease is considered to be any abnormal disturbance of function or structure of the human body. The term pathogenesis refers to the origin and development of a disease, which leads to noticeable changes or manifestations (signs and symptoms). Physicians use signs and symptoms as key indicators of disease or injury. Once a diagnosis has been made, the physician may be able to give a prognosis (duration and outcome) of the disease.

Physicians use signs, which are objective in nature, to arrive at a probable diagnosis. Patients present with both objective and subjective information about their condition. An objective sign or symptom is a manifestation that can be seen, heard, or measured by any observer. Examples include such conditions as swelling, fever, bruising, hemorrhage, and so on. While objective signs and symptoms are evident to the observer, the physician also considers the patients' subjective account. A subjective sign or symptom is one that is known by the patient but cannot be seen or measured by the physician. An example of a subjective sign is when the patient states that they have had nausea and vomiting for the past three days.

Signs and symptoms are important diagnostic indicators since their presence or absence provides key information allowing differentiation between diseases and the extent and stage of the disease. When a patient has no symptoms, they are referred to as asymptomatic.

When evaluating symptoms, a physician will consider the beginning date and nature of the onset and whether any causative factors were present. Other considerations include the nature, location, severity, and timing of symptoms as well as aggravating or relieving factors associated with the presenting symptom(s).

An iatrogenic disease is one that is caused by the medical treatment itself. When the underlying cause of a disease is unknown, it is referred to as idiopathic. Acute diseases that have a fast onset but last a short period of time are referred to as acute diseases. An example of an acute disease is chickenpox, caused by the varicella virus. A chronic disease usually has a slow onset but may last for an extended length of time. Examples of common chronic diseases include diabetes, emphysema, and hypertension.

The human body reacts to pathogenic processes. These reactions allow physicians to use diagnostic tools, such as imaging procedures and laboratory tests, to discover the cause and to arrive at a diagnosis and treatment. A few of the basic human responses to pathogenic processes include inflammation, edema, ischemia and infarction, hemorrhage, and abnormal cell growth.

Inflammation is the body's response to invasion by microorganisms such as viruses, bacteria, and fungi. The human body responds to invasion by attempting to localize the injurious entity with the inflammation process. There are various forms of inflammation ranging from acute to chronic. The five clinical signs that indicate acute inflammation are redness, heat, swelling, pain, and loss of function. Infection is an inflammatory process in response to a disease-causing organism. Edema, ascites, and hydrocephalus are terms referring to an abnormal accumulation of fluid.

Edema is the accumulation of abnormal amounts of fluid in the intercellular tissue spaces or body cavities. Edema can be localized (e.g., trauma to the knee or ankle joint), or generalized with swelling of the subcutaneous tissues throughout the body (anasarca).

Ascites is the term used for fluid accumulation within the peritoneal cavity. Hydrocephalus refers to dilation or widening of the ventricles and is associated with increased intracranial pressure.

The presence of any abnormal accumulation of fluid (edema, ascites, and hydrocephalus) within a body cavity results in increased tissue density (thickness) and generally requires an increase in the technical x-ray exposure factors.

Ischemia and infarction are terms that are used in reference to the cardiovascular system. Ischemia is the disruption of the blood supply to an organ or part of an organ depriving cells and tissues of oxygen and nutrients. Ischemia may occur if a blood clot (thrombus) or foreign substance, such as a cholesterol plaque or fat (embolus) lodges in a vessel. Infarction is a localized area of necrosis (death) resulting from a sudden insufficiency of arterial or venous blood supply. The most common types of infarction also referred to as occlusion are myocardial and pulmonary.

Hemorrhage refers to rupture of a blood vessel, either an artery or a vein. Hemorrhage may be external or internal within a body cavity. An abnormal accumulation of blood within the tissues, joint spaces, or body cavities causes increased tissue density. Whenever a pathological process results in increased tissue density (e.g., edema and ascites), the limited radiographer will generally need to make adjustments in the technical x-ray exposure factors.

Terminology associated with changes in the size and quantity of cells include atrophy, aplasia, hypertrophy, hyperplasia, and dysplasia. Atrophy refers to a wasting or decrease in the size of tissues, organs, or the entire body. Atrophy can occur due to the reabsorption of cells, diminished cellular growth, pressure, ischemia, malnutrition, decreased cellular function, or hormonal changes. A similar but different term is aplasia, which refers to the failure of a body part or organ. The term also refers to the congenital absence of an organ or tissue. Hyperplasia refers to excessive proliferation of normal cells in the normal tissue arrangement of an organ.

Hypertrophy refers to the general increase in bulk or size of a part or organ and is not related to tumor formation. Hypertrophy often develops in response to increased use or function of the part or organ. For example, in response to certain cardiovascular diseases, the heart size often increases as it attempts to compensate for a decline in heart muscle functioning. Dysplasia is abnormal tissue development that often results from prolonged chronic irritation or inflammation.

Additive and Destructive Pathology

As the human body responds to various diseases and conditions the affected tissues, organs, and systems may either increase or decrease in composition (i.e., density/thickness). It is important for the limited radiographer to recognize which diseases and conditions may cause such changes as it may be necessary to make adjustments in the technical x-ray exposure factors.

Additive diseases and conditions cause increased tissue density and usually require an increase in the technical x-ray exposure factors. Diseases that cause a decrease in tissue density are referred to as destructive. Figure 11-1 lists common examples of additive and destructive diseases and conditions.

As certain diseases progress, the number and/or types of atoms in the affected tissue may change. These changes can have a direct influence on the attenuation (absorption) of the x-ray beam by the affected tissue, and ultimately the selection of the technical x-ray exposure factors. In destructive type diseases, a decrease in the affected body tissue occurs, thus less attenuation (absorption) of the x-ray beam.

If the limited radiographer is aware of the patient's medical history or a possible diagnosis, prior to the x-ray examination, a change in the technical x-ray exposure factors can be made, thus reducing the number of unnecessary retake examinations. If a destructive disease is present, the limited radiographer can decrease the technical x-ray exposure factors. Likewise if an additive disease condition is present, the radiographer can increase the technical x-ray exposure factors.

Additive (increased attenuation) Disease & Conditions
- Acromegaly
- Congestive heart failure
- Hydrocephalus
- Paget's disease
- Pulmonary edema

Destructive (decreased attenuation) Diseases & Conditions
- Active tuberculosis
- Atrophy (either from disease or lack of use)
- Multiple myeloma
- Osteporosis

FIGURE 11-1 Additive and destructive diseases and conditions
Source: Delmar, Cengage Learning.

To summarize, additive type disease processes generally require an increase in the technical x-ray exposure factors in order to adequately penetrate the anatomic area; whereas, destructive diseases generally require a decrease in the technical x-ray exposure factors.

The 15% kilovoltage (kVp) rule may be used to make the technical x-ray exposure factor adjustments. For example, if the limited radiographer has information that indicates an additive condition exists in the part being examined, an increase in the kVp may be used. According to the 15% kVp rule, a 15% increase in kVp is equivalent to doubling the milliamperage-seconds (mAs). Also, according to the 15% kVp rule, a 15% decrease in kVp is equivalent to decreasing the mAs by half or 50%. If adjustments in the technical x-ray exposure factors are needed for skeletal radiographic procedures the 15% kVp rule is the preferred method. Kilovoltage controls the penetrability of the x-ray beam and ultimately the visible scale of contrast on the radiograph. Changes in the technical x-ray exposure factors for skeletal x-ray examinations usually do not require more than 5 to 10 kVp, and thus do not significantly alter the visible scale of contrast on the radiograph.

To review, the 15% kVp rule is generally applied to radiographs of the skeleton, whereas increases in technical x-ray exposure factors for chest radiographs are made with the milliamperage (mA). For additional information on the 15% kVp rule and other technical factor adjustments, refer to Chapter 9, Fundamentals of Radiographic Exposures, and Chapter 10, Digital Radiography and Picture Archiving and Communication System (PACS).

Unless the limited radiographer has access to previous radiographs with recorded technical x-ray exposure factors the initial x-ray exposures should be made using a standardized technique chart. The exception to this statement is when the limited radiographer has information about the presence of an additive or destructive disease. In this situation, it is best for the radiographer to start with the technical x-ray exposure factors on a standardized technique chart and make adjustments as necessary to the technical x-ray exposure factors.

The presence, stage, and extent of disease processes may not be known prior to performing the x-ray examination. Many variables make it difficult and sometimes impossible to predict how the presence of pathological processes will affect the production of a diagnostic radiograph. The limited radiographer must carefully review the x-ray examination request, obtain as much information as possible about the patient's history, and observe and evaluate the patient in order to select proper technical x-ray exposure factors. During the pre-examination period, the limited radiographer should evaluate the patient to determine if adjustments in the standard positioning routines might be necessary.

The American College of Radiology (ACR) is a professional organization that includes radiologists, radiation oncologists, medical physicists, interventional radiologists, and nuclear medicine physicians. For more than 75 years the ACR has had as its goal safety in imaging. A few of the other ACR objectives include serving patients and society by maximizing the value of imaging, advancing the science of radiology, and improving the quality of patient care.

Leading the way in radiology, ACR committees consisting of esteemed members develop guidelines designed to assist physicians in providing appropriate radiological care for patients. These guidelines are intended to establish a legal standard of care and as such can serve to guide the limited radiographer in performing x-ray examinations. *The ACR Practice Guideline for General Radiography* states that, "the goal of radiography is to establish the presence or absence and nature of disease by demonstration of the disease process itself or the effects of the disease process on the normal anatomy" (American College of Radiology [ACR], 1996). All involved in the performance of general radiography should conduct imaging studies with the minimal radiation dose necessary to achieve a diagnostic radiograph. Limited radiographers should conduct all imaging procedures using the ALARA concept (i.e., as low as reasonably achievable). The ACR encourages all imaging facilities to have policies and procedures to reasonably attempt to identify pregnant patients prior to any imaging procedures involving ionizing radiation (ACR, 1996). For additional information about ALARA and x-ray examination during pregnancy, refer to Chapter 16, Radiation Protection.

The limited radiographer should be provided with a written or electronic request for x-ray examinations. This request should provide sufficient information that includes signs and symptoms and/or relevant history (including known diagnoses) (ACR, 1996). Also the ACR lists the following minimum requirements for general radiography that should be followed in order to render a diagnostic radiographic image (ACR, 1996):

- All radiographs should be permanently labeled with the patient and facility information, examination date, image orientation, and the side (right or left) of the anatomic site being examined.
- All facilities performing general radiography should have routines for standard projections of each anatomic area to be radiographed.
- Appropriate collimation should be used to limit x-ray exposure to the anatomic area of interest.
- A technique chart listing technical x-ray exposure factors that will reliably produce diagnostic radiographs of anatomic parts of patients of different sizes should be available.
- All radiographs should be reviewed for positioning and diagnostic quality at the facility before the patient is released.
- Repeat radiographs should be performed when necessary for diagnostic quality and repeat rates should be part of the quality control process.

- All facilities producing radiographs should have policies and procedures for appropriate shielding of patients.
- All facilities should have immobilization and assistance procedures appropriate for the age and size range of patients to be imaged; including patients who are unable to cooperate, or unable to be positioned in the usual manner due to age or physical limitations, and without unnecessary irradiation of staff (ACR, 1996).

Plain radiography without the use of a contrast agent has its role in imaging pathologic processes and is often the first choice in imaging modalities. Specialized imaging modalities provide additional information that the physician uses to diagnose diseases. These imaging include ultrasound (US), computed tomography (CT), and magnetic resonance imaging (MRI). Nuclear medicine and positron-emission tomography (PET) are also used when indicated to aid in diagnosis of human diseases. For additional information on other diagnostic imaging modalities and procedures, refer to Chapter 14, Imaging Specialties.

Etiology

Advances in medical research are continuing to discover the cause of diseases, also referred to as etiology. The list of causes of diseases is extensive; however, the most common causes are viruses, bacteria, environmental pollutants or chemicals, genetic triggers, and trauma. Diseases can also be grouped into several categories that includes congenital and hereditary, inflammatory, degenerative, metabolic, traumatic, and neoplastic.

The word congenital originates from Latin, meaning born together or present at birth. A hereditary disease is defined as having genetic characteristic(s) transferred from parent to offspring. A heredofamilial disease refers to any disease that occurs in families due to an inherited defect or process. Health care professionals have known for a long time that common diseases (e.g., heart disease, cancer, and diabetes), and rarer diseases (e.g., hemophilia, cystic fibrosis, and sickle cell anemia), can run in families (U.S. Surgeon General's Family History Initiative, 2008). Family members share their genes, as well as their environment, lifestyles, and habits. The key features of a family history that may increase risk are:

- Diseases that occur at an earlier age than expected (10 to 20 years before most people get the disease;
- Disease in more than one close relative;
- Disease that does not usually affect a certain gender (e.g., breast cancer in a male); and
- Certain combinations of diseases within a family (e.g., breast and ovarian cancer or heart disease and diabetes) (Centers for Disease Control and Prevention [CDC], 2008a).

Individuals in families with a history of particular diseases may help delay or prevent such diseases by participating in increased medical surveillance and testing.

Inflammatory diseases develop when the body reacts to an invading agent (e.g., bacteria, virus, etc.). Reactions to toxic substances, environmental pollutants, and allergies to various substances may also cause inflammatory diseases. When inflammation is caused by a disease-causing pathogen, infection occurs.

Degenerative diseases are generally associated with the aging process although may develop following a traumatic injury. Current medical research is focused on the aging process and the role of hereditary and genetics, diet, lifestyle, and environmental factors in the development of degenerative diseases.

Metabolic diseases are those that interfere with the normal physiologic function of the body. Examples of metabolic diseases include osteoporosis and cystic fibrosis.

Traumatic injuries result from impacts on the body. Such impacts come from outside forces that crush, twist, or distort the body. Injuries resulting from exposure to extreme temperatures, cold and hot, as well as burns (chemical, electrical, lighting strike, and fire) are also considered to be traumatic injuries.

Neoplastic diseases are those in which a new, abnormal growth occurs in the body. Such abnormal growths may be benign or malignant, noninvasive or invasive. For simplicity, benign neoplasms generally remain localized whereas malignant neoplasms often invade and destroy adjacent structures. Also, a characteristic of malignant neoplasms is that they spread to distant locations, referred to as metastasis.

Chest and Bony Thorax Pathology and Imaging Considerations

The chest x-ray is the most common medical imaging examination with 68 million chest x-rays performed each year in the United States (American Society of Radiologic Technologists [ASRT], 2008; Pelsoci, 2008). Radiography of the chest and bony thorax provides important diagnostic information about the soft tissues, bone, pleura, mediastinum, lung tissue, and significant cardiovascular structures. Also, chest imaging contributes to information concerning heart size and shape and serves to monitor the progression of certain diseases and to determine the effectiveness of treatments and therapies.

Specialized imaging modalities used to diagnose chest and body thorax diseases and conditions include CT, MRI, and US imaging. CT and MRI are also used to further evaluate and stage the severity of certain diseases and are frequently used during the pre-treatment and pre-surgical planning stages.

Anatomy Overview of the Bony Thorax and Chest

The bony thorax consists of twelve pairs of ribs encircling and protecting the pulmonary and cardiovascular organs. Anteriorly, the first seven pairs of ribs are attached to the sternum by costal cartilage. Posteriorly the ribs articulate with the thoracic vertebrae (Figure 11-2).

The bony thorax is widest at approximately the eighth through the ninth ribs. The sternoclavicular and acromioclavicular joints are the two major sets of joints of the thorax. The acromion process is located posteriorly on the scapula and overhangs the shoulder joint. Both sets of joints are inspected when determining whether the patient's body was improperly positioned for the posterior–anterior (PA) projection chest x-ray examination (Figure 11-3).

The person reviewing the PA projection chest radiograph will look to see if both sternal ends of the clavicles appear symmetrical in relationship to the vertebral spine. If the reviewer can see both the right and left sternal ends of the clavicles at the same distance from the centerline of the vertebral spine, then no rotation

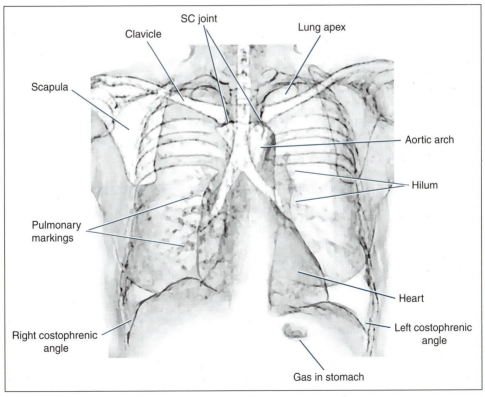

FIGURE 11-2 Anatomy of a posterior–anterior (PA) chest
Source: Delmar, Cengage Learning.

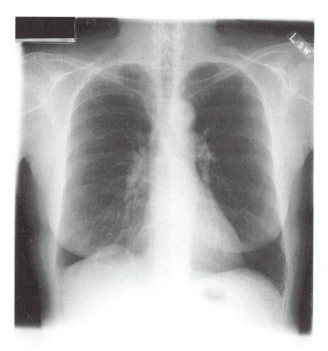

FIGURE 11-3 Posterior–anterior (PA) projection chest radiograph
Source: Delmar, Cengage Learning.

of the patient's body, has occurred. The direction of the patient's rotation can be determined by observing which sternal end of the clavicle is closest to the vertebral spine. Likewise, the distance between each of the sternoclavicular joints should appear symmetrical on the PA chest radiograph.

The diaphragm, a dome-shaped muscle, separates the thoracic and abdominal cavities and is the primary muscle of inspiration. During inspiration, the diaphragm moves downward, and during expiration it moves upward. Chest x-ray examinations are taken immediately after the patient has been instructed to "take in a deep breath," thus moving the diaphragm downward. If the patient has successfully inhaled and no movement exists, the lateral borders (costophrenic angles) of the diaphragm will appear sharp and pointed on the PA chest radiograph. A well-defined appearance of both the right and left costophrenic angles is significant to the physician, because if either or both appear blunted, it may be a sign of pathology (Scheffer and Tobin, 1997).

The mediastinum or middle septum is divided into anterior, middle, and posterior portions. The mediastinal region extends from the base of the neck above to the diaphragm below and lies between the sternum in front and the thoracic vertebrae behind. The anterior portion of the mediastinum contains the thyroid and thymus glands. The middle portion of the mediastinum contains the heart, great vessels, esophagus, and trachea. The posterior portion of the mediastinum contains the descending aorta and vertebral spine.

Visible radiographic changes in the mediastinum are signs of pathology. A shift of the mediastinum is a visible displacement of the heart, trachea, aorta, and hilar vessels. Mediastinal shift indicates an imbalance of pressures between the two sides of the thorax and indicates to the physician which side is abnormal. An aspirated foreign body that is obstructing a mainstem bronchus is a common cause of mediastinal shift toward the normal side.

Widening of the mediastinum is also an important radiographic sign of pathology. To determine the cause of mediastinal widening, the physician will begin with the identification of as many normal structures as possible. A thymoma is the most common primary tumor of the anterior mediastinum and is more frequent in individuals ranging from 45 to 50 years of age. A thymoma radiographically appears as a well-circumscribed mass.

The trachea divides into the right and left primary bronchus with the right primary bronchus leading to the right lung and the left leading to the left lung. The right primary bronchus is wider, shorter, and more vertical than the left. This difference is significant because food particles or other aspirated objects are more likely to enter and lodge in the right primary bronchus (Figure 11-4).

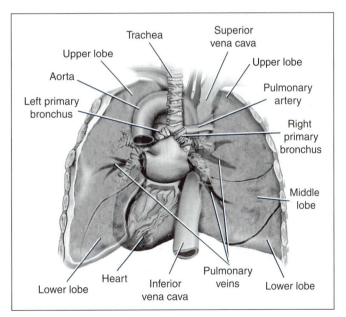

FIGURE 11-4 Lungs and right and left bronchus and structures of the mediastinum
Source: Delmar, Cengage Learning.

The right and left lungs are the organs of respiration and occupy the right and left chest cavities, separated by the mediastinum. Each lung is cone-shaped with a pointed end or apex at the top, reaching about 1 inch above the clavicle. The hilum is a depression on the medial surface of each lung where vessels and bronchi enter. The lower end or base rests upon the upper convex surface of the diaphragm. Normal lung tissue will radiographically appear translucent with markings representative of the blood-filled pulmonary vessels.

The cardiovascular system delivers oxygen, nutrients, and other substances to all the cells of the body. The system is also responsible for removal of the waste products of metabolism. The circulatory system includes the heart, arteries, arterioles, capillaries, venules, veins, and lymph vascular structures including the spleen and bone marrow.

The heart is the pump for the circulatory system and is located in the lower anterior chest in the middle mediastinum, and rests upon the left diaphragm. The top of the heart, or base, is located below the second rib with about two-thirds of the heart located to the left of the body's midline.

A normal sized heart, as visualized on a PA chest radiograph, should have a transverse diameter that is less than 50% of the transthoracic diameter. An additional factor that may mimic cardiac enlargement in chest radiography includes incorrect source-to-image distance (SID), poor inspiration, abdominal distension, pectus excavatum, and large fat pads.

Plain Chest X-Ray Examination

A plain (non-contrast) chest x-ray examination is often performed as part of a routine physical examination. The procedure may also be performed to reveal or rule out conditions such as pneumonia, congestive heart failure, tuberculosis, or lung and heart conditions (ACR, 1993).

According to the American College of Radiology *ACR Practice Guidelines for the Performance of Pediatric and Adult Chest Radiography*, there are several indications for requesting a chest radiograph and these are listed below (ACR, 1993).

- Evaluation of signs and symptoms potentially related to the respiratory, cardiovascular, and upper gastrointestinal systems, as well as musculoskeletal system of the thorax;
- Need for information about thoracic disease processes, including systemic and extrathoracic diseases that secondarily involve the chest. Because the lungs are a frequent site of metastases, chest radiography can be useful in staging extrathoracic, as well as thoracic, neoplasms;
- Follow-up of known thoracic disease processes to assess improvement, resolution, or progression;

- Monitoring of patients with life-support devices and patients who have undergone cardiac or thoracic surgery or other interventional procedures;
- Compliance with government regulations that mandate chest radiography. Examples include surveillance PA chest radiograph for active tuberculosis or occupational lung disease or exposures and other surveillance studies; and,
- Preoperative radiographic evaluation when cardiac or respiratory symptoms are present or when there is significant potential for thoracic pathology that could compromise the surgical result or lead to increased peri-operative morbidity or mortality (ACR, 1996).

Since chest and bony thorax radiographs are used to determine heart size and shape as well as to visualize pathology, disease processes, and trauma, the limited radiographer must control factors that might otherwise distort the image. Such factors include patient posture, degree of inspiration, correct positioning, and the proper selection of technical x-ray exposure factors (Figure 11-5).

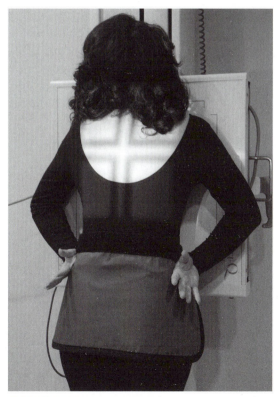

FIGURE 11-5 PA chest radiograph
Source: Delmar, Cengage Learning.

Subtle changes in pulmonary and vascular structures can be easily obscured by a slight shift of the patient's body or inaccurate exposure factors. A chest x-ray examination taken at less than a 72-inch SID results in visible magnification of the heart and mediastinal structures on the radiograph, thus possibly leading to an erroneous diagnosis. Also, if during inspiration, the patient takes in less than a full breath and poor expansion of the lungs results, an inaccurate diagnosis may be rendered.

Radiography of the chest requires high kVp techniques. Kilovoltage ranges between 110 and 125 kVp are used to create the long scale of contrast required to produce diagnostic quality chest radiographs. A fast exposure time is also necessary during chest radiography to avoid motion, which results in blurring of the anatomic structures on the radiograph. Such motion degrades the diagnostic quality of the radiographic imaging and may contribute to unnecessary retake examinations.

Because chest radiography requires a high kVp and a fast exposure time, the limited radiographer should make necessary adjustments to the technical x-ray exposure factors with the mA control.

The limited radiographer should be aware of the patient's suspected diagnosis and alert to the patient's clinical signs and symptoms. This information may alert the limited radiographer that the technical x-ray exposure factors and standard positioning routines may need to be modified or adapted. The following are key clinical indicators in the form of patient history type questions that may alert the limited radiographer that such modifications and adaptations are needed.

Key Clinical Indicators

- **Is the patient in congestive heart failure?**
  This may indicate that abnormal amounts of pulmonary fluid may be present in the chest cavity. The heart may be enlarged and the patient may have dyspnea.

- **What is the cause of the patient's chest pain?**
  Will the patient require emergency measures while undergoing the chest x-ray examination?

- **Does the patient have pneumonia?**
  This may indicate that abnormal amounts of pulmonary fluid may be present in the chest cavity and there may be areas of increased density in the lungs due to the inflammation process.

- **Does the patient have a lung tumor?**
  This may indicate that abnormal amounts of pulmonary fluid may be present in the chest cavity or areas of increased density in the lungs may be present due to the inflammation process.

- **Has the patient had previous chest surgery, radiation therapy, or mastectomy?**
  If the answer is yes to any one of these, the limited radiographer should expect alteration in the normal attenuation of the chest structures which may affect the attenuation of the x-ray beam.

Although most people undergoing a plain chest x-ray examination will be able to come into the imaging department or medical office, those unable to do so may have a portable chest x-ray examination, also referred to as bedside radiography. About one-half of all chest x-ray examinations are taken at the patient's bedside to evaluate line and tube placement (Katai, Lofgren, and Meholic, 2006).

"The portable chest x-ray examination is the imaging modality of choice for evaluation of cardiopulmonary diseases in patients under certain circumstances and in select patient populations (e.g., critically ill, postoperative, newborn)" (ACR, 1993). Additional implications for portable chest x-ray examinations include, but are not limited to, the evaluation of patients with cardiopulmonary symptoms following cardiac or thoracic surgery, trauma, patients with monitoring and/or life support devices, and patients who are critically ill or medically unstable (ACR, 1993).

Proper patient positioning is essential to obtaining diagnostic chest radiographs. The limited radiographer's main responsibility during the examination is to ensure that the patient is properly positioned and that all technical factors are correct. Although the physical condition of the patient and the attending physician's preferences are factors in the type of projections requested for any given anatomic area, there are certain standards that are considered optimum in delivering radiography services. The ACR recommends that the following specifications be considered as the minimum standards to be met when performing plain chest x-ray examinations.

A standard chest x-ray examination should include an erect PA and left lateral projection made during full inspiration (ACR, 1993). Many experts recommend that the x-ray exposure be made on the second breath hold, which generally provides a deeper inspiration and moves the diaphragm down out of the lower lung fields. The chest x-ray examination may be modified by the physician or qualified technologist depending on the clinical circumstances (e.g., when young children are not yet able to stand, supine images are performed) other patient positions that may be used occasionally include supine, oblique, decubitus, or lordotic (Figures 11-6A and B) (ACR, 1993).

In some cases a single view such as an anterio-posterior (AP) or PA projection may provide sufficient diagnostic information.

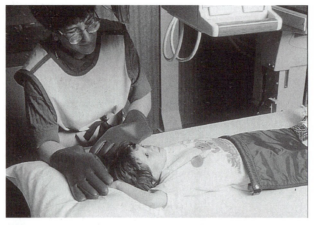

(A)

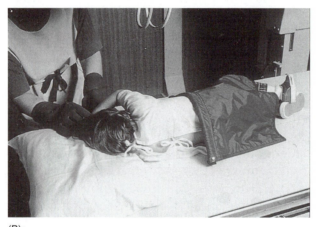

(B)

FIGURE 11-6 (A) AP and (B) lateral chest—child
Source: Delmar, Cengage Learning.

On inspection, chest radiographs should include both of the lung apices and costophrenic angles. The mid-thoracic vertebral bodies and the left retrocardiac vertebral bodies and the left retrocardiac pulmonary vessels should also be visible. The scapulae should be positioned off of the lungs on the PA projection, and the arms should be elevated for the lateral position (Figure 11-7).

The vertebral column should be centered between the clavicles. The examination should conducted with at least a 72-inch SID for routine upright projections to minimize magnification of the anatomic structures.

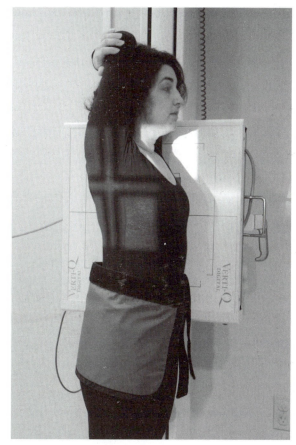

FIGURE 11-7 Lateral chest (arms overhead)
Source: Delmar, Cengage Learning.

The lateral projection is crucial in identifying abnormalities in the posterior costophrenic angles, within the mediastinum, and in areas related to the spine (Katai, Lofgren, and Meholic, 2006). If due to the patient's condition (e.g., unable to stand or sit upright), an AP projection x-ray examination of the chest is taken, the heart and mediastinum will appear about 15% wider than on a PA projection of the same area (Katai, Lofgren, and Meholic, 2006). The limited radiographer should be aware that an AP portable chest x-ray examination should be conducted as close to the standard 72-inch SID as possible to reduce the effects of image magnification. Obtaining a 72-inch SID during portable radiography is often impossible to achieve due to various constraints of space accommodation around the patient's bedside. Portable x-ray examinations acquired with less than the standard SID should be marked to indicate the actual SID used.

Lateral decubitus projection x-ray examinations of the chest may be requested when the physician suspects that the patient may have pleural effusion. Oblique positions of the chest and the use of chest fluoroscopy can be helpful in evaluation of pulmonary nodules. Expiratory views may also be requested to detect pneumothorax and endobrochial obstruction.

A basic understanding of what the interpreting physician is reviewing when inspecting chest radiographs can help the limited radiographer when performing the procedure. The following list provides examples of what the physician inspects during the evaluation and diagnostic interpretation of chest radiographs.

PA Projection
- Ribs: posterior and anterior ribs, axillary margin, vertebral spine, clavicles, and scapula.
- Mediastinum: aortic arch.
- Hilum: relative height and size of the right and left hilum and the hilar angle.
- Heart: apex configuration, calcifications, and left atrium.
- Diaphragms/pleura: contour, including costophrenic angels, upper abdomen, and apices.
- Parenchyma: entire lung field.

Lateral Projection
- Bones: vertebral spine and sternum.
- Mediastinum: retrosternal space, tracheal air column, and retrotracheal space.
- Hilum: interlobar arteries size and shape and posterior wall of the bronchus intermedius.
- Heart: retrosternal space and the posterior margin (including inferior vena cava junction).
- Diaphragm/pleura: pleural fissures, contour, including costophrenic angles, and upper abdomen.

Radiographic Pathology of the Chest

It is important for the limited radiographer to understand that variations and deviations from the normal anatomic architecture of the bony thorax and the respiratory and circulatory organs are key indicators of pathological processes. Certain disease processes produce characteristic radiographic findings, and these will be briefly discussed.

The silhouette sign is present if the border of a structure normally seen on a chest radiograph (e.g., the heart or aorta) is obscured by fluid or abnormal tissue. An example is when the lung, which is normally filled with air, becomes filled with fluid. Wherever the fluid-filled lung touches another structure they blend together and any existing distinct border is no longer visualized. When the border of a normal structure is obscured a silhouette sign is present. The silhouette sign is used to evaluate radiographs for such conditions as atelactasis, pleural fluid, tumors, and pneumonia. Increased opacities in the lungs indicate increased attenuation of the x-ray beam and can be caused by abnormalities in the mediastinum, pleura, or parenchyma. These can often be distinguished by **air bronchograms**, which occur when air-filled bronchi are outlined by fluid-filled alveoli. The **ground glass sign** refers to an increased opacity of the lung parenchyema that is not dense enough to obscure underlying pulmonary vessels. The term is more commonly used in interpretation of CT studies where the hazy areas of increased lung opacity have the same translucent appearance as glass that has been mechanically ground.

Lucent areas within the lung fields indicate areas where there is increased penetration by the x-ray beam. This causes the lungs to appear abnormally dark or black. These areas may have definable borders that can be described as ring shadows, cysts, or cavities. A few of the possible reasons for the areas of increased darkness may be attributed to abnormalities of the chest wall (e.g., mastectomy), or may reflect obstructive or vascular lung disease.

Pneumonia. Pneumonia is a common disease of the lungs that can be fatal if not diagnosed and treated properly (Wilkins and Wilkins, 2005). Pneumonia is an inflammation of the lungs usually due to infection with bacteria, viruses, or other pathogenic organisms. Approximately 50% of pneumonia cases are believed to be caused by viruses and tend to result in less severe illness than bacteria-caused pneumonia (American Lung Association, 2007). There are two broad categories of pneumonia: community-acquired pneumonia (CAP) and nosocomial pneumonia. CAP is a disease that affects individuals who have not recently been hospitalized, whereas nosocomial pneumonia and infections are a result of treatment in a hospital or a health care setting, but secondary to the patient's original condition (Merck Manual's Online Medical Library, 2009a and b). Infections are considered nosocomial if they first appear 48 hours or more after hospital admission or within 30 days after discharge (Merck Manual's, 2009b). This type of infection is also known as hospital-acquired infection or health care–associated infection. The delivery of medical care has increasingly shifted from hospital-based to home care, and more people are residing in nursing homes or extended-care facilities; thus a new name, health care–acquired pneumonia (HCAP) (Merck Manual's, 2009a). Other groups of people who may be at risk for HCAP include patients who are admitted as day cases for hemodialysis or intravenous infusion (e.g., chemotherapy) (Merck Manual's, 2009a).

Pneumonia is often a complication of a pre-existing condition or infection and triggered when a patient's immune system is weakened, especially the elderly (over age 65). Certain diseases, such as tuberculosis, chronic obstructive pulmonary disease (COPD), diabetes mellitus, congestive heart failure, and sickle cell anemia also predispose someone to pneumonia. Pneumonia can also be caused by the inhalation of food, liquid, gases, or dust. One type is caused by fungi is *pneumocystis carinii* pneumonia (PCP) which primarily affects patient with acquired immunodeficiency disease (AIDS) (American Lung Association, 2007; Merck Manual's, 2009a and b). *Streptococcus pneumoniae* or pneumococcal pneumonia are the most common cause of bacterial pneumonia acquired outside of hospitals. Pneumonia and influenza together are ranked as the eighth leading cause of death in the United States (American Lung Association, 2007).

The symptoms of viral pneumonia are similar to influenza symptoms and include fever, dry cough, headache, muscle pain, weakness, fever, and increasing breathlessness. The development of bacterial pneumonia can vary from a gradual to a sudden onset. Patients may present with chills, severe chest pains, sweats, cough that produces rust-colored or greenish mucus, **tachypnea** (increased respiration rate), **tachycardia** (increased heart rate), and bluish-colored lips or nails due to lack of oxygen. There are no generally effective treatments for most types of viral pneumonia; however, if bacterial pneumonia is diagnosed early in the disease progression, effective antibiotics can be prescribed. Unfortunately, like some types of drug-resistant tuberculosis, some drugs have become ineffective in treating pneumococcal pneumonia.

The pneumococcal polysaccharide vaccine (PPC) is recommended for anyone over 65, those with serious long-term health problems, anyone with a compromised immune system, all Alaskan Natives, and certain Native American populations (American Lung Association, 2007). The vaccine protects against 23 types of pneumococcal bacteria and is effective in 80% of healthy adults (American Lung Association, 2007). The pneumococcal conjugate vaccine (PCV) is recommended for children less than 2 and children between 2 and 5 who have serious long-term health problems, compromised immune systems, are Alaskan Native, Native American, African American, or attend a group day care center (American Lung Association, 2007). These vaccines are generally given once, although revaccination after 3 to 5 years is recommended for children with nephritic syndrome, asplenia, or sickle cell anemia who would be less than 11 years old at revaccination (American Lung Association, 2007). Revaccination is also suggested for adults at high risk who received their first vaccination six years ago or more (American Lung Association, 2008d). Influenza vaccination is also recommended because pneumonia often occurs as a complication of the flu (American Lung Association, 2008d). Additional information about pneumonia and influenza vaccination and prevention measures may be found on the Centers for Disease Control and Prevention's website (http://www.cdc.gov) and the American Lung Association's website (http://www.lungusa.org).

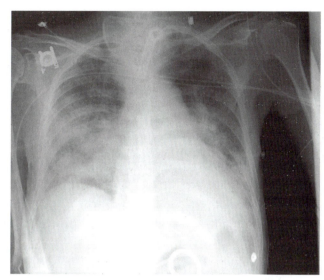

FIGURE 11-8 Pneumonia
Source: Delmar, Cengage Learning.

The chest radiograph is often used in the diagnostic workup for suspected pneumonia but is frequently found to be negative regardless of the patient's age (Wilkins and Wilkins, 2005). The clinical definition of pneumonia includes both the presence of an abnormal opacity on the chest radiograph and signs and symptoms (Wilkins and Wilkins, 2005).

The physician uses the clinical signs and symptoms as well as laboratory and radiographic findings to make a definitive diagnosis. On chest radiographs, pneumonia appears as a soft, patchy, ill-defined alveolar infiltration or abnormal pulmonary densities (Figure 11-8).

Legionnaire's Disease. Legionnaire's Disease is a type of severe bacterial pneumonia that achieved its name when four people attending an American Legion convention in Philadelphia in 1976 were stricken and died (CDC, 2008c). The infective agent *Legionella pneumophilia* is responsible for the hospitalization of between 8,000–18,000 people in the United States each year (CDC, 2008c). The symptoms of Legionnaire's disease are similar to those accompanying pneumonia and both demonstrate patchy infiltrates throughout the lungs on chest radiographs (Kowalczyk and Mace, 2009).

Tuberculosis. Tuberculosis (TB) is a pulmonary infection caused by inhalation of the *mycobacterium tuberculosis* (American Lung Association, 2008k). The disease is mainly spread through the air when people who have the disease cough, sneeze, speak, laugh, or sing, and in doing so give off tiny drops of moisture that contain the TB bacterium. Generally the TB bacterium affects the lungs, but it can occur in other places in the body. On a chest radiographs, the lung lesions most commonly associated with TB are usually seen in the apices of the lungs on chest radiographs (Figure 11-9) (Kowalczyk and Mace, 2009).

Tuberculosis was often a fatal disease in past centuries; however, during the 1940s and 1950s drugs to treat the disease were discovered. After the 1960s very few cases of TB were recorded in the United States. TB was not eradicated in many Third World countries, but since 1990, reported cases of TB have been increasing. The resurgence is attributed to several factors: global travel, an increase in the number of immunonocompromised patients, and an increase in the number of individuals with acquired immunodeficiency disease (AIDS) (CDC, 2007). People who are susceptible to TB include those who are infected with the human immunodeficiency virus (HIV), the virus that causes AIDS; those who have AIDS; drug and/or alcohol abusers; and those with compromised immune systems (American Lung Association, 2008k; CDC, 2007).

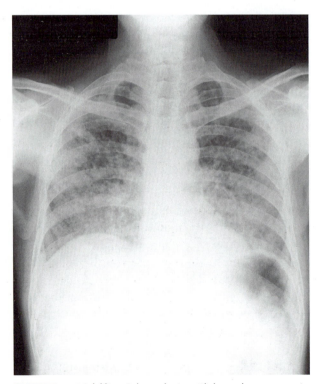

FIGURE 11-9 Miliary tuberculosis with bronchopneumonia
Source: Delmar, Cengage Learning.

Today, the most serious problem concerning the treatment of TB is that the organism has the ability to become multi-drug resistant, making the current two-drug treatment regimen ineffective.

The Centers for Disease Control and Prevention (CDC) recommend that limited radiographers and others who provide care for persons who have compromised immune systems should have a TB skin test (The Mantoux test) every six months (CDC, 2007). Also, those in direct contact with a patient who has TB should wear a mask and wash their hands often (CDC, 2007). For additional information, limited radiographers are encouraged to read the *Guidelines for Preventing the Transmission of Mycobacterium tuberculosis in Health Care Settings* (*2006 MMWAR 54/RR*) available at the CDC website (http://www.cdc.gov).

Acute Respiratory Distress Syndrome.   Acute respiratory distress syndrome (ARDS) is the sudden failure of the respiratory system. It can occur in anyone over the age of 1 who is critically ill (American Lung Association, 2008b). ARDS can be life-threatening because the normal gas exchange process fails to occur due to severe fluid buildup in both lungs. The condition is characterized by tachypnea, dyspnea (difficult breathing), and low oxygen levels in the blood. Approximately 25% to 40% of ARDS cases are fatal (American Lung Association, 2008b). Death usually results from multi-system organ failure due to lack of oxygen, rather than lung failure alone.

ARDS is caused mainly by extensive lung inflammation and small blood vessel injury due to sepsis (bacterial infection of the blood), trauma, and/or a severe pulmonary infection such as pneumonia. ARDS can also result from inhalation of salt water, smoke inhalation of toxic chemicals, aspiration, narcotics, sedatives, and shock.

ARDS is diagnosed in people who are already critically ill from shock, sepsis, or other trauma, but otherwise exhibit no major underlying lung disease (American Lung Association, 2008b).

The diagnosis is made when there is difficulty in providing adequate oxygenation and diffuse abnormalities are visible on a chest radiograph. The chest radiograph usually demonstrates diffuse interstitial and patchy air-space fibrosis that may appear as a coarse reticular pattern (American Lung Association, 2008b and h).

Treatment of ARDS involves intensive supportive care with supplemental fluids, oxygen, and mechanical ventilation. Those who survive may benefit from pulmonary rehabilitation and support from others who have experienced the condition (American Lung Association, 2008b).

Interstitial lung disease (ILD).   Interstitial lung disease (ILD) is a general term that includes a variety of chronic lung disorders (American Lung Association, 2008h). The origin of ILD is not always clearly known but it appears to occur in the following manner. First, the lung tissue is damaged, and then the walls of the air sacs in the lung become inflamed. Finally, scarring (**fibrosis**) begins in the interstitium (tissue between the air sacs), and the lung becomes less elastic, or stiff. Other similar conditions include air-space disease and atelectasis.

Because it is often difficult for the interpreting physician to distinguish between these conditions on a plain chest radiograph, additional imaging studies may be ordered. ILD affects the tissue surrounding the alveoli and capillaries within the lung, but does not infiltrate into the alveoli. On chest radiographs, the conditions can be differentiated because in ILD air remains in the alveoli, whereas in air-space disease, air is not present. The most common radiographic signs of ILD are the presence of **Kerley's B lines**. Kerley's B lines are small septations in the lung that contain lymphatics and venules and are visible on chest radiographs only when they are abnormally thickened. These lines form short (1 to 2 cm), horizontal lines that connect with the pleura along the lateral margins of the lung. **Kerley's A lines** are less common and form longer lines that radiate from right and left pulmonary hilum (Katai, Lofgren, and Meholic, 2007; Kowalczyk and Mace, 2009).

Air-Space Disease.   Air-space disease primarily affects the alveoli of the respiratory bronchioles. The air bronchogram sign is one of the key radiographic findings of air-space disease and results when airless alveoli outline air-filled bronchi and are seen on chest radiographs as a dark branching pattern within the opaque lung parenchyma (Katai, Lofgren, and Meholic, 2007; Kowalczyk and Mace, 2009).

Air bronchograms are produced when the alveoli are filled with blood, pus, water, or cells. Air bronchograms can be caused by a number of conditions including congestive heart failure, ingestion of water (i.e., drowning), and blood due to trauma (Katai, Lofgren, and Meholic, 2007).

Atelectasis.   Atelectasis is the incomplete expansion of a portion of the lungs and is similar to air-space disease in that it produces airless alveoli. Atelectasis occurs when the air in the alveoli is absorbed and not replaced by fluid or cells and results in a loss of lung volume. As the lung loses volume, pulmonary structures change positions causing the fissures and intrapulmonary vessels to shift and crowd together. This shifting of pulmonary structures is considered the classical radiographic sign of atelectasis (Katai, Lofgren, and Meholic, 2007).

Chronic Obstructive Pulmonary Diseases (COPD) and Related Conditions.   Chronic obstructive pulmonary disease (COPD) refers to two lung diseases, chronic bronchitis and emphysema (American Lung Association, 2008d). COPD is characterized by obstruction to airflow that interferes with normal breathing. Both of these conditions frequently co-exist, but it does not include other obstructive diseases such as asthma. COPD is the fourth leading cause of death in American and more women die from the disease than do men (American Lung Association, 2008d). Smoking is the primary risk factor for COPD; however other risk factors such as exposure to air pollution, secondhand smoke and occupational dust, and chemicals have been implicated (American Lung Association, 2008d).

Chronic Bronchitis.   Chronic bronchitis is the inflammation and eventual scarring of the lining of the bronchial tubes, the major airways into the lungs. When the bronchi are inflamed and/or infected, less air is able to flow to and from the lungs and heavy mucus or phlegm is coughed up. Once the bronchial tubes are scarred and are constantly irritated, airflow may be hampered, and the lungs become scarred. Females are more likely than males to be diagnosed with chronic bronchitis (American Lung Association, 2008).

Chronic bronchitis is defined by the presence of a mucus-producing cough most days of the month, three months of a year for two successive years without other underlying disease to explain the cough. Bronchitis may be caused by a variety of bacteria and viruses and may be primary or secondary to an upper respiratory infection, pertussis (whooping cough), or long-term exposure to air pollution or cigarette smoking. The most common radiographic indication of bronchitis is a generalized increase in bronchovascular markings, especially in the lower lungs (Katai, Lofgren, and Meholic, 2007; Kowalczyk and Mace, 2009).

Emphysema.   Emphysema is a condition in which the walls between the alveoli lose their ability to stretch and recoil, causing the alveoli to become weak and break. As the lungs lose their elasticity, air is trapped in the alveoli resulting in a decrease in the free exchange of oxygen and carbon dioxide. Those with emphysema present with shortness of breath, cough, and a limited exercise tolerance. Emphysema and chronic bronchitis frequently co-exist together to comprise COPD. Cigarette smoking is the most common cause of emphysema and is responsible for 80% to 90% of deaths due to COPD (American Lung Association, 2008f). In addition, the American Lung Association (ALA) estimates that 100,000 Americans living today were born with a deficiency of a lung protein known as alpha 1-antitrypsin (AAT) (American Lung Association, 2008f). In the absence of AAT, an inherited form of emphysema called alpha 1-antitrypsin deficiency-related emphysema is almost inevitable (American Lung Association, 2008f).

The classic radiographic sign of emphysema is overinflation of the lungs with flattening of the domes of the diaphragm (Figure 11-10) (Katai, Lofgren, and Meholic, 2007; Kowalczyk and Mace, 2009).

On the lateral chest radiograph, another important sign is increased size and lucency of the retrosternal air space and the distance between the posterior side

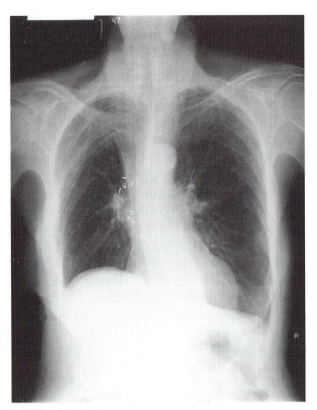

FIGURE 11-10 Emphysema
Source: Delmar, Cengage Learning.

of the sternum and the anterior wall of the ascending aorta (Katai, Lofgren, and Meholic, 2007; Kowalczyk and Mace, 2009). The limited radiographer may have to reduce the technical x-ray exposure factors, with imaging patients with advanced pulmonary emphysema where a large amount of air may be trapped in the lungs.

Asthma. Asthma is an inflammatory condition of the lungs that makes it difficult to breathe. Asthma is a chronic condition, even when there are no noticeable symptoms. Each person with asthma has his or her own provoking triggers that initiate the inflammation, causing the airways to tighten or restrict. These series of events produce airway obstruction, chest tightness, coughing, and wheezing that can lead to asthma attacks. If severe, asthma causes severe shortness of breath and low levels of oxygen in the blood. A recent study conducted by researchers at the National Institutes of Health (NIH) found that more than 50% of current asthma sufferers in the United States can attribute their attacks to specific allergies (American Lung Association, 2008c). Secondhand smoke exposure in both adults and children is a risk factor for new asthma cases (American Lung Association, 2008c). Outdoor pollutants known to trigger asthma attacks include ozone, particulate matter, nitrogen dioxide, and sulfur dioxide. Work-related exposure to vapors, dust, and smoke also can increase the risk of developing asthma.

Findings on chest radiographs are inconclusive as a diagnostic aid in the early stages of the asthma. However, in people with chronic asthma, especially those with a history of frequent and repeated episodes of illness, thickening of the bronchial walls may be evident on chest radiographs (Katai, Lofgren, and Meholic, 2007; Kowalczyk and Mace, 2009).

Occupational Lung Diseases

Occupational lung disease is the number one cause of work-related illness in the United States in terms of frequency, severity, and preventability (American Lung Association, 2008j). Many occupational lung diseases are related to a specific occupation or exposure to hazardous materials, such as asbestosis, coal workers' pneumoconiosis (black lung), silicosis (exposure to fine sand as in ceramic workers), berylliosis, byssinosis or brown lung (exposure to raw cotton), and farmer's lung. Workplace exposures can cause or worsen adult-onset asthma, COPD, and lung cancer.

Asbestosis. Asbestosis is a progressive lung disease that involves scarring of lung tissue as a result of exposure to asbestos. Asbestos was a material used between 1999 and 2004 in the construction industry because of its properties as a good insulator and fire retardant material (American Lung Association, 2008j). An estimated 1.3 million employees in the construction industry had significant exposure (American Lung Association, 2008j). According to a study by the Environmental Working Group, almost 10,000 deaths per year in the United States, or close to 30 deaths per day, are due to asbestos-related diseases, including mesothelioma, asbestosis, lung cancer, and gastrointestinal cancer (American Lung Association, 2008j).

Mesothelioma. Mesothelioma is a rare cancer of the lining of organs in which 70% to 80% of the cases are directly attributed to asbestos exposure. The disease has a long latency period, with symptoms appearing 30 to 50 years after the exposure. Mesothelioma affects men five times more than women and is more common in Whites (American Lung Association, 2008j).

Pleural mesothelioma is a highly malignant tumor that radiographically appears as an irregular scalloped or nodular density within the pleural space. The tumor may be accompanied by a large pleural effusion that may obscure the underlying pathology (Katai, Lofgren, and Meholic, 2007; Kowalczyk and Mace, 2009).

Coal Worker's Pneumoconiosis (Black Lung Disease). Coal worker's pneumoconiosis, more commonly called black lung disease, is a chronic condition caused by inhaling coal dust that then becomes imbedded in the lungs. When this happens, the lungs loose their elasticity and harden over time, making it difficult for the lungs to expand and for the victim to breathe. Each year between 1999 and 2004, an average of 355 people died from black lung disease (American Lung Association, 2008j).

In the early stages of the disease, chest radiographs illustrate nodules that tend to be ill-defined densities. As the disease progresses, the radiographs may illustrate a pattern of increasing massive fibrosis that appear as one or more masses of fibrous tissue with smooth, well-defined borders. These gradually migrate toward the hilum of the lung, leaving an area of overinflated lung between them and the chest wall (Katai, Lofgren, and Meholic, 2007; Kowalczyk and Mace, 2009).

Silicosis. Silicosis is caused by exposure to free crystalline silica, which is primarily found in industries such as mining, foundry, and sandblasting. Inhalation of the fine dust can cause swelling in the lungs and eventual lung tissue scarring (fibrosis). Like many of the other occupational lung conditions, exposure to the dust generally occurs over a period of time, and the onset of the disease is gradual.

The classic radiographic appearance of silicosis is multiple nodular shadows scattered throughout the lungs. Over time, these nodules may be circumscribed and of uniform density and may become calcified. As the condition progresses, the pulmonary nodules increase in size and may join to form large masses in the lungs. Radiographic signs are usually bilateral, relatively symmetric, and usually restricted to the upper half of the lungs.

Hypersensitivity Pneumonitis. Hypersensitivity pneumonitis also called farmer's lung is caused by repeated exposure to organic dusts, fungus, mold, or other substances (American Lung Association, 2008j). Moldy hay, bird droppings, contamination in humidifiers or air conditioners, and certain chemicals may also cause this condition. When these agents are inhaled, a hypersensitivity reaction occurs within the lung's parenchyma. The reaction causes the alveoli in the lungs to become inflamed, eventually leading to fibrous scarring of the lungs. The radiographic findings vary depending on the stage of the disease; however, in acute stages, opacities within the lungs form an ill-defined nodular pattern (Katai, Lofgren, and Meholic, 2007; Kowalczyk and Mace, 2009).

Sick Building Syndrome. Sick building syndrome has been attributed to a large number of people complaining about illnesses that are difficult to trace to a specific origin (American Lung Association, 2008j). The sick building syndrome is thought to arise from the energy conservation movement. In an effort to contain rising energy costs, many building owners tightly sealed the structures, while the ventilation systems mostly recycled indoor air. According to the National Institute of Allergy and Infectious Disease (NIAID), lack of adequately ventilated office spaces aids in the transmission of the organism that causes pneumonia (American Lung Association, 2008j).

Sick building syndrome and other occupational-related lung diseases are leading causes of lost work productivity. The direct costs (e.g., medical expenses of occupational injuries and illnesses) are estimated at $45.8 billion, and indirect costs (e.g., lost wages) may range up to $229 billion (American Lung Association, 2008j). Additional information about occupational lung diseases and its prevention can be found on the American Lung Association's website: http://www.lungusa.org.

Lesser-Known Lung Diseases

The list of lesser-known diseases that primarily affect the lungs is a lengthy one. Among the more familiar that the limited radiographer may encounter are those briefly described in the following section.

Histoplasmosis. Histoplasmosis a systemic infection caused by a fungus *Histoplasma capsulatum* found in soil, especially that contaminated by bird or bat excreta. The fungus is common in most of the Central and Eastern United States. The illness occurs in two forms, acute and chronic (American Lung Association, 2008i and g). The acute form has been described as like a mild case of influenza. The chronic form, which is less common, may resemble the symptoms associated with TB.

The radiographic signs of histoplasmosis often mimic the appearance of tuberculosis. Chest radiographs may demonstrate single or multiple areas of pulmonary infiltration, most often seen in the lower lung. A common radiographic finding in adults is a solitary, sharply circumscribed granulomatous nodule most often in a lower lobe. Chronic cases of histoplasmosis are radiographically demonstrated by zones of parenchymal consolidation, often with a large loss of lung volume, usually in the upper lobe. Cavitation is possible and progressive fibrosis in the mediastinum has been demonstrated (Katai, Lofgren, and Meholic, 2007; Kowalczyk and Mace, 2009).

Coccidioidomysosis. Coccidioidomysosis, also called valley fever, is an infection in the lungs caused by inhaling spores of the fungus *Coccidioides immitis*. The fungus thrives in semiarid soil found the Southwestern United States, California, and parts of Central and South America. Of the estimated 150,000 infections reported per year, approximately 60% occur in Arizona (American Lung Association, 2008i). Many of those infected with the fungus have no symptoms or apparent illness.

Others report an influenza-like syndrome with fever, weakness, achy joints, cough, and chest pain. Although most cases are mild, in a very small percentage, the disease may result in pneumonia and may spread to other areas of the body such as brain, spinal cord, bones, skin, and other tissue. Coccidioidomycosis infections occurring outside the lungs are generally associated with those with impaired immune systems, pregnant women, and non-Whites.

Infections with fungal organisms result in focal air-space disease, more likely to cause hilar adenopathy. Resolving infections often leave behind nodules that if calcified can be easily distinguished on follow-up chest radiographs (Katai, Lofgren, and Meholic, 2007; Kowalczyk and Mace, 2009).

Hantavirus Pulmonary Syndrome (HPS). Hantavirus pulmonary syndrome (HPS) appeared as a mysterious disease in the spring of 1993, affecting people in the Southwestern United States (i.e., Arizona, Colorado, New Mexico) (American Lung Association, 2008i). It was discovered that rodents harbor hantaviruses, especially rats and mice, and approximately three-fourths of those affected lived in rural areas.

The HPS infection cannot be transmitted from one person to another but must be contracted by inhaling airborne saliva or fecal matter from infected animals. HPS triggers an illness similar to influenza and accompanied by its classical symptoms. Those with HPS, however, rapidly progress to severe respiratory distress and acute respiratory distress syndrome (ARDS). The CDC has published guidelines for the prevention and control of HPS infections and this information may be obtained from the Centers for Disease Control and Prevention's website: http://www.cdc.gov.

Severe Acute Respiratory Syndrome (SARS). Severe Acute Respiratory Syndrome (SARS) first made its worldwide appearance in 2003 with the most recent cases occurring in China. SARS is caused by a virus from the coronoviruses group and symptoms include fever higher than 100.4 degrees Fahrenheit, chills, muscle soreness, headache, and general malaise. Most people who are affected with SARS develop pneumonia with approximately 10% to 20% of these progressing to a level of respiratory difficulty so severe that a mechanical respirator is required (American Lung Association, 2008i).

The radiographic appearance of SARS varies with the degree of severity of the disease, but bilateral ground glass opacities or consolidation area are apparent (Katai, Lofgren, and Meholic, 2007; Kowalczyk and Mace, 2009).

Lung Cancer

Lung cancer is the leading cancer killer in both men and women in the United States. While the lung cancer rate appears to be dropping among White and African-American men in the United States, it continues to rise among both White and African-American women (American Lung Association, 2006).

There are two major types of lung cancer: non-small cell lung cancer and small cell lung cancer. The non-small cell lung cancer is much more common and usually metastases to different parts of the body more slowly than small cell lung cancer. Squamous cell carcinoma, adenocarcinoma, and large cell carcinoma are three types of non-small cell lung cancer (American Lung Association, 2006; National Institutes of Health [NIH]; National Cancer Institute, 2008a). Without treatment, small cell lung cancer has the most aggressive progress of any type of pulmonary tumor. The median survival time from diagnosis is generally only two to four months (NIH National Cancer Institute, 2008b).

Smoking is considered to be the major cause of lung cancer. Inhalation of radon gas is the second leading cause of lung cancer (American Lung Association, 2006). According to the Environmental Protection Agency (EPA), radon, a naturally occurring radioactive gas found in the soil, can enter buildings and homes through cracks in the foundation. Once inside, the gas can become concentrated and the particulate radiation given off by radon gas can be inhaled. The EPA recommends that all homeowners test their home for radon gas and if the level exceeds 4 picocuries per liter of air (pCi/L) on a yearly average, the home should be mitigated to reduce the levels. In most states, schools and workplaces are required by regulation to be tested for radon gas levels and mitigated if elevated levels are found.

Unfortunately, there are few symptoms of early lung cancer so when symptoms occur, the cancer is often in an advanced stage. Symptoms of lung cancer include chronic cough, hoarsenes, hemoptysis, weight loss, dyspnea, wheezing, chest pain, fever with an unknown origin, and repeated episodes of bronchitis or pneumonia. These symptoms are common to many other lung conditions, so all complaints must be investigated.

Many physicians advise smokers and former smokers and others who may be at high risk for lung cancer to participate in a low-radiation dose high-resolution computed tomography (HRCT) screening study of the lungs (American Lung Association, 2006; ACR, 2008). Population-wide HRCT lung screening of the at-risk groups is controversial because it is highly sensitive and leads to many false positives, which must be further investigated. The ACR has published a list of indications for the use of HRCT and the most frequently used is for the evaluation of diffuse pulmonary disease discovered on chest radiography (ACR, 2008).

The limited radiographer may find additional information on lung cancer on the Centers for Disease Control and Prevention's website and *ACR Practice Guideline for the Performance of High-Resolution Computed tomography (HRCT) of the Lungs in Adults* on the American College of Radiology's website previously cited.

Respiratory and Cardiovascular Diseases and Conditions

There are many respiratory and cardiovascular diseases and conditions that the limited radiographer may encounter. The list below provides a brief index of terminology that may benefit the limited radiographer in providing continuity of care during x-ray examinations.

A Brief Index of Terminology

- *Aneurysm* is a localized dilation of an artery that most commonly involves the aorta.
- *Atherosclerosis* is the major cause of vascular disease of the extremities resulting from fatty deposits (plaques) in the intima. These plaques produce progressive narrowing and often completely occlude large and medium-sized arteries.
- *Bronchiectasis* is a condition involving abnormal widening of the bronchial tubes and the formation of small pockets of infection. It usually occurs as a complication of primary infections such as bronchitis, pneumonia, pertussis, or tuberculosis.
- *Bronchiolitis* is a condition in which bronchioles, the smaller airways within the lungs, become inflamed. It is most common in early infancy and often occurs due to viral infections.
- *Coarctation of the aorta* refers to a narrowing, or constriction, of the aorta and most commonly occurs just beyond the branching of the blood vessels to the head and arms.
- *Congestive heart failure (CHF)* occurs when the heart is unable to circulate blood at a sufficient rate and volume to provide adequate blood supply to the tissues.
- *Cystic fibrosis* is a disease resulting from a defective autosomal recessive gene that affects the endocrine glands and involves the respiratory system and many other organs. The disease affects approximately 30,000 people in the United States and its progression is tracked by chest x-ray examinations (American Lung Association, 2008e). Chest radiographs demonstrate the extent of bronchial thickening and hyperinflation and are useful in staging the progress of the disease and in diagnosing respiratory complications (Katai, Lofgren, and Meholic, 2007; Kowalczyk and Mace, 2009). Patients with cystic fibrosis are at increased risk of pulmonary infections, recurring respiratory infections, and pneumonia.
- *Embolism* is all or part of a thrombus that becomes detached from a vessel wall and enters the bloodstream.
- *Empyema* is an accumulation of pus in the pleural cavity.
- *Hypertension*, also called high blood pressure, may be benign or malignant. The benign form is characterized by a gradual onset and a prolonged course. When hypertension causes increased intra cranial pressure it is called malignant

hypertension. Blood pressure is an indication of cardiac function relating to the amount of blood pumped per minute by the heart, and the total peripheral resistance. For additional information, refer to Chapter 4, Medical Asepsis and Patient Care.

- *Hyaline membrane disease,* also known as respiratory distress syndrome (RDS), affects premature infants who suffer from incomplete maturation of the surfactant-producing system. Chest radiographs demonstrate the air-bronchogram sign (Katai, Lofgren, and Meholic, 2007; Kowalczyk and Mace, 2009).
- *Lung abscess* is a localized area of dead (necrotic) tissue surrounded by inflammatory debris.
- *Pertussis (whooping cough)* is a highly contagious disease caused by the bacteria *Bordetella pertussis* and can be prevented with a vaccine. The disease can last for weeks and typically causes severe coughing.
- *Pleurisy* is an inflammation of the pleura.
- *Pleural effusion* results when excess fluid collects in the pleural cavity. A pleural effusion containing blood is called a hemathorax. These conditions are generally classified as additive (increased density) and require increases in the technical x-ray exposure factors.
- *Pulmonary edema* is an abnormal accumulation of fluid in the extravascular tissues. A few of the most common causes of pulmonary edema are left-sided heart failure, pulmonary venous obstruction, lymphatic blockage, and ARDS.
- *Tetrology of Fallot* is the most common cause of cyanotic congenital heart disease in infants and consists of four abnormalities: (1) high ventricular septal defect, (2) pulmonary stenosis, (3) overriding of the aortic orifice above the ventricular defect, and (4) right ventricular hypertrophy.
- *Thrombus* is an intravascular clot.

The Bony Thorax

Rib fractures are one of the most common thoracic injuries that the limited radiographer may encounter in the medical office or immediate medical care outpatient facility. These injuries are often sustained following blunt chest trauma and approximately 10% of all patients must ultimately receive hospital care (Eiff, Hatch, and Calmbach, 2003; Doty, 2008).

The most common causes of rib fractures in the elderly is a fall whereas in adults, motor vehicle accidents (MVA) are the most common mechanism of injury (Eiff, Hatch, and Calmbach, 2003; Doty, 2008). Certain types of rib fractures are associated with an increased risk of pulmonary and cardiovascular organ damage. Medical care providers must be alert to the signs and symptoms of pneumothorax, hemothorax, and vascular or abdominal organ laceration in those presenting with suspected rib fractures (Eiff, Hatch, and Calmbach, 2003; Doty, 2008). Ribs commonly fracture at the point of impact or at the posterior angle, and ribs four through nine are the most commonly fractured. Child abuse must be considered in children who present with multiple rib fractures or with fractures in different stages of healing (Doty, 2008).

The ribs form a somewhat circular or cage-like structure around the pulmonary and cardiovascular organs. Trauma and pathology can occur to either the posterior or anterior portions, or both (Figure 11-11). This portion to be radiographically investigated is important for the limited radiographer to know in

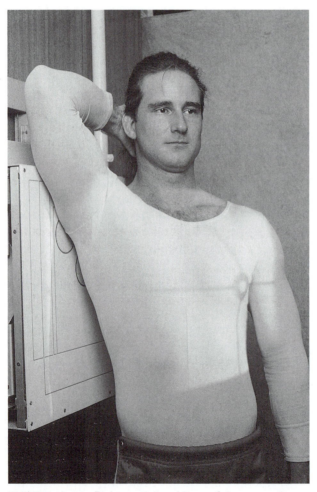

FIGURE 11-11   Right posterior oblique of the upper rib cage
Source: Delmar, Cengage Learning.

Area of Trauma	Projections/Positions	Instructions
Posterior Ribs Ribs 1–9/10	AP projection (above diaphragm) Erect position	Patient instructed to "take in a deep breath and hold it."
Posterior Ribs Ribs 11–12 Trauma	AP projection (below diaphragm) Erect position	Patient instructed to "take in a deep breath. Let it out. Hold it out. Don't breath or move."
Anterior Ribs Ribs 1–9/10 Trauma	PA projection Erect position (above diaphragm)	Patient instructed to "take in a breath. Let it out. Take in another breath and hold it. Don't breathe or move."
Anterior Ribs Ribs 11–12 Trauma	PA projection Erect position (below diaphragm)	Patient instructed to "take in a deep breath. Let it out. Hold it out. Don't breath or move."
Anterior Rib Trauma	Oblique positions Erect position Right anterior oblique (RAO) Left anterior oblique (LAO)	The patient's breathing technique will be dependent on whether the injury is above or below the diaphragm.
Posterior Rib Trauma	Oblique positions Erect position Right posterior oblique (RPO) Left posterior oblique (LPO)	The patient's breathing technique will be dependent on whether the injury is above or below the diaphragm.

FIGURE 11-12 Standard projections of ribs
Source: Delmar, Cengage Learning.

order to properly position the patient and to give correct breathing instructions. Figure 11-12 provides the standard projections and breathing instructions for each area of the rib cage.

In addition to the projections listed above, a standard chest x-ray examination (an erect PA and lateral) is also usually requested when a patient has suspected rib fractures. Additional studies such as CT and angiography may also be required.

Extremities: Pathology and Imaging Considerations

The upper and lower extremity x-ray examinations are performed to detect conditions such as fractures, soft tissue damage, arthritis, and tumors. The upper extremity includes the fingers, hands, wrists, elbows, forearms, upper arms, and shoulders. The lower extremity includes the toes, feet, ankles, lower legs, knees, upper legs, and hips.

Introduction

Data released by the National Center for Health Statistics cite deformities or orthopedic impairments as the most frequent chronic condition reported with almost 35 million conditions. These conditions along with arthritis and heart disease caused the highest numbers of restricted activity days and bed disability days per year for the time period of the analysis (CDC, 2008d). Based on this information, the limited radiographer may find that they are engaged in performing as many or more x-ray examinations of the extremities as plain chest x-ray examinations.

The ACR has issued guidelines and indications for the performance of radiography of the extremities. These guidelines suggest that the following are but a few of the clinical indications for radiography of the extremities:

1. Trauma;
2. Suspected physical abuse in infants and young children;
3. Metabolic diseases, nutritional deficiencies, and osseous changes from systemic disease;
4. Neoplasms, benign and malignant;
5. Primary non-neoplastic bone pathology;
6. Arthopathies;
7. Infections;
8. Preoperative or postoperative and/or follow-up studies;
9. Congenital syndromes and developmental disorders;
10. Vascular lesions;
11. Evaluation of soft tissue in an extremity (e.g., suspected foreign body);
12. Pain; and,
13. Correlation of abnormal skeletal findings on other imaging studies (ACR, 2003).

In addition to plain (non-contrast) radiographs of the extremities, additional diagnostic studies may be used. These include CT, MRI, radionuclide bone scan, arthroscopy, and laboratory tests.

Radiography textbooks devoted to radiography anatomy and positioning provide information about basic or standard projections and positions of the extremities. For any anatomic area, supplemental (non-standard) projections and positions are suggested when specific anatomy or pathology needs to be radiographically visualized. In preparing for the limited radiography profession, students will complete a course devoted to radiographic anatomy and positioning; therefore, this section is intended to supplement that information.

Figure 11-13 provides a list of the ACR's minimum recommendations for upper and lower extremity x-ray examinations in routine circumstances (ACR, 2003). The projections and positions may be modified for any given clinical situation and

Anatomic Area	Projections and Positions
Fingers	PA, lateral, and oblique
Hand	PA, oblique, and lateral (fanned fingers)
Wrist	PA, lateral and oblique
Forearm	AP and lateral
Elbow	AP and lateral
Humerus	AP and lateral
Shoulder	AP views in internal and external rotation and orthogonal projections in appropriate clinical situations
Acromioclavicular Joints	**Upright AP**
Clavicle	AP and AP angulated view
Scapula	AP and lateral
Toes	AP, lateral, and oblique
Foot	AP, lateral, and oblique
Os Calcis	Lateral and axial
Ankle	AP, lateral and oblique (mortise)
Lower leg	AP and lateral
Knee	AP and lateral
Patella	AP, lateral and sunrise view
Femur	AP and lateral
Hip	AP and lateral

FIGURE 11-13 American College of Radiology (ACR) minimum recommendations for upper and lower extremity x-ray examinations in routine circumstances
Source: Delmar, Cengage Learning.

as previously mentioned, additional radiographs may be warranted as part of or in addition to the initial examination. The physician may request additional imaging examinations after evaluation of the initial radiographs.

Trauma Radiography

Radiography of a patient who has been injured is often referred to as trauma radiography. Medical personnel who work daily in emergency care facilities are often more experienced in the care of patients with life-threatening injuries; however, regardless of the type of medical facility, limited radiographers should expect to encounter patients who have injuries resulting from trauma.

The limited radiographers' knowledge of standard positioning is often challenged in obtaining radiographs of patients who have injuries. Because of the nature and extent of the injury, the limited radiographer may have to adapt the routine to avoid further damage and to minimize the patient's discomfort and pain. For example, when x-ray examinations are requested of several different areas of the body, to avoid unnecessary movement of the patient, the limited radiographer can take all of the AP projections first. Any additional x-ray examinations can then be taken after the attending physician has reviewed the initial radiographs and gives permission to move the patient and to adjust the position.

Many medical facilities have standard operating procedures regarding moving trauma patients. One such procedure was just mentioned. When a patient arrives and has restricted mobility, initial "scout" radiographs are taken of the part "as is" after which, the attending physician reviews the radiographs before the patient is moved or their position adjusted.

Osteoarthritis

Osteoarthritis is the most common type of arthritis and is referred to as a degenerative joint disease (NIH National Institute of Arthritis and Musculoskeletal and Skin Diseases, 2002). It affects the cartilage that covers the ends of bones that meet to form a joint. As osteoarthritis progresses, the surface layer of cartilage breaks down and wears away allowing the bones under the cartilage to rub together, causing pain, swelling, and loss of motion of the joint. Over time, the joint may lose its normal shape. Also, small deposits of bone, osteophytes, may develop on the edge of the joints. Unlike other forms of arthritis, such as rheumatoid arthritis, osteoarthritis affects only joint function and does not affect skin tissue, the lungs, the eyes, or the blood vessels. Rheumatoid arthritis, the second most common form of arthritis, causes the immune system to attack the tissues of the joints, leading to pain, inflammation, and eventual joint damage and malformation. Compared to osteoarthritis, which is considered a disease of the elderly, rheumatoid arthritis typically begins at a younger age (NIH National Institute of Arthritis and Musculoskeletal and Skin Diseases, 2002).

Osteoarthritis most often occurs in the hands (at the ends of the fingers and thumbs), spine (neck and lower back), knees, and hips. The warning signs of osteoarthritis include:

- Stiffness in a joint after getting out of bed or sitting for a long time;
- Swelling in one or more joints; and,
- Crunching feeling or the sound of bone rubbing on bone.

Plain (non-contrast) x-ray examinations of the affected joint or joints is the imaging modality of choice for the initial diagnosis of osteoarthritis. Radiographic findings include osteophyte formation, joint space narrowing, sclerosis, and cysts (Figure 11-14) (Katai, Lofgren, and Meholic, 2007; Kowalczyk and Mace, 2009).

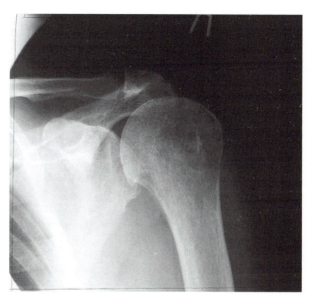

FIGURE 11-14 Osteoarthritis of the shoulder
Source: Delmar, Cengage Learning.

Magnetic resonance imaging is often used to assess the extent of soft-tissue involvement and arthroscopy examinations may also be used to further assess the joint.

The Upper Extremity

The upper extremities include the fingers, hands, wrists, elbows, forearms, upper arms, and shoulders.

The Hand and Fingers

Radiographs of the hand should include the proximal carpal bones, all five phalanges, and the distal tips. There are 19 bones in the hand consisting of 14 phalanges (proximal, middle, and distal portions) and 5 metacarpals that form the palm (Figures 11-15A and B). The hand also may have one or more sesamoid bones that lie in the tendons of the hand. The most common fractures occurring in the hand are in the phalanges (Eiff, Hatch, and Calmbach, 2003).

Occult fractures and bone bruises occur most commonly at the carpal scaphoid and the ribs (Eiff, Hatch, and Calmbach, 2003). Such bone fractures and bruises may not be visible on a radiograph immediately following trauma but may

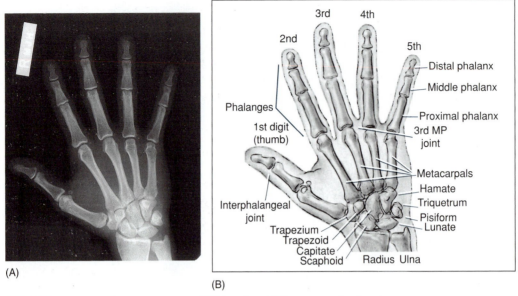

FIGURE 11-15 (A) Posterior-anterior (PA) hand and (B) anatomic landmarks
Source: Delmar, Cengage Learning.

be radiographically demonstrated about ten days after the incident. This is thought to result from bone resorption or displacement at the fracture site.

There are many reasons leading to fractures of the phalanges. In children up to nine years old, the majority of these injuries are related to compression trauma such as catching a finger in a door. Between the ages of 10 to 40, the most common cause of phalangeal injury results from sports activities. At around age 30, many of the hand injuries are related to machinery accidents (Eiff, Hatch, and Calmbach, 2003). As the patient ages, falling is the most common accident resulting in fractures to the fingers.

Many fractures and joint injuries are not well visualized because of inadequate radiographs often caused by a combination of factors. It is the responsibility of the limited radiographer to overcome factors such as patient motion, inadequate part positioning due to the injury, and poor selection of the technical x-ray exposure factors.

The most common fractures occurring in the hand and fingers are described as follows.

A **Boxer's fracture** is a very common injury that involves the neck of the fifth metacarpal. This injury results from direct trauma to the hand with axial loading or compression; often occurring when the individual punches an object that does not move upon impact.

The **Bennett's fracture/dislocation** is the most common injury to the thumb, often as a result of a fistfight. It occurs when a direct blow is received on the hand with the metacarpophalangeal (MCP) joint of the thumb partially flexed.

A deformity known as **gamekeeper's thumb** results from an abduction injury to the thumb in which avulsion of the ulnar collateral ligament is torn from the base of the proximal phalanx. **Avulsion** occurs when a fragment of bone is literally pulled away from the bone shaft.

Avulsion fractures usually occur around joints due to muscle, ligament, and tendon tearing. The most common metacarpal fracture occurs at the base of thumb (first metacarpal).

Other conditions can also be evaluated with x-ray examinations of the fingers and hand. For example, a **mallet finger** is a very common malady. The abnormality is visible where the fingertip is curled downward and the patient cannot straighten the finger out. The deformity occurs at the distal interphalangeal (DIP) joint and is usually the result of injury that damages the tendon or tears it away from the bone. Like a mallet finger, the **trigger finger** is a condition where a finger intermittently becomes locked in a bent position. The patient is able to force the finger to straighten back into normal position, but the finger cannot return to normal position on its own. This type of injury is often due to overuse and x-ray examinations are conducted to rule out fractures or other underlying pathology before treatment is started.

The Wrist. The wrist is a joint consisting of eight small bones arranged in two rows (Figures 11-16A and B).

Proximal Row	Distal Row
Scaphoid	Trapezium
Lunate	Trapezoid
Triquetrum	Capitate
Pisiform	Hamate

The carpal bones are held together by ligaments which allow movement and flexion. Carpometacarpal joints exist between the distal rows of carpals and the metacarpals. Intercarpal joints are found between each of the carpal bones. The radiocarpal joints are found between the proximal row of carpals, primarily the scaphoid and lunate, and the radius bone of the forearm. The hands and wrist are very sensitive, containing many bones, ligaments, tendons, and muscles, which may suffer fractures, strains, and sprains.

Falling is the leading cause of unintentional injury among Americans 65 and older; however, no one is exempt from slipping, stumbling, or tripping (CDC, 1996). It is a human instinct to reach out and try to catch oneself during a fall and this often

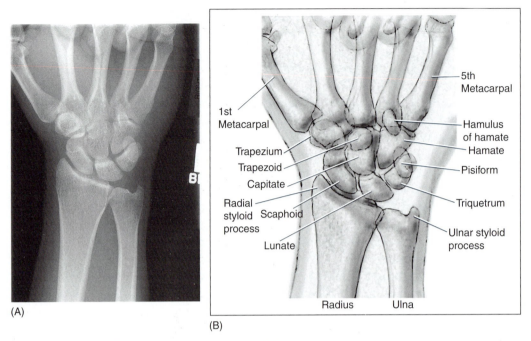

(A)

(B)

FIGURE 11-16 (A) PA radiograph of the wrist and (B) anatomic landmarks
Source: Delmar, Cengage Learning.

results in fractures of the wrist. The **Colles' fracture** is the most common fracture of the wrist resulting from falling on an outstretched hand (Figure 11-17).

The fracture occurs at the distal radius with dorsal displacement of the distal fracture fragment. A **Smith's fracture** of the wrist is a basically a reverse Colles' fracture with the distal fracture fragment displacing toward the palmar side of the wrist rather than a dorsal displacement. A **Barton's fracture** is an intra-articular fracture of the distal radius that involves the styloid and articular surface of the distal radius. A **chauffeur's fracture** is an intra-articular fracture of the distal radius primarily involving the styloid of the radius. The fracture is caused by axial compression that is transmitted through the scaphoid bone.

The limited radiographer should always include the entire anatomic area of interest on any radiographic projection or position. The requested joint or long bone should be placed on the center of the cassette or image receptor (IR) and the central ray (CR) directed to the mid-point of the area or to the designated point of entry. The mid-shaft of long bones is generally placed in the center of the cassette or IR and the CR directed to mid-shaft. In situations where there is no obvious injury or pain in a long bone, the limited radiographer should attempt to include both joints on all radiographs. When this is not possible, each joint should be demonstrated on at least one of the routine projections or positions.

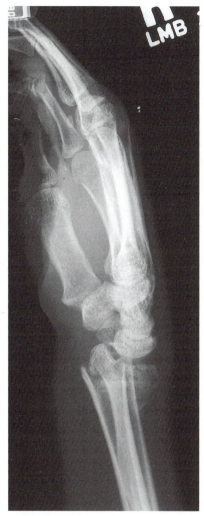

FIGURE 11-17 Colles' fracture of the wrist
Source: Delmar, Cengage Learning.

Carpal tunnel syndrome often occurs when an individual is involved in repetitive work that compresses a key nerve in the wrist (NIH National Institute of Neurological Disorders and Stroke, 2008). If the median nerve, which runs from the forearm into the hand becomes pressed or squeezed at the wrist, a sharp, piercing pain shoots through the wrist and up the arm. The carpal tunnel is a narrow, rigid passageway of ligament and bones at the base of the hand and houses the

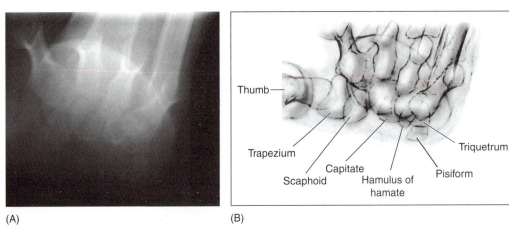

(A)   (B)

FIGURE 11-18   (A) Carpal canal radiograph and (B) anatomic landmarks
Source: Delmar, Cengage Learning.

median nerve and tendons. The result may be pain, weakness, or numbness in the hand and wrist, radiating up the arm.

Initial symptoms of carpal tunnel syndrome are gradual, starting with frequent burning, tingling, or itching numbness in the palm of the hand and the fingers, especially the thumb and the index and middle fingers. As symptoms worsen, people report feeling the tingling during the day and resulting decreased grip strength.

A special radiographic projection may be useful in demonstrating carpal tunnel syndrome and is referred to the carpal canal or tunnel projection, tangential, or inferosuperior projection of the wrist (Figures 11-18A and B).

When the patient is properly positioned for this projection, the carpals are demonstrated in a tunnel-like, arched arrangement.

The Forearm.   The forearm consists of two long bones, the radius and the ulna (Figures 11-19A and B). Processes on the ends of the two bones are important to both wrist and elbow radiography. Both the radius and ulna have a rounded disk-shaped head and a styloid process at the distal ends. At the proximal end of the forearm, the ulna is the larger of the two bones and has a large, palpable olecranon process. The large, crescent-shaped semilunar or trochlea notch curves anteriorly to form a pointed, beak-like projection called the coronoid process. At its upper or proximal end, the radius articulates with the capitulum of the humerus at the elbow, and with the ulna (superior radioulnar joint). The head of the radius articulates at a small depression on the ulna, the radial notch, to form the proximal radioulnar joint. Other components of the forearm include blood vessels and soft tissue.

Forearm fractures account for most limb fractures (Patient UK, 2008b). These fractures can be classified as proximal, middle, or distal and can affect one or both

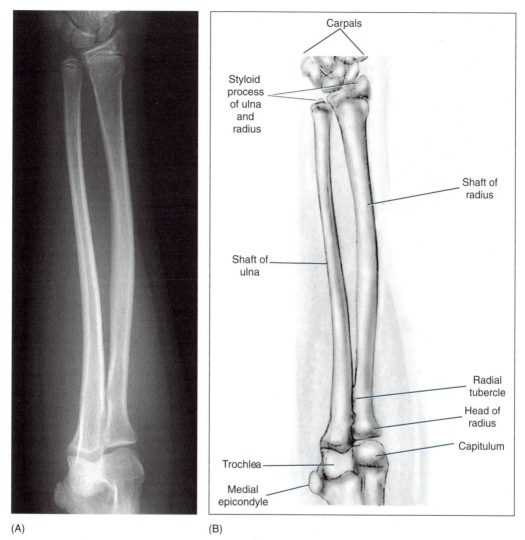

FIGURE 11-19 (A) AP forearm radiograph and (B) anatomic landmarks
Source: Delmar, Cengage Learning.

of the forearm bones. Forearm fractures are further classified as either open or closed. If the bone penetrates the skin, it is an open type fracture. This type of fracture provides easy access for pathogens to enter, possibly causing inflammation and infection and either preventing or delaying the healing process. If the skin is not penetrated, it is a closed fracture. Proximal forearm fractures may involve the elbow joint and distal forearm fractures may involve the wrist.

In adults, the mechanism of injury is usually significant force, most commonly occurring in motor vehicle accidents, direct blow, fall from a height, or during participation in sports. In children, the cause of forearm injury is usually indirect (e.g., falling on an outstretched hand). Often children suffer a **greenstick-type fracture**, in which the cortex breaks on one side without separation or breaking of the opposing cortex (Figure 11-20) (Mayoclinic.com, 2008). The result is similar to that of trying to break a green twig.

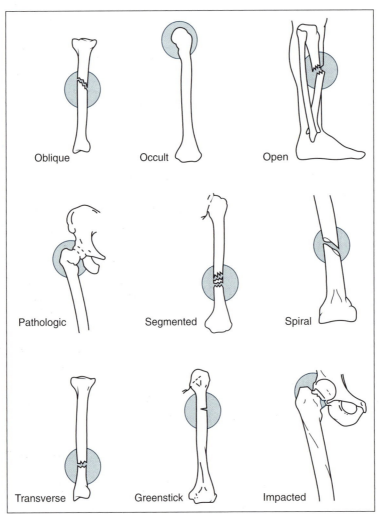

Oblique Occult Open

Pathologic Segmented Spiral

Transverse Greenstick Impacted

FIGURE 11-20 Examples of bone fractures
Source: Delmar, Cengage Learning.

A Galleazzi fracture is commonly caused by a fall on an extended, pronated wrist. The fracture consists of a solitary break in the distal one-third of the radius with accompanying subluxation or dislocation of the distal radioulnar joint.

A night-stick fracture occurs at the mid-shaft of the ulna. It usually results from a direct blow to the forearm. A Monteggia fracture occurs at the proximal third of the ulna with anterior dislocation of the radial head. It is usually caused by a fall onto an outstretched, extended, and pronated elbow or direct blow.

Often, repetitive flexion-extension of the elbow or pronation–supination of the wrist can lead to overuse injuries. Sports injuries such as tennis and golfer's elbow are examples of overuse injuries. Such injuries may result in a sprain or in some cases a stress fracture (NIH National Institute of Arthritis and Musculoskeletal and Skin Diseases, 2004; American Academy of Orthopaedic Surgeons [AAOS], 2008d). A sprain is any trauma to a joint and its associated ligaments and results in pain and disability (AAOS, 2008d). Common signs of a sprain are pain, rapid swelling, limited function, and localized warmth over the area. Sprains can also occur to muscles, ligaments, or other spinal structures and are often associated with stretching and small fractures.

Stress fractures occur when a person is subjected to repetitive trauma and are generally located at the point of muscle attachment (AAOS, 2008d). Stress fractures are a common injury to the lower extremity and occur when the bone bends almost to the point of breaking. The result may be a hairline crack that is too fine to be demonstrated on a radiograph but causes pain in the patient. Stress fractures are usually tender before they are painful and the area of tenderness is well defined (AAOS, 2008d). Normally a stress fracture affects only part of the bone, but if the patient continues to subject the area to pressure, the hairline fracture can become a complete fracture. During healing, the physician may request progressive x-ray examinations to determine the rate of healing and monitor evidence of further damage.

The Elbow Joint.　　The humerus, radius, and ulna combine to form the elbow joint (Figures 11-21A and B). The elbow joint is supported by strong ligaments and a tough capsule and surrounded by pads of fat and several bursa containing joint fluid. The elbow is a very stable joint and dislocates less frequently than the shoulder joint; however it is the joint most frequently examined in emergency clinics (Goswami, 2002). The most common fracture in the adult elbow involves the radial head. A radial head fracture involves the elbow joint. Fractures of the radial neck occur most often in children (Patient UK, 2008a).

Trauma to the elbow can occur from a fall on an outstretched hand and the outcome results in a radial head fracture. This type of fracture is often occult (hidden, not visible) and the interpreting physician may use the "fat pad sign" in examining images of the elbow (Goswami, 2002; Hobbs, 2005).

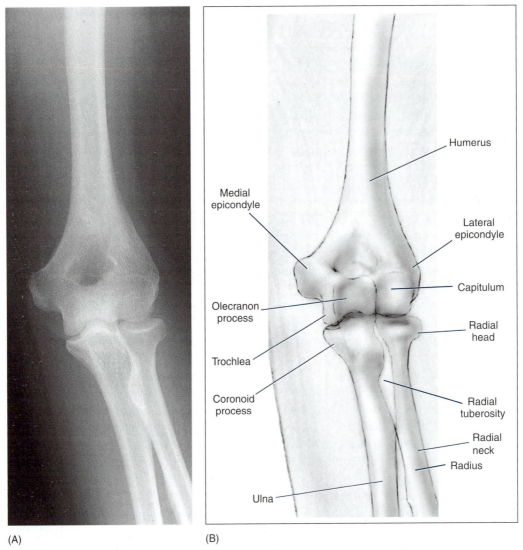

FIGURE 11-21 (A) AP radiograph of the elbow and (B) anatomic landmarks
Source: Delmar, Cengage Learning.

Fat pads are small masses surrounding the elbow joint and can be seen on a properly positioned lateral radiograph. The anterior and posterior fat pads are in close proximity to the radial, coronoid, and olecranon fossae. The anterior fat pad can be demonstrated on a lateral radiograph of the elbow as a superimposition of fat over the radial and coronoid fat pads. The posterior fat pad, located deep within the concavity of the olecranon fossa, is not normally seen on a properly aligned lateral position (Goswami, 2002; Hobbs, 2005).

It is important for the limited radiographer to understand that the fat pad sign may demonstrate a false positive if the elbow is improperly positioned or aligned in the lateral position. Proper positioning and alignment of the elbow requires a 90-degree flexion of the elbow joint (Figure 11-22).

In a lateral examination of a non-injured elbow joint, the posterior fat pad should not be visible on the radiograph because it is hidden within the olecranon process (Goswami, 2002; Hobbs, 2005).

A positive fat pad sign may indicate an occult fracture. Accessory x-ray examinations of the traumatized elbow may be required because plain x-ray examinations may not demonstrate subtle fractures of the radial head. Furthermore, it is often difficult to perform x-ray examinations on patients with limited mobility. Examples of non-routine elbow projections are the trauma AP projection and axial lateral projections. In the trauma AP projection, if the patient cannot partially extend the elbow and it remains flexed near 90 degrees, the limited radiographer should angle the central ray 10 to 15 degrees into the joint. If the elbow is flexed more than 90 degrees, the Jones position can be acquired (Bontrager and

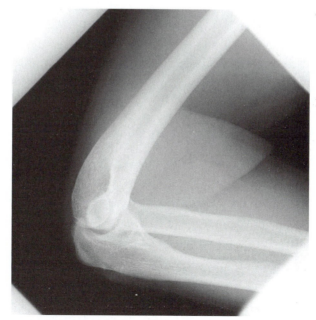

FIGURE 11-22 Failure to flex the elbow 90°
Source: Delmar, Cengage Learning.

Lampignano, 2005). These and other alternative radiographic projections of the traumatized elbow joint are available when the standard projections cannot be obtained. The limited radiographer should consult available textbooks dedicated to radiographic positioning to learn about additional methods of imaging patients with limited mobility.

The Humerus, Shoulder Joint, Scapula, and Clavicle.   The humerus is the second largest bone in the body. Its smooth, round, proximal head articulates with the glenoid cavity or fossa of the scapula. The anatomic neck of the humerus is located obliquely and adjacent to the humeral head. The humeral head has two processes, the greater and lesser tubercles, separated by the intertubercular sulcus or bicipital groove. The shoulder joint is made up of three bones: the scapula, clavicle, and the humerus (Figures 11-23A and B). These bones are joined together by soft tissues (ligaments, tendons, muscles, and joint capsule) to form a platform for arm mobility. The shoulder consists of three joints: glenohumeral joint, acromioclavicular joint, and sernoclavicular joint and one articulation, which together form the relationship between the scapula and the chest wall. Several layers of soft tissues cover the bones of the shoulder. The top layer is the deltoid muscle, which gives the shoulder a rounded appearance. The deltoid muscle allows the arm to be lifted overhead. Directly beneath the deltoid muscle is the sub-deltoid bursa, a fluid-filled sac.

The scapula is one of the largest flat bones in the body and has a triangular shape that creates three borders (superior, medial, and lateral) and three angles (superior, inferior, and lateral). The superior border contains a deep indentation called the scapular notch and the lateral angle contains the glenoid fossa, which articulates with the humeral head. This articulation is called the glenohumeral joint. The acromion process lies on the superior aspect of the scapula, projecting posteriorly and superiorly with the lateral end forming an articulation with the clavicle, the acromioclavicular joint. The posterior surface of the scapula has ridges and spines, which serve as important attachments for shoulder muscles.

The clavicle serves to attach the bones of the arm to the axial skeletal. The lateral end articulates with the acromion process of the scapula to form the acromioclavicular joint. The medial end articulates with the sternum to form the sternoclavicular joint.

According to the American Academy of Orthopaedic Surgeons (AAOS), in 2003, approximately 13.7 million people went to the doctor's office for shoulder problems, including 3.7 million visits for shoulder and upper arm sprains and strains (AAOS, 2008c). Injuries to the humerus and shoulder are frequently caused by athletic activities that involve excessive, repetitive, overhead motion, such

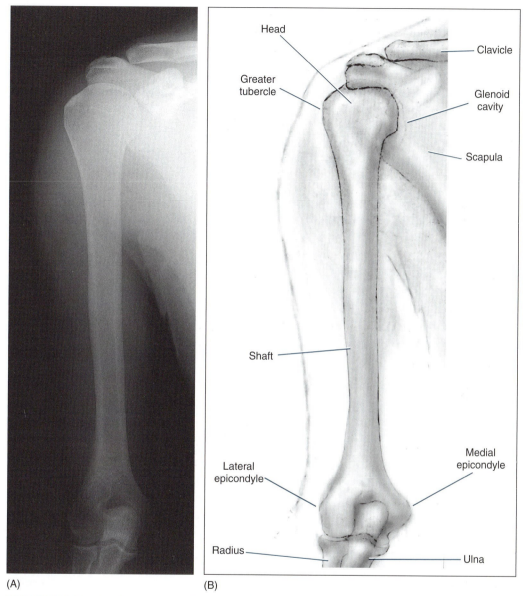

FIGURE 11-23 (A) AP humerus radiograph and (B) anatomic landmarks
Source: Delmar, Cengage Learning.

as swimming, tennis, pitching, and weight lifting. The AAOS lists the following as patient history type questions that may indicate a shoulder injury (AAOS, 2008c).

- Is the shoulder stiff?
- Can the arm be rotated in all of the normal positions?
- Does the shoulder feel like it could pop out or slide out of the socket?
- Does the shoulder lack strength to carry out normal daily activities? (AAOS, 2008c).

Most problems in the shoulder involve the muscles, ligaments, and tendons but when fractures of the humerus do occur they are either distal at the elbow joint or proximal near the shoulder (AAOS, 2009). A mid-shaft fracture of the humerus is most likely to be related to a fall or motor vehicle accident. Humeral fractures usually follow physeal lines of the humerus which divide it into four parts: the humeral head, greater tuberosity, lesser tuberosity, and the humeral shaft (AAOS, 2008c and 2009). Proximal humerus injuries are generally evaluated with standard radiographic projections of the shoulder.

Because the chest protects the scapula and surrounding muscles, the scapula is not easily fractured but is often associated with injuries to the chest.

Dislocations occur when the bones on opposite sides of a joint do not line up. Dislocations can involve any of three different joints of the shoulder girdle. The following are examples of shoulder girdle dislocations (AAOS, 2009):

- A dislocation of the acromioclavicular joint is called a "separated shoulder."
- A dislocation of the sternoclavicular joint interrupts the connection between the clavicle and the sternum.
- The glenohumeral joint can be dislocated anteriorly or posteriorly (AAOS, 2009).

An anterior dislocation of the shoulder is generally caused by the arm being forcefully twisted outward (external rotation) when the arm is above the level of the shoulder. A posterior dislocation of the shoulder is less common than anterior dislocations and may occur from seizures or electric shocks when the muscles of the front shoulder contract and forcefully tighten (AAOS, 2009).

Soft-tissue injuries are tears of the ligaments, tendons, muscles, and joint capsule of the shoulder, such as rotator cuff tears and labral tears. The rotator cuff is one of the most important components of the shoulder and is comprised of a group of muscles and tendons that hold the bones of the shoulder joint together. When the rotator cuff is injured, the victim may not recover the full function of the shoulder. Tendinitis of the shoulder refers to inflammation of a tendon in the shoulder. Bursitis is inflammation of the bursa sacs that protect the shoulder. Repeated bouts of tendinitis and bursitis may irritate and wear down the tendons, muscles, and surrounding structures (NIH National Institute of Arthritis and Musculoskeletal and Skin Diseases, 2001).

The clinical presentation of shoulder girdle injuries is generally pain, swelling and bruising at the site of trauma, and the inability to freely move the shoulder. As previously mentioned, whenever a patient presents with trauma to a joint or long bone, the limited radiographer may have to resort to non-standard projections and positions to obtain the necessary diagnostic radiographs. Limited radiographers should never attempt to manipulate or force the patient to assume a position that is uncomfortable or obviously painful.

The Lower Extremity

The lower extremities includes the toes, feet, ankles, lower legs, knees, upper legs, and hips.

The Foot and Toes

The lower limbs and pelvis provide weight-bearing support for the body and enable the body to move. The toes, feet, and ankles are particularly subject to sprains, strains, and fractures because of their continual use and weight load. The foot is comprised of 26 bones, consisting of three groups, phalanges, metatarsals (head, base, and shaft), and the tarsals. The seven tarsal bones of the ankle joint and proximal foot include the calcaneus, talus, cuboid, navicular, and three cuneiform bones. The calcaneus is also referred to as the heel and is the largest of the tarsal bones (Figure 11-24).

Like the phalanges in the hand, the phalanges of the foot also have a proximal, middle, and distal phalanx. The joints between the phalanges are referred to interphalangeal (IP) joints and are classified as diarthrodial hinge-type joints. The great toe like the thumb is considered the first digit and sesamoid bones may also be found in the tendons within the foot.

Primary medical care facilities report treating a broad range of fractures that involve the toes (Eiff, Hatch, and Calmbach, 2003). Almost all toe fractures result from either a stubbing injury or a heavy object being dropped on the toe. Standard radiographic projections of the toes include an AP, lateral, and oblique (Bontrager and Lampignano, 2005). Because most toe fractures are minimally displaced, the oblique position often provides the best image of the traumatized area. Dislocations of the IP joints are relatively common and are usually obvious on inspection of the radiographic images (Eiff, Hatch, and Calmbach, 2003).

Foreign objects (e.g., metal, wood splinters, etc.) entering the sole of the foot are common sources of injuries particularly in people who do not wear shoes. Soft tissue projections of the foot and toes may be requested to demonstrate low-density objects, such as wood, glass, plastic, that may be embedded in the soft tissues. This

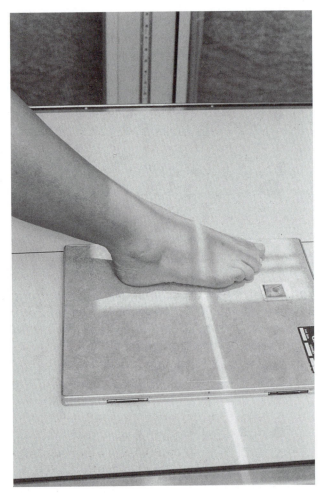

FIGURE 11-24 AP foot
Source: Delmar, Cengage Learning.

is often referred to as "soft-tissue" technique and requires maintaining the standard mAs value but reducing the kVp to decrease the x-ray beam penetration of the soft tissues.

Heel or calcaneus pain is an extremely common complaint and often begins without any prior history of injury or trauma. Inflammation of the connective tissue on the sole of the foot (plantar fascia) where it attaches to the heel bone is the most common cause of pain (AAOS, 2009). Calaneal pain may also be associated with a

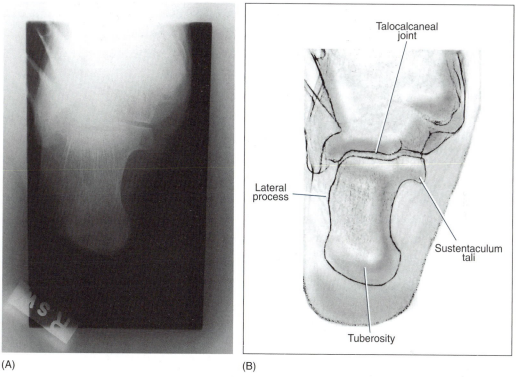

(A)   (B)

FIGURE 11-25 (A) Axial calcaneus radiograph and (B) anatomic landmarks
Source: Delmar, Cengage Learning.

spur or bony protrusion. A lateral positioned radiograph of the calcaneus provides good visualization of the bone (Figures 11-25A and B).

The navicular bone is subject to stress fractures in those engaged in weight-bearing activities such as running and long-distance walking. Stress fractures are not easily identified on plain x-ray examinations; however, MRI is useful in identification of this problem (Eiff, Hatch, and Calmbach, 2003). Most stress fractures occur in the weight-bearing bones of the lower leg and foot.

The Ankle, Leg, and Knee

The ankle joint is formed by the talus, tibia, and fibula. The distal ends of the tibia and fibula create a mortise (socket) for the trochlea of the talus. The mortise is formed by the distal ends of the fibula (lateral malleolus) and the tibia (medial malleolus), each extending downward on either side of the trochlea (Figures 11-26A and B).

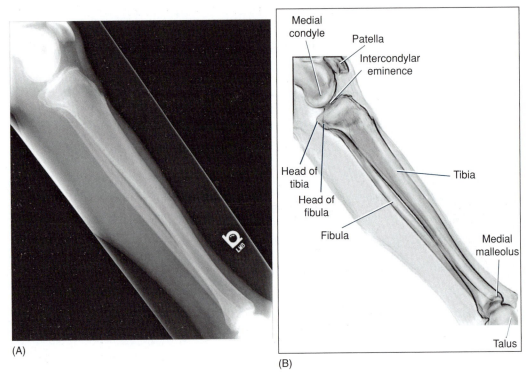

FIGURE 11-26 (A) AP lower leg and (B) AP radiograph
Source: Delmar, Cengage Learning.

The lower leg has two bones, the tibia and the fibula. The tibia or shinbone is located medially near the midline of the body. The tibial tuberosity is located anteriorly at the proximal end of the tibia. This roughened area of bone serves as the attachment for the patellar tendon. The medial and lateral tibial condyles form an articular facet for the head of the fibula. The fibula is the slender bone in the lower leg and is located laterally to the midline of the body.

The knee is the largest joint in the body and the kneecap or patella is the largest sesamoid bone. The patella articulates with the distal femur forming the patellofemoral joint. As previously mentioned, the knee is a common site of arthritis, osteoarthritis, rheumatoid arthritis, and other associated diseases. Chondromalacia, also called chondromalacia patellae, refers to softening of the articular cartilage of the kneecap. This condition occurs most often in young adults and can be caused by injury, overuse, misalignment of the patella, or muscle weakness (NIH National Institute of Arthritis and Musculoskeletal and Skin Diseases, 2008d).

Ankle, leg, and knee disorders can be the result of disease or injury. Injuries may occur as the result of a direct blow, sudden movement, fall, or may occur from repetitive injury and continued use over a long time period. According to the AAOS, ankle fractures occur in 184 per 100,000 persons per year and account for nearly 1.2 million emergency room visits (AAOS, 2008a). A severe ankle sprain may elicit the same clinical symptoms as a fracture, so every injury must be thoroughly evaluated. Common complaints include immediate and severe pain, swelling, bruising, tenderness, non-weight-bearing, and an "out of usual place" deformity of the area (NIH National Institute of Arthritis and Musculoskeletal and Skin Diseases, 2008d). CT or MRI imaging may be requested because of suspected soft tissue, muscle, and ligament injuries.

The **Pott's fracture** is the most common fracture of the lower leg and involves the medial malleolus (Eiff, Hatch, and Calmbach, 2003). In this fracture, the medial malleolus of the tibia is associated with an outward and backward dislocation of the foot.

The tibial spine (anterior cruciate) can be involved in avulsion type injuries. Most commonly the anterior tibial spine is sheared away from the bone. This injury usually occurs in children or adolescents as a result of a fall from a bicycle (Eiff, Hatch, and Calmbach, 2003). Patella fractures generally result from a direct blow to the bone, such as in a fall.

Meniscal injuries may cause a partial or total tear and the seriousness of the injury depends on the location and extent of the tear. Cruciate ligament injuries are sometimes referred to as sprains; however it usually refers to when the ligament is stretched or torn (or both) by a sudden twisting motion or a direct impact. The medial collateral ligament of the knee is more easily injured than the lateral collateral ligament and frequently occurs in contact sports like football or hockey.

Growth plate injuries are caused by a fall or blow to the limb and can also be caused from overuse. Although many growth plate injuries are caused by accidents that occur during play or athletic activity, growth plates are also susceptible to other disorders, such as bone infection. Shin splints, Achilles tendon injuries, and stress fractures are all included in the multiple disorders that may occur to the growth plates of the bones of children (NIH National Institute of Arthritis and Musculoskeletal and Skin Diseases, 2008b).

Osgood-Schlatter disease is a condition caused by repetitive stress on part of the growth area of the upper tibia and is characterized by inflammation of the patellar tendon and surrounding soft tissue.

Osteochrondritis dissecans results from a loss of the blood supply to an area of bone underneath a joint surface. Although the knee joint is the most frequently affected, any joint can be involved as a result of a slight blockage of a small artery or unrecognized injury or hairline fracture that damages the overlying cartilage.

Contusions can occur to any part of the body and often result from a direct blow. A contusion to bone usually results from a kick occurring directly over a bone. In this case, the bone usually will not fracture but bleeding under the bone may occur. Swelling lifts nerve endings away from the bone, causing extreme tenderness and pain, and discoloration. Compression on the area, plus elevation of the limb and application of ice are often recommended to reduce swelling.

The Femur, Hip, and Pelvis

The femur or thighbone is the longest, strongest, and heaviest bone in the body. Located on the proximal end of the femur are the greater and lesser trochanters, neck, and head. In anatomy, the hip is the bony projection of the femur, which is known as the greater trochanter, and the overlying muscles and fat. The hip joint is between the femur and acteabulum of the pelvis and its primary function is to support the weight of the body in both static (e.g., standing) and dynamic (e.g., walking or running) postures.

The hip joint is a synovial joint formed by the articulation of the rounded head of the femur and the cup-like acetabulum of the pelvis and is classified as a ball-and-socket joint. The hip joint has a strong fibrous capsule that permits a great range of motion, comparable in movement only to the shoulder joint.

The pelvic girdle serves as an attachment for the bones and muscles of the leg and also provides support for the viscera of the lower abdominal region. The entire pelvis consists of four bones: two hipbones, one sacrum, and one coccyx (Figure 11-27).

Each hipbone has three divisions; ilium, ischium, and pubis, which are separate bones that fuse into one bone in late adolescence. The ilium is the uppermost part of the pelvic girdle. The upper edge of the ilium is the iliac crest, which, if followed anteriorly, ends in the anterior superior iliac spine (ASIS). Both the iliac crest and the ASIS are important radiographic positioning landmarks. Inferiorly, a wing-shaped portion of the ilium, the ala, forms part of the superior acetabulum. The ischium is the lower portion of the pelvic girdle and has an enlarged roughened area, the ischial tuberosity, upon which the body rests when seated. Anteriorly, the tuberosity and the inferior ischial ramus join the inferior public ramus to form the lower border of the obturator foramen. The obturator is a large opening formed by the ramus and body of each ischium and by the pubis and is the largest obturator foramen in the body. The symphysis pubis in the lower anterior part of the pelvic girdle forms when the opposing pubis bones meet.

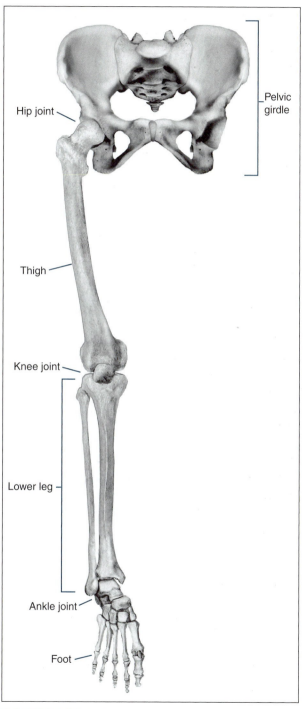

Hip joint

Pelvic girdle

Thigh

Knee joint

Lower leg

Ankle joint

Foot

FIGURE 11-27 Pelvis and lower limb
Source: Delmar, Cengage Learning.

Femoral Shaft and Hip Fractures. Femoral shaft fractures are usually seen in young adults as the result of motor vehicle accidents (MVA) or gunshot wounds. Fractures of the femur are the most common long bone fracture in the patient who suffers from multiple injuries due to MVA. Complications of the shaft fracture includes significant blood loss (2 to 3 units) and venous thromboses.

According to the *Morbidity and Mortality Weekly Report* (MMWR) issued by the U.S. Department of Health and Human Services, an estimated 850,000 fractures occur annually in the United States among persons age 65 and older (CDC, 2008b). Of this estimate a great percentage are hip fractures related to falling, most often by falling sideways onto a hip (Figure 11-28).

In 1990, the Centers for Disease Control and Prevention estimated that the number of hip fractures would exceed 500,000 by the year 2040. About one out of five hip fracture patients dies within a year of their injury. About 78% of all fractures occur in women and osteoporosis increases a person's likelihood of sustaining

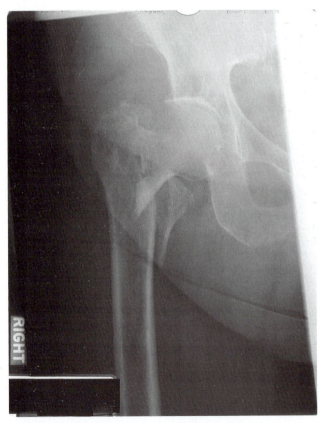

FIGURE 11-28 Intertrochanteric fracture of the hip
Source: Delmar, Cengage Learning.

a hip fracture (2008b). The femoral neck of the femur is a common fracture site for older people who have fallen. The classic physical sign for such a fracture is the external rotation of the involved foot, where the lesser trochanter is clearly visible in profile. During positioning the patient, the limited radiographer should never attempt to rotate the leg or foot, rather a pelvis radiograph should be taken "as is" without movement of the part.

Dislocation or luxation is the complete loss of articular contact of bones forming a joint. The most common dislocations in skeletal radiography are of the hip, patella, thumb, shoulder, and fingers. Persons presenting with a dislocation may demonstrate pain and abnormality in shape or misalignment in the area of dislocation. Subluxation is a partial or incomplete dislocation.

Osteoporosis

The National Osteoporosis Foundation (NOF) estimates that more than 30 million Americans have osteoporosis, 80% of whom are women. In the United States today, 10 million people already have the disease and 20 million more have low bone mass (osteopenia), placing them at increased risk for osteoporosis (National Osteoporosis Foundation, 2008). Osteoporosis is an under-diagnosed and silent condition that has financial, physical, and psychosocial consequences. The World Health Organization (WHO) Study Group defined osteoporosis in 1994 as a systemic skeletal disease characterized by low bone mass and microarchitectural deterioration of bone tissue, resulting in an increase in bone fragility and susceptibility to fracture (World Health Organization [WHO], 1994).

The National Institutes of Health (NIH) defines osteoporosis as "a skeletal disorder characterized by compromised bone strength predisposing an individual to an increased risk of fracture" (NIH Osteoporosis and Bone-Related Diseases National Resources Center, 2008). The NIH definition recognizes factors that prevent people from achieving optimal bone mass and conditions that lead to bone loss later in life. The NIH also states that bone strength is the combination of bone density and bone quality (Figures 11-29 and 11-30).

Typically, those with osteoporosis have no pain or indication of the disease process until they break a hip, wrist, or sustain spinal fracture(s) that may leave a dowager's hump or reduce their height by a few inches. A broken hip or crushed vertebrae may begin an initial downward spiral of lost mobility and illness, culminating in death.

The WHO and other medical research organizations have identified the following factors that may contribute to risk of developing osteoporosis:

- Family history of osteoporosis and bone fracture;
- White or Asian ethnicity;

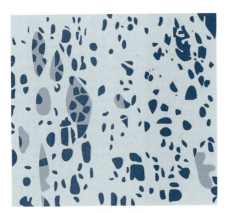

FIGURE 11-29 Normal bone
Source: Delmar, Cengage Learning.

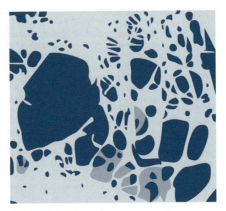

FIGURE 11-30 Osteoporotic bone
Source: Delmar, Cengage Learning.

- Thin or small body frame with a premenopausal body weight of less than 127 pounds;
- Smoking;
- Excessive alcohol consumption;
- Sedentary lifestyle;
- Calcium-deficient diet (either at the present or as a child);
- Certain medications, such as steroids commonly used to treat asthma and arthritis and high dosages of thyroid hormone;
- Early menopause before the age of 45; and,
- Other pathologies.

Lower risk factors for developing osteoporosis include:

- White women with a dark complexion;
- Women of African or Black ancestry;
- Women who are overweight;
- Women who eat large amounts of dairy products and vegetables; and,
- Women who exercise regularly (WHO, 1994; NIH Osteoporosis and Bone-Related Diseases National Resource Center, 2008).

Areas of bones affected by osteoporosis will radiographically appear spongelike and may show osteopenia (abnormal decrease in bone mass). Because osteoporosis is a destructive bone disease, the usual kVp exposure ranges will easily penetrate the porous bone; therefore, a reduction in kVp may be required to produce diagnostic radiographs in areas of osteoporotic bone.

Prevention of osteoporosis requires a lifetime of many healthy-living activities that include good nutrition, adequate intake of nutrients (e.g., calcium, vitamins, and minerals), daily weight-bearing exercise, and avoidance of smoking and alcohol.

Many people think that there is nothing that can be done after a diagnosis of osteoporosis has been made (NHI Osteoporosis and Bone-Related Diseases National Resource center 2008). The good news is that the Federal Drug Administration (FDA) has approved bone-rebuilding drugs; however, more potentially effective drugs are always being developed.

After osteoporosis has been diagnosed, a physician prepares a treatment plan designed to help maintain the patient's current bone mass and prevent additional bone loss. Treatment usually involves a long-term program that includes medication, diet, exercise, and regular serial bone mineral density (BMD) monitoring. It is important that serial BMD measurements used to monitor a patient's response to treatment be precise and accurate in order to detect small changes in BMD.

Because osteoporosis is a silent disease and signs and symptoms may not be evident in the early stages, a bone density test may be used to determine bone mass.

BMD measurements can be useful in diagnosis and treatment of osteoporosis and also in tracking how successful the prescribed treatments are in curbing additional bone loss. During routine medical visits or health screening examinations, completion of a risk assessment questionnaire may be used to identify potential victims of osteoporosis.

The International Society for Clinical Densitometry (ISCD) publishes official positions listing indications for BMD testing. These ISCD's position statements change, as new research becomes available. The following indications are current as of October 2007 and additional information about BMD testing and revised ISCD position statements may be obtained at the ISCD website (www.ISCD.org).

ISCD 2007 Official Indications for BMD testing
- Women aged 65 and older;
- Postmenopausal women under age 65 with risk factors for fracture;
- Women during the menopausal transition with clinical risk factors for fracture, such as low body weight, prior fracture, or high-risk medications use;
- Men aged 70 and older;
- Men under age 70 with clinical risk factors for fracture;
- Adults with a disease or condition associated with low bone mass or bone loss;
- Adults taking medications associated with low bone mass or bone loss;
- Anyone being considered for pharmacologic therapy;
- Anyone being treated, to monitor treatment effect; and,
- Anyone not receiving therapy in whom evidence of bone loss would lead to treatment (International South for Clinical Densitometry [ISCD], 2007).

The Vertebral Spine

The vertebral column is divided into five sections and within each section the vertebrae have distinct characteristics (Figure 11-31).

The distinctive characteristics and curves of each section require specific radiographic positioning and central ray placement. Certain terms often associated with the vertebral curvature include lordosis, kyphosis, and scoliosis

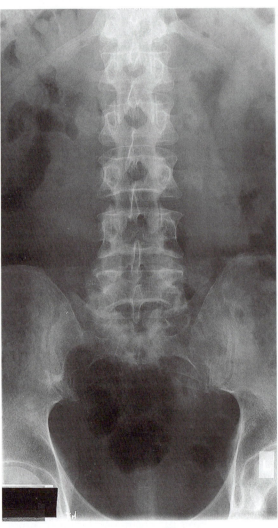

FIGURE 11-31 Lumbar spine, AP projection
Source: Delmar, Cengage Learning.

(Figure 11-32). **Lordosis** simply means "bent backward" and describes the normal anterior concavity of the lumbar and cervical spine. The term lordosis may also be used to describe an abnormally increased curvature or "sway-back" of the lumbar spine section. An abnormal or exaggerated thoracic "humpback" curvature with increased convexity is called **kyphosis**. An abnormal or exaggerated lateral curvature of the vertebral spine is called **scoliosis**.

The vertebral column provides flexible support for the trunk and upper body and provides a protective housing for the spinal cord. The spinal canal follows the curves of the vertebral spine beginning at the base of the skull and extending into the sacrum.

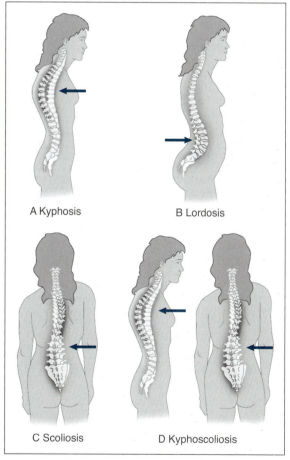

FIGURE 11-32 Illustration of kyphosis, lordosis, scoliosis, kyphoscoliosis
Source: Delmar, Cengage Learning.

Standard X-Ray Examinations of the Vertebral Spine

Standard x-ray examinations of the vertebral spine are made to identify or exclude anatomic abnormalities or disease processes of the spine. The *ACR Practice Guideline for the Performance of Spine Radiography in Children and Adults* has established minimum criteria for imaging for each section of the vertebral spine. The following information has been condensed from this guideline document (ACR, 2007).

Cervical Spine Examination in Adults

- The entire cervical spine from the craniocervical junction to the superior end plate of thoracic 1 should be included on the radiograph;
- A standard examination includes AP, lateral, and open mouth (odontoid) projections;
- A swimmer's lateral position should be performed if necessary to assess the lower cervical segments and C7–T1 alignment;
- In cases of significant clinical suspicion of cervical spine injury, cross-table lateral, AP, open mouth odontoid or submental views may be obtained prior to moving the patient for further examination; and,
- Additional projections and imaging with CT and MRI may be necessary (ACR, 2007).

Cervical Spine Examination in Infants and Children

- A standard examination includes AP, odontoid, and lateral projections; and,
- Additional projections and imaging with CT and MRI may be necessary (ACR, 2007).

Thoracic Spine Examination

- A standard examination includes AP and lateral projections. In these radiographs, the lower cervical or upper lumbar anatomy should be visualized to assure accurate numbering of thoracic levels; and,
- Additional projections that may be required include; swimmer's lateral position of the upper thoracic region, oblique positions, and thoracolumbar or other spot-type projections (ACR, 2007).

Lumbosacral Spine Examination

- A standard examination includes AP and lateral projections. A PA projection may be used instead of the AP to reduce radiation dosage; and,
- Additional projections that may be required include both oblique positions, spot-type lateral projection of L5–S1, angled AP projection of L5–S1, and flexion and extension lateral positions (ACR, 2007).

Scoliosis Examination

- A standard scoliosis examination includes erect PA or AP of the entire thoracolumbar spine that demonstrates the iliac crests (ACR, 2007).

Sacrum and Coccyx Examination

- The upper part of the sacrum is visible on the lumbosacral examination;
- For specific investigation of either the sacrum or coccyx, a standard examination includes a cephalad-angled AP projection of the sacrum and a lateral position of the sacrum and coccyx; and,
- For specific investigation of the sacroiliac joints, bilateral oblique positions may be used (ACR, 2007).

Soft-tissue structures are not usually visible on plain radiographs of the vertebral spine but the disk spaces between the vertebrae may be seen. Additional imaging studies may be used to fully evaluate the vertebral spine, spinal cord, and surrounding soft tissue structures.

Some figures estimate that nearly 253,000 people in the United States live with a disability related to a spinal cord injury (French, et al., 2007). Some of the most common causes of injuries to the vertebral column include direct trauma, hyperextension-flexion injuries, osteoporosis, and metastatic destruction. Lower back injuries account for many occupational injuries and result in loss of work, wages, and productivity (French, et al., 2007). An abbreviation associated with trauma to the cervical spine is SCIWORA (spinal cord injury without radiographic abnormality) and is used when there is the presence of neurological symptoms in the absence of radiographic findings.

Trauma and fractures to any portion of the vertebral spine can be life-threatening and represents a potential medical emergency situation. The degree of severity of the injury depends on two major factors: the type of injury and the level of the injury. A complete injury means that there is no function below the level of the injury; whereas, an incomplete injury means that there is some functioning. Some of the more common mechanisms of injury include certain types of forces on the vertebral column.

1. *Compression forces* on the neck can cause facet jamming and fixation.
2. *Shear forces* disrupt the ligaments and produce anterior or posterior subluxation.
3. *Hyperextension and hyperflexion forces* occur when there is excessive forward and backward movement that causes a whipping type motion of the vertebral spine.
4. *Lateral hyperflexion and hyperrotary forces* occur from side to side and a looking-back-over-the-shoulder type movement.

A few of the more common fractures of the vertebral spine include the following.

The **hangman's fracture** is associated with hanging type injuries and often results after a motor vehicle accident in which the person's chin strikes the dashboard. It results from a hyperextension injury that can be easily missed on plain x-ray examinations of the cervical spine area. A hangman's injury results in a bilateral pedicle fracture involving the arch of the second cervical vertebral body.

An anterior subluxation or dislocation is often associated with this type of injury.

A **teardrop fracture** is a caused by a severe hyperflexion injury of the cervical spine that results in anterior compression fracture of the vertebral body and disruption of the posterior ligament. The **clay shoveler's fracture** occurs in the lower cervical spine. The injury is the result of hyperflexion and was first identified in workers attempting to throw a shovel full of clay with the shovel stuck in the clay. This type of injury has also been identified in individuals engaged in weight lifting and football.

Whiplash is a general term encompassing soft tissue neck injuries from a variety of causes. A herniated nucleus pulposus (HNP), commonly called "slipped disk," is a condition that occurs when injury to one of the intervertebral disks causes the soft inner part to protrude into the spinal canal. The protrusion exerts pressure on the spinal cord and spinal nerves located in the spinal canal, which may result in severe pain and may cause numbness in the extremities.

Plain (non-contrast) x-ray examinations are the most common imaging modality used to assess low back pain because of the visibility of vertebral fractures, subluxation, erosion of the vertebral bodies, and other conditions such as osteoporosis. Myelography may be requested when vertebral disk disorders are suspected. MRI and CT imaging are superior in demonstrating the spinal cord, nerve roots, subarachnoid and epidural spaces, and vertebral disks. CT is the imaging modality of choice when the clinical evaluation indicates a vertebral fracture with possible spinal cord involvement.

The Abdomen

The abdomen is the area located below the thoracic cavity and directly above the pelvic cavity. The abdomen contains many of the vital organs of the digestive and urinary systems. Four important terms associated with the abdominal cavity include the peritoneum, mesentery, omentum, and mesocolon. Most of the abdominal structures and organs as well as the wall of the abdominal cavity are covered by the peritoneal membrane. The peritoneum forms large folds that bind the abdominal organs to each other and to the walls of the abdomen. Double folds of peritoneum are called the mesentery, which loosely connects the small intestines to the posterior abdominal wall. The omentum is a specific type of double-fold peritoneum that extends from the stomach to other organs. The lesser omentum extend superiorly from the lesser curvature of the stomach to portions of the liver. The greater omentum connects the transverse colon to the greater curvature of the stomach inferiorly. The mesocolom refers to the peritoneum that attaches the colon to the posterior abdominal wall.

X-Ray Examination of the Abdomen

The World Health Organization (WHO) indicates that the peak incidence of abdominal trauma occurs in persons aged 14 to 30 years (ACR, 2002). Abdominal trauma can result from either blunt forces or penetrating injuries. Blunt abdominal injuries can result from either compression (secondary to a direct blow or against a fixed external object), or from deceleration forces. The liver and spleen are the most frequently damaged organs resulting from blunt force injuries.

Penetrating abdominal trauma implies that either a gunshot, shrapnel, or stab wound has entered the abdominal cavity. Any type of abdominal injury should be considered as life threatening until the complete scope of the injuries has been evaluated. A mnemonic for remembering the key elements in taking a medical history when the patient presents with suspected abdominal injuries is AMPLE which means:

- Allergies;
- Medications;
- Past medical history;
- Last meal or other intake; and,
- Events leading to the presentation.

Identifying serious intra-abdominal pathology on plain (non-contrast) radiographs can be a challenge to the physician since the abdominal organs do not provide optimum visible contrast (Figure 11-33). CT imaging has increased the positive identification of most abdominal injuries resulting from trauma. Initial focused abdominal ultrasound for trauma may be performed at the patient's bedside.

The *ACR Practice Guideline for the Performance of Abdominal Radiography* suggests that the minimum standard projections of the abdomen consist of a supine AP and/or horizontal beam (upright, decubitus, or cross-table lateral) projections (ACR, 2002). The supine radiograph should include the area from the symphysis pubis, inferiorly, to the upper abdomen, or at least to the superior margin of the kidneys, and ideally to the level of the diaphragm. The upright, decubitus, or cross-table lateral x-ray examination is obtained with the x-ray beam parallel to

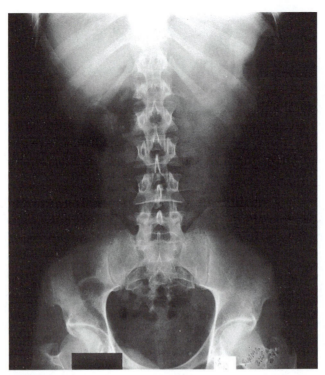

FIGURE 11-33 AP abdomen radiograph
Source: Delmar, Cengage Learning.

the floor and perpendicular to the film or IR, to optimize the visualization of small amount of pneumoperitoneum. The upright examination may be obtained in the AP or PA projection and the film should be centered 2 inches above the iliac crest in the adult patient. The left lateral decubitus position is obtained in the AP projection. The most superior part of the right side of the abdomen from the right hemidiaphragm to the pelvis must be centered and included on the radiograph. If the patient cannot be placed on the left side, the right lateral decubitus position may be used as an alternative. The cross-table lateral examination is seldom used for adults and older children, except for critically ill patients when an upright or decubitus film cannot be obtained. A standard plain chest x-ray examination is also usually requested when the patient presents with abdominal trauma. An acute abdominal series may be requested and includes x-ray examinations made in AP supine and erect AP abdominal position and a standard PA chest radiograph taken with the patient in the erect position, whenever possible. Specific indications for an acute abdominal series include post-operative complications, intra-abdominal mass, perforated organ, ascites, and ileus. Additional examples of conditions that may require abdominal x-ray examinations include bowel obstruction and/or performation, volvulus, ileus ulcerative colitis, Crohn's disease, and appendicitis.

Metabolic Diseases

Metabolic diseases are caused by a disturbance of the normal physiologic function of the body. Disorders and diseases of the endocrine system and disturbances of fluid and electrolyte balance are included in this category. Metabolic disease may be inherited or the onset may be of unknown origin. The scope of metabolic diseases has been limited to those that have a direct impact on the skeletal system and are likely to be encountered by the limited radiographer.

Gout

Gout is a painful condition that occurs when the product of uric acid is deposited as needle-like crystals in the joints and/or soft tissues. Once deposited in the joints, the uric acid crystals cause inflammatory arthritis, which leads to intermittent swelling, redness, heat, pain, and stiffness in the joints.

Gout is more frequent in men and affects joints at any location, but in many people initially affects the joints of the big toe (podagra) (NIH National Institute of Arthritis and Musculoskeletal and Skin Disease, 2008a). Gout also affects other joints and areas around the joints such as the ankles, heels, knees, wrists, fingers, and elbows. Uric acid crystals can also collect in the kidneys and cause kidney stones. Radiographically, the bony changes associated with gout include erosion of the joint with overhanging edges.

Osteoporosis, Osteomalacia, and Paget's Disease

Osteoporosis, osteomalacia, and Paget's disease are also metabolic disorders that have radiographic significance. Osteoporosis has already been covered in the chapter; however, is mentioned here because it is considered a metabolic disorder.

Osteomalacia. Osteomalacia is characterized by increasing softness of bones, so that they become flexible and brittle, thus causing deformities. Osteomalacia is caused by a lack of calcium in the tissues generally occurring from inadequate intake or absorption of calcium, phosphorus, or vitamin D. If osteomalacia occurs before the growth plate closes it is called rickets. Osteomalacia may be present in people with chronic diseases such as hepatic disease, pancreatitis, resections of the gastrointestinal tract, and in certain renal diseases.

Because this condition causes a decrease in calcium deposits in the tissues, the limited radiographer may have to decrease the technical x-ray exposure factors.

Paget's Disease.   Paget's Disease, osteitis deformans, named after a British surgeon Sir James Paget (1814–1899), is a skeletal disease of the elderly with chronic inflammation of bones. The disease process causes thickening and softening of bones and the bowing of long bones. Paget's disease is more common in men than women and generally begins in the fifth decade of life (NIH National Institute for Arthritis and Musculoskeletal and Skin Diseases, 2008a). The pelvis, spine, skull, and long bones are the most frequently affected bones.

The progression of Paget's disease is in two stages. In the first stage bone is destroyed (osteolytic stage), but is replaced by abnormally soft, poorly mineralized bone (osteoblastic stage). Normal bone is gradually replaced by osteoid material, which is very porous and bulky with increased vascularity. Soft, porous consistency in the weight-bearing bone leads to stress-induced deformities and fractures. A complication of Paget's disease is the development of osteogenic sarcoma.

Radiographically, Pagetic bone appears with cortical thickening, radiolucent and radiopague areas.

Acromegaly

Acromegaly is a progressive metabolic disorder caused by excessive secretion of growth hormone from the pituitary gland (Kowalczyk and Mace, 2009). It generally affects middle-aged persons and is characterized by elongation and enlargement of bones of the extremities, frontal bone, and mandible. An enlargement of the nose and lips with thickening of the facial soft tissue is also evident. Persons with acromegaly present with prominent facial features in the forehead and jaw, widened teeth, and abnormally large, spadelike fingers. Visible radiographic changes in the cranium include an enlarged sella turcia and changes in the dimensions of the calvarium (Kowalczyk and Mace, 2009).

Bone Tumors

Bone tumors may be either benign or malignant. The most common benign bone tumors are osteoma, osteochondroma, and giant cell tumor. The most common malignant bone tumors are osteosarcoma and myeloma (i.e., types of chondrosarcoma) and Ewing's tumor (Furlow, 2001). Bone tumors may be diagnosed through radiographic interpretation and involves the visual appearance and pattern of bone destruction, location of the tumor, and its position within the bone. These factors along with the patient's age are important in the radiographic diagnosis. Osteoma, a benign bony tumor of bonelike structure, develops on the bone and occasionally at other sites.

Osteochondroma

Osteochondroma, another benign bone tumor, typically strikes more males than females and arises from the growth zone between the epiphysis and diaphysis of long bones. Giant cell tumor or osteoclastoma may be either benign or malignant. 50% of the diagnosed giant cell tumors will be benign with 15% being malignant and generally more prevalent in individuals between the ages of 20 and 30 years (Kowalczyk and Mace, 2009).

Ewing's Sarcoma

Ewing's sarcoma, a malignant bone tumor, generally occurs between the ages of 5 to 15 years and rarely after the age 30. This neoplastic disease is more common in males than females and more frequent in Caucasian population (Furlow, 2001). This tumor arises from the medullary canal and involves the bone diffusely and may involve the entire shaft of the bone.

Chondrosarcoma

Chondrosarcoma, a malignant tumor, arising from cartilaginous origin, constitutes only a very small percentage of the malignant skeletal bone tumors. More males than females are affected by chondrosarcoma with the most common sites being the pelvis, shoulder, and ribs (Kowalczyk and Mace, 2009; Furlow, 2001).

Neoplastic diseases of the vertebral spine occur in people of all ages. The most common benign tumors are osteoma, osteochondroma, and giant cell tumor. The primary malignant bone tumors are osteosarcoma, Ewing's tumor, and myeloma.

Imaging and Abuse

Abuse of any kind is disturbing but unfortunately occurs all too frequently. Victims represent all socio-economic, cultural, and ethnic backgrounds and no one is exempt. Abuse victims are usually children, the elderly, disabled, and those incapable of defending themselves, but anyone may become the next target. Evidence of abuse must be investigated thoroughly in order that its perpetrators may be stopped and victims protected (Bilchik, 2007).

Diagnostic imaging studies may provide the first clues to physical abuse. Such studies often prove critical in determining whether abuse has occurred. All medical staff serve as the watchdogs for the signs and symptoms of abuse and become the voice for those unable or unwilling to ask for help.

With the advancements in diagnostic imaging along with nuclear medical imaging, US, CT, and MRI, the scope of imaging abnormalities due to abuse and neglect were finally able to be fully visualized. These studies have not only served to catalog the various manifestations of inflicted injury, but correlation with surgical and autopsy findings have provided insights into the mechanisms responsible for these injuries (Kleinman, 1998).

The goal of diagnostic imaging is to achieve optimal sensitivity and specificity.

"Because most forms of abuse tend to be cyclic, there is a high risk of repetitive injury, particularly in infants and young children. A missed diagnosis carries the risk that a child will be subjected to further assaults. In infants, these attacks tend to escalate in severity and culminate with life-threatening central nervous system injury" (Kleinman, 1998).

All staff in the primary care and emergency department should be proficient in triage of children and adults with suspected abuse or neglect. Clear and precise information will allow the physician to make decisions regarding examinations, tests, and treatment as well as whether to make a report to CPS (Lorenzetti, 2007).

All 50 states have child abuse reporting statutes. These statutes have as their primary purpose the identification of child abuse and neglect and, secondarily, the protection of children through state monitoring of families and the provision of services. Also, many medical centers have an interdisciplinary crisis assistance team composed of a primary care physician, nurse, social worker, psychiatrist, and radiologists to review and evaluate all suspected or confirmed cases of abuse.

The basis for notification of state authorities is not knowledge but reasonable suspicion or belief. That is, a person does not need to know that abuse or neglect exists in order to report. A mandated reporter must report if the given medical or social data indicates abuse or neglect.

The role of the radiologist and limited radiographer in cases of suspected abuse is usually that of a consultant acting with limited clinical and laboratory information. When findings indicate the possibility of abuse, the radiologist or film-reading physician has the responsibility to indicate this in the written report as well as in direct verbal communication to the referring physician or physician representative (Kleinman, 1998). If the referring or attending physician is unwilling to file a report, the radiologist or film-reading physician has the legal responsibility to do so. Limited radiographers are also held accountable to report suspected or confirmed child abuse. In this situation, the limited radiographer should prepare written documentation of any such communication to the supervising physician. This is an important step in the legal chain in order to protect oneself from a legal charge of failure to report.

Diagnostic imaging studies may provide the first clues to physical abuse (Baker, 2007). The attending triage physician may be the first to suspect abuse and should convey this information to radiology staff with the imaging request. In many cases, the radiologist or reading-physician may be the first to detect an abnormality that might indicate potential abuse or non-accidental trauma.

Skeletal injuries are the most common physical abuse injuries observed in the radiology setting; however, all staff must be alert to less obvious signs of abuse and neglect. Fractures of the skull, long bones, and ribs are the most frequent sites requiring radiographs of the specific bones and joints involved. The radiographic skeletal survey is the method of choice for global skeletal imaging in cases of suspected abuse and may be requested in place of or in addition to specific bone radiographs (American Academy of Pediatrics, 2000).

REVIEW QUESTIONS

1. The term pathology originates from the Greek term *pathos* which means:
   a. pain
   b. trauma
   c. suffering
   d. disease

2. When the underlying cause of a disease is unknown it is referred to as:
   a. iatrogenic
   b. idiopathic
   c. irrespective
   d. introspective

3. _____is a generalized swelling of the subcutaneous tissues throughout the body.
   a. Anasarca
   b. Ascites
   c. Ischemia
   d. Aplasia

4. The failure of a body part or organ to reach normal size or development is:
   a. anasarca
   b. ascites
   c. ischemia
   d. aplasia

5. **All** of the following are examples of an additive disease or condition, **except**:
   a. Paget's disease
   b. Osteoporosis
   c. Acromegaly
   d. Hydrocephalus

6. According to the 15% kilovoltage (kVp) rule, a 15% increase in kVp is equivalent to doubling the milliamperage-seconds (mAs).
   a. True
   b. False

7. Key features of a family history that may increase risk are:
   a. diseases that occur at an earlier age than expected
   b. disease in more than one close relative
   c. certain combinations of disease within a family
   d. all of the above

8. The most common medical imaging examination in the United States is _____ x-ray.
   a. abdomen
   b. chest
   c. knee
   d. hand

9. The body thorax is widest at approximately the ___ through the ___ ribs.
   a. second-third
   b. fourth-fifth
   c. sixth-seventh
   d. eighth-ninth

10. During expiration, the diaphragm moves downward.
    a. True
    b. False

11. The ___ is a depression on the medial surface of each lung where vessels and bronchi enter.
    a. apex
    b. crest
    c. hilum
    d. base

12. A ___ inch source to image distance (SID) is required for routine chest x-ray examinations.
    a. 36
    b. 48
    c. 60
    d. 72

13. The lateral projection of the chest is crucial in identifying abnormalities in the:
    1. posterior costophrenic angle
    2. mediastinum areas
    3. areas related to the spine

    Possible Responses
    a. 1 and 2
    b. 1 and 3
    c. 2 and 3
    d. 1, 2, & 3

14. The ___ sign is present if fluid or abnormal tissue obscures the border of a structure normally seen on a chest radiograph.
    a. ground glass
    b. sail
    c. silhouette
    d. air bronchogram

15. Approximately ___% of pneumonia cases are believed to be caused by viruses.
    a. 15
    b. 25
    c. 50
    d. 75

16. Tachypnea refers to increased:
    a. respiration
    b. blood pressure
    c. urine output
    d. pulse

17. The Centers for Disease Control and Prevention (CDC) recommends that limited radiographers and others who provide care for persons who have compromised immune systems should have a tuberculosis test every:
    a. three months
    b. six months
    c. year
    d. two years

18. Kerley's B lines are the most common radiographic signs of:
    a. pneumonia
    b. Legionnaire's disease
    c. air-space disease
    d. interstitial lung disease

19. The air bronchogram sign is one of the key radiographic findings of:
    a. pneumonia
    b. Legionnaire's disease
    c. air-space disease
    d. interstitial lung disease

20. Pertussis is also commonly called:
    a. croup
    b. emphysema
    c. whooping cough
    d. asthma

21. Coal worker's disease is also called:
    a. pneumoconiosis
    b. asbestosis
    c. berylliosis
    d. byssinosis

22. Histoplasmosis is a systemic infection caused by a fungus that thrives in:
    a. water
    b. soil
    c. sewage
    d. hay

23. Hantavirus pulmonary syndrome (HPS) appeared as a mysterious disease in the spring of:
    a. 1963
    b. 1975
    c. 1986
    d. 1993

24. The major cause of lung cancer is:
   a. cigarette smoking
   b. radon gas
   c. automobile exhaust
   d. genetic inheritance

25. **All** of the following are true regarding x-ray examination of a patient with trauma to the right posterior chest in the region of ribs 1–9, **except**:
   a. standard chest x-ray examination
   b. posterior-anterior (PA) projection with above diaphragm breathing instructions
   c. patient instructions are to take on expiration
   d. posterior oblique projection

26. The American College of Radiology (ACR) minimum recommendations for x-ray examination include:
   1. anterior-posterior (AP) projection
   2. posterior-anterior (PA) projection
   3. lateral
   4. oblique

   Possible Responses
   a. 1 and 2
   b. 1 and 3
   c. 2 and 3
   d. 3 and 4

27. Osteophytes are small deposits of bone that may develop on the edge of joints.
   a. True
   b. False

28. There are ___ bones in the hand.
   a. 28
   b. 19
   c. 12
   d. 8

29. **All** of the following carpal bones are arranged in the proximal row, **except**:
   a. scaphoid
   b. lunate
   c. hamate
   d. pisiform

30. _____ fracture is the most common fracture of the wrist:
   a. Barton's
   b. Colles'
   c. Chauffeur's
   d. Smith's

31. The second largest bone in the body is the:
   a. tibia
   b. fibula
   c. femur
   d. humerus

32. There are ___ tarsal bones in the foot.
   a. 5
   b. 7
   c. 9
   d. 12

33. Typically "soft-tissue" technique requires a reduction in:
   a. exposure time
   b. milliamperage
   c. kilovoltage
   d. distance

34. In 1990, the Centers for Disease Control and Prevention estimated that by 2040, the number of hip fractures would exceed:
   a. 5,000
   b. 15,000
   c. 50,000
   d. 500,000

35. Those at lower risk for developing osteoporosis include:
   1. White women with a dark complexion
   2. those with a sedentary lifestyle
   3. overweight women
   4. those of African or Black ancestry

   Possible Responses
   a. 1 and 3
   b. 3 and 4
   c. 1, 3, & 4
   d. 2, 3, & 4

36. ___ is an abnormal or exaggerated lateral curvature of the vertebral spine.
    a. Lordosis
    b. Scolosis
    c. Kyphosis
    d. Mylosis

37. The World Health Organization (WHO) indicates that the peak incidence of abdominal trauma occurs in persons aged:
    a. 5–10
    b. 14–30
    c. 35–45
    d. 55–65

38. ___ is a disease associated with uric acid crystals deposited in the joints and/or soft tissue.
    a. Gout
    b. Acromegaly
    c. Osteoporosis
    d. Rickets

39. Abuse victims are usually:
    a. children
    b. elderly
    c. disabled
    d. all of the above

REFERENCES

American Academy of Orthopaedic Surgeons. (2008a). *Ankle fractures*. Retrieved from http://orthoinfo.aaos.org

American Academy of Orthopaedic Surgeons. (2008b). *Common foot problems*. Retrieved from http://orthoinfo.aaos.org

American Academy of Orthopaedic Surgeons. (2008c). *Common shoulder injuries*. Retrieved from http://orthoinfo.aaos.org

American Academy of Orthopaedic Surgeons. (2008d). *Stress fractures*. Retrieved from http://orthoinfo.aaos.org

American Academy of Orthopaedic Surgeons. (2009). *Common shoulder injuries*. Retrieved from http://orthoinfo.aaos.org

American Academy of Pediatrics: Section on Radiology. (2000, June). *Diagnostic imaging of child abuse*, American academy of Pediatrics initial published in Pediatrics (1991; 87–262–264) *105*(6). Retrieved from aapolicy.aapublications.org

American College of Radiology. (1993, Revised 2006). ACR practice guideline for the performance of pediatric and adult portable (mobile unit) chest radiography. Retrieved from www.ACR.org

American College of Radiology. (1996, Amended 2007). *ACR practice Guideline for the performance of general radiography*. Retrieved from www.acr.org

American College of Radiology. (2002, Revised 2006) *ACR practice guideline for the performance of abdominal radiography*. Retrieved from http://www.acr.org

American College of Radiology. (2003, Amended 2006). *ACR practice guideline for the performance of radiography of the extremities*. Retrieved from www.acr.org

American College of Radiology. (2007). *ACR practice guideline for the performance of spine radiography in children and adults*. Retrieved from http://www.acr.org

American College of Radiology. (2008). *ACR practice guideline for the performance of high-resolution computed tomography (HRCT) of the lungs in adults*. Retrieved from www.acr.org

American Lung Association. (2006, November). *Facts about lung cancer*. Retrieved from www.lungusa.org

American Lung Association. (2007) *Pneumonia fact sheet*. Retrieved from http://www.lungusa.org

American Lung Association. (2008a). *Acute bronchitis*. Retrieved from http://www.lungusa.org

American Lung Association. (2008b). *Acute respiratory distress syndrome (ARDS)*. Retrieved from www.lungusa.org

American Lung Association. (2008c). *Asthma*. Retrieved from http://www.lungusa.org

American Lung Association. (2008d). *Chronic obstructive pulmonary disease (COPD) fact sheet*. Retrieved from http://www.lungusa.org

American Lung Association. (2008e). *Cystic fibrosis (CF) fact sheet*. Retrieved from www.lungusa.org

American Lung Association. (2008f). *Emphysema*. Retrieved from http://www.lungusa.org

American Lung Association. (2008g). *Histoplasmosis*. Retrieved from www.lungusa.org

American Lung Association.(2008h). *Interstitial lung disease and pulmonary fibrosis*. Retrieved from http://www.lungusa.org

American Lung Association. (2008i). *Lesser-known lung disease*. Retrieved from www.lungusa.org

American Lung Association. (2008j). *Occupational lung diseases*. Retrieved from www.lungusa.org

American Lung Association. (2008k). *Tuberculosis fact sheet*. Retrieved from www.lungusa.org

American Society of Radiologic Technologists. (2008). *Radiography of the chest*. Retrieved from https://www.asrt.org

Baker, A. (2007). *Forensic pathologists & pediatric radiologists: Partners in seeking the truth*. Retrieved from www.pedrad.org

Bilchik, S. (2007). Portable guides to investigating child abuse—Diagnostic imaging of child abuse. Retrieved from http://www.ncjrs.gov

Bontrager, K. W., & Lampignano, J. P. (2005). *Textbook of radiographic positioning and related anatomy* (5th ed.). St Louis, MO: Mosby-Year Book Inc.

Centers for Disease Control and Prevention. (1996). *Morbidity and Mortality Weekly Report.* October 18, 1996/Vo. 45/No. 41. Retrieved from www.cdc.gov

Centers for Disease Control and Prevention. (2007) *Tuberculin skin testing fact sheet.* Retrieved from www.cdc.gov

Centers for Disease Control and Prevention. (2008a). *Family history is important for your health.* Retrieved from http://www.cdc.gov

Centers for Disease Control and Prevention. (2008b). *Hip fractures among older adults.* Retrieved from www.cdc.gov

Centers for Disease Control and Prevention.(2008c). *Patient facts: Learn more about legionnaire's disease.* Retrieved from www.cdc.gov

Centers for Disease Control and Prevention. National Center for Health Statistics. (2008d). *Prevalence of selected chronic conditions: United States, 1990–92.* Retrieved from http://www.cdc.gov

Doty, C. I. (2008). *Fracture, Rib.* EMedicine from WebMD. Retrieved from http://www.emedicine.com

Eiff M. P., Hatch, R. L., & Calmbach W. L. (2003). *Fracture management for primary care.* Philadelphia: Saunders.

French, D. D., Campbell R., Sabharwal, S., Nelson, A., Palacios, P., & Gavin Dreschnack, D. (2007). *Health care costs for patients with chronic spinal cord injury in the veterans health administration.* Retrieved from www.pubmedcentral.nih.gov

Furlow, B. (2001). Radiography of bone tumors and lesions. *Radiologic Technology 72*(5), 455–469.

Greathouse, JS. *Radiographic Positioning & Procedures: A Comprehensive Approach. 2006.* Clifton Park, NY: Thomson Delmar Learning.

Goswami, G. K. (2002). The fat pad sign. *Radiologic Technology 222*:419–420.

Hobbs, D. L. (2005). Fat pad signs in elbow trauma. *Radiologic Technology 77*(2).

Katai, L. H., Lofgren, R., & Meholic, A. (2006). *Fundamentals of chest radiology* (2nd ed.). Philadelphia: Elsevier, Inc.

Kleinman, P. K. (1998). *Diagnostic imaging of child abuse* (2nd ed.). St. Louis, MO: Mosby, Inc.

Kowalczyk, N., & Mace, J. D. (2009). Radiographic pathology for technologists (5th ed.). St. Louis, MO: Mosby Elsevier.

Lorenzetti, J. P. (2007). A voice for the voiceless: The role of the radiology professional in child abuse cases. *RT Image 20*(2).

MayoClinic.com. (2008). *Children's health. Greenstick fractures.* Retrieved from http://www.mayoclinic.com

National Institutes of Health. National Institute of Arthritis and Musculoskeletal and Skin Diseases. (2001, May Revised March 2006.) *Shoulder problems.* NIH Publication No. 06-4865. U.S. Department of Health and Human Services.

National Institutes of Health. National Institute of Arthritis and Musculoskeletal and Skin Diseases. (2002, Revised May 2006) *Osteoarthritis.* Retrieved from www.niams.nih.gov

National Institutes of Health. National Institute of Arthritis and Musculoskeletal and Skin Diseases. (2004). *Sports injuries.* (NIH Publication No. 04-5278). U.S. Department of Health and Human Services.

National Institutes of Health. National Institute of Neurological Disorders and Stroke. (2008). *Carpal tunnel syndrome fact sheet.* Retrieved from www.ninds.nih.gov

National Institutes of Health. Osteoporosis and Bone-Related Diseases National Resource Center. (2008). *Osteoporosis overview.* Retrieved from www.osteo.org

National Osteoporosis Foundation. (2008). *Osteoporosis: A debilitating disease that can be treated.* Retrieved from www.nof.org

National Institutes of Health. National Institute of Arthritis and Musculoskeletal and Skin Diseases. (2008a). *Gout.* Retrieved from www.naims.nih.gov

National Institutes of Health. National Cancer Institute. (2008a) (Last modified August 1, 2008). *Non-small cell lung cancer.* Retrieved from www.cancer.gov

National Institutes of Health. National Institute of Arthritis and Musculoskeletal and Skin Diseases. (2008b). *Growth plate injuries.* Retrieved from www.niams.nih.gov

National Institutes of Health. National Cancer Institute. (2008b) (Last modified May 28, 2008). *Small cell lung cancer.* Retrieved from www.cancer.gov

National Institutes of Health. National Institute of Arthritis and Musculoskeletal and Skin Diseases. (2008c). *Information for patients about Paget's disease of bone.* Retrieved from www.niams.hih.gov

National Institutes of Health. National Institute of Arthritis and Musculoskeletal and Skin Diseases. (2008d). *Joint basics.* Retrieved from www.niams.nih.gov

Patient UK. (2008a). *Elbow injuries and fractures.* Retrieved from http://www.patient.co.uk

Patient UK. (2008b). *Forearm injuries and fractures.* Retrieved from http://www.patient.co.uk

Pelsoci, T. M. (2008). Low-cost manufacturing process technology for amorphous silicon detector panels: Applications in digital mammography and radiography. *National Institute of Standards and Technology GCR* 03(844), 19. Retrieved from www.atp.nist.gov

Scheffer, K. J., & Tobin, R. S. (1997). *Better x-ray interpretation.* Philadelphia: Springhouse Corporation.

The International Society for Clinical Densitometry. (2007). Pediatric official positions of the International Society for Clinical Densitometry. Retrieved from http://www.iscd.org.

The Merck Manuals Online Medical Library. (2009a). Community-acquired pneumonia. Retrieved from http://www.merck.com

The Merck Manuals Online Medical Library. (2009b). Infections. Retrieved from http://www.merck.com

U.S. Surgeon General's Family History Initiative. (2008). Retrieved from http://www.hhs.gov

Wilkins, T. R., & Wilkins, R. L. (2005). Clinical and radiographic evidence of pneumonia. *Radiologic Technology* 77(2): 106–110.

World Health Organization. (1994). *Assessment of fracture risk and its application to screening for postmenopausal osteoporosis.* Report of a WHO study group. WHO Technical Report Series 843, 1–29.

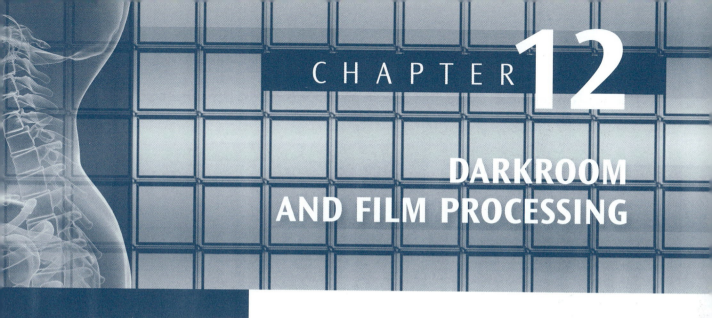

CHAPTER 12

DARKROOM AND FILM PROCESSING

Key Terms

Artifacts
Automatic Film Processing
Developer
Film Base
Film Emulsion
Film Fog
Fixer
Intensifying Screens
Latent Image
Light Absorption
Manifest Image
Radiographic Film
Screen Film
Sensitivity Speck
Sensitometry
Silver Halide Crystal
Silver Recovery
Speed

Chapter Outline

Objectives

Upon completion of the chapter, the student will meet the following objectives by verifying knowledge of the facts and principles presented through oral and written communication at a level deemed competent.

- Identify appropriate responses related to processing-area location, construction, and function.
- Describe the composition of screen film and explain the function of each part.
- Recall three characteristics of screen film.
- Identify proper procedures for handling and storing radiographic film.
- Outline the procedure for checking safelight illumination.
- Explain the purpose of intensifying screens.
- Identify the difference between calcium-tungstate and rare-earth screens.
- Outline the procedure for proper care and cleaning of intensifying screens.
- Discuss basic automatic processing.
- Describe the steps in film processing.
- Explain the purpose of replenishment of processing chemicals.
- Recognize common film artifacts and identify causative factors.
- Demonstrate competence in each task listed. Refer to the appendix for the individual procedure/performance guides.

Introduction

Processing a film or image today is specific to how the image is produced. Processing, however, does require a chemical reduction of the image. Manual processing of the film/screen image is rarely used today because automatic processing is commonly available. This is helpful because manual processing is time consuming and subject to a high degree of error. Without assumption of usage, manual processing is discussed here to provide a foundation of background knowledge for the new student.

When information is needed, it may be accessed from manufacturers of radiographic processing–related products.

Processing Area Considerations

A processing area should offer an environment in which the necessary functions can be carried out safely and efficiently, without providing hazards that would compromise the diagnostic quality of finished radiographs. The processing area actually requires "safe" artificial light rather than total blackness. However, the processing area is still commonly called "the darkroom," and this term will be used throughout the chapter.

Location of the Darkroom

Whether they are located in an office or in a hospital, most processing areas today are automated. To save time, darkrooms are generally located near the radiographic rooms. The distance between the darkroom and radiography rooms is more important in a multi-doctor clinic or large hospital, where the patient volume may require a full-time person to perform film processing and equipment maintenance.

Darkroom ventilation should provide a constant flow of fresh air with a temperature between 60°F and 70°F. The relative humidity level should be maintained at between 40% and 60%. This prevents a buildup of chemical odors, yet allows enough air moisture to prevent static electricity that can discharge to the film and cause artifacts. A well-ventilated darkroom is also important for a healthy work environment. A film-viewing area may be adjacent to the darkroom where radiographs can be viewed (Figure 12-1). The darkroom should be large enough to provide space for loading and unloading cassettes, film storage bin, processing equipment, and related accessories.

Walls adjacent to the radiographic rooms should be shielded with 1.6 mm (¹⁄₁₆ in) lead all the way to the ceiling to protect unexposed film from radiation exposure. Passboxes may be built into the walls to allow passage of cassettes between the darkroom and radiographic room. A typical passbox has two sets of doors to allow such passage between rooms and an interlock system on each set of doors to prevent accidental light exposure should both be opened at the same time (Figure 12-1). Each set of doors will have two compartments, one for exposed and one for unexposed cassettes. The ideal location for a passbox is near the film-loading bench in the darkroom.

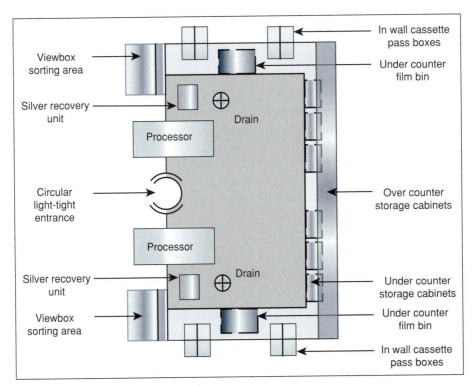

FIGURE 12-1 A typical darkroom plan
Source: Delmar, Cengage Learning.

Darkroom walls and floor should be covered with a non-porous, chemical- and stain-resistant surface (e.g., Formica®). A radiographic processing area should have a single entrance door that allows for absolute lighttight fittings. Variations on the single entrance are: (1) a maze-type entry (Figure 12-2), (2) a revolving door (Figure 12-3) and (3) an electric interlocking door system. Whatever the entrance design, the purpose is to protect radiographic film from being struck by light and/or radiation and being fogged. Processing-area lighting consists of safelight, radiographic illumination, and regular lighting.

Radiographic Film

A radiograph is a permanent image created when ionizing radiation passes through matter and onto photographic film. The latent image is invisible, and will become manifest image, or visible, after the film is processed. The recording medium, or radiographic film, plays a very critical role in the production of diagnostic

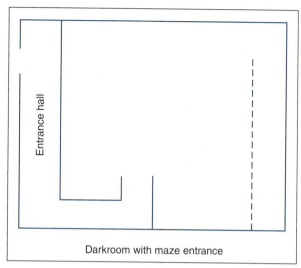

Darkroom with maze entrance

FIGURE 12-2 Darkroom with maze entrance
Source: Delmar, Cengage Learning.

radiographs. If the film is defective, or has been improperly stored or handled, the final diagnostic image may be less than perfect. Also, many things can happen during the film-processing stage that may detract from the diagnostic value of the radiograph. To avoid these problems, it is helpful to learn about radiographic film construction, latent image formation, types of film, and proper film handling and storage.

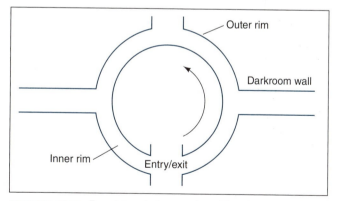

FIGURE 12-3 Revolving darkroom door. The outer rim is built into the wall and has two openings: one into the darkroom and one to the outside. The door's inner rim is suspended, which allows it to rotate on a central bearing. The inner rim's opening can be turned to coincide with the outer rim's openings.
Source: Delmar, Cengage Learning.

Radiographic film consists of two parts, the base and the emulsion, surrounded by a protective covering of gelatin called the supercoating. The film base is constructed of a polyester that provides a rigid yet flexible support for the emulsion. A subcoating of adhesive covers the base and serves to bind the emulsion to the base polyester. The film emulsion consists of a mixture of gelatin and silver halide crystals. Usually, 95% of the silver halide consists of silver bromide with the remainder being silver iodide.

Most radiographic film is coated on both sides and thus is called double emulsion film. The film emulsion is the most important layer of the film because it contains the crystals that will hold the latent image formation. The gelatin in the emulsion allows for an even distribution of the silver halide crystals. Its properties allow for rapid softening in the developer solution and quick hardening in the fixer solution. Refer to Figure 12-4, for a cross section of radiographic film. The emulsion reaction to ionizing radiation can be altered by the way the crystals are manufactured and their mixture. Each manufacturer of film closely guards the unique formulas that are responsible for its film characteristics. Film characteristics include speed, contrast, and resolution. Each of these areas will be included in the discussion on film types.

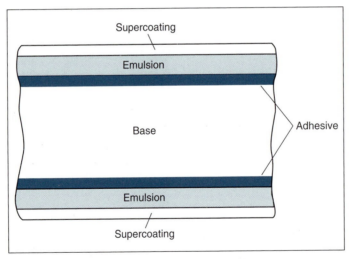

FIGURE 12-4 Cross section of radiographic film
Source: Delmar, Cengage Learning.

Latent Image Formation

As ionizing radiation exits from matter and strikes radiographic film, energy is deposited in the emulsion. The transfer of information between the radiation and film emulsion is by photoelectric interaction. Each silver halide crystal has on its surface **sensitivity specks** of tiny particles of atomic silver and silver sulfide. When these specks are struck by ionizing radiation, ionization of the silver halide crystals results in positively charged silver ions and negatively charged bromine ions, expressed as:

$$AgBr + radiation \longrightarrow Ag^+ + Br^-$$

These sensitized specks will react to the developer chemicals during film processing. Silver halide crystals that have been ionized (radiated) will be changed into black grains through the development process. Silver halide crystals that have not been ionized will remain in crystal form and will not be changed during the development stage of film processing. These unexposed, undeveloped silver halide crystals will react to the fixer chemicals and will be released from the emulsion in the fixation step of processing and recovered through a silver-recovery chamber.

Types of X-Ray Film

Many different types of film are manufactured for medical radiography. This variety reflects the diversity of radiographic procedures requiring special application film, such as those used in mammography, cardiography, dental radiography, and so forth. The major differences between the types of film are the thickness of the film emulsion and its response to both x-ray and light emitted from the intensifying screen.

Direct exposure film responds best to x-ray. Direct exposure film is rarely used today because (1) its increased emulsion-silver content makes it more costly and (2) it requires a much higher x-ray exposure. *Because direct exposure film requires an increase in x-ray exposure, its use does not justify the increase in radiation exposure to the patient.* By using screen-type film, the radiation exposure to the patient can be reduced. This is possible because **screen film** (sensitive to light) is used with intensifying screens that emit light during the x-ray exposure, thereby allowing a reduction in the x-ray exposure.

Screen film has three characteristics that are routinely considered: contrast (high or low), speed (sensitivity), and light absorption. Each film manufacturer produces screen film with a certain level of contrast. This level may be high-contrast, which produces a very black-and-white shaded image, or low-contrast, which produces a gray shaded image. The film contrast of a particular brand of film is directly related to the latitude or range of exposure factors (mA, time, kVp) that will produce an acceptable image. Usually film manufacturers provide two or more latitudes, referred to as medium- or high-contrast film. The physician who is responsible for interpreting the radiographic image may wish to select the level of film contrast to be used for most radiographic procedures.

Screen film is also available in different speeds or sensitivity. The speed of a screen film refers to how fast the silver halide crystals in the emulsion respond to the light emitted from the intensifying screens. High-speed (fast) screen film contains a thick emulsion, large crystals, or a higher concentration of crystals in the emulsion. Visibility of anatomic detail on the finished radiograph may be decreased with the use of high-speed screen film. An advantage, however, of this type of film is the faster exposure times can be used. Film-speed and contrast-level selection should be a collective effort of the radiographer and physician.

Spectral absorption, commonly called spectral matching, refers to the use of film whose sensitivity is correctly matched to the light spectrum emitted from the intensifying screen. Calcium-tungstate intensifying screens emit blue and blue-violet light and should be matched to silver halide emulsion film or blue-sensitive film. Rare-earth intensifying screens should be matched to screen film that is sensitive to green light. However, they may also be compatible with blue-sensitive film. Correct spectral matching is also referred to as film-screen combination or spectral system. Selecting the correct combination is very important because if the match is incorrect, the film will not respond properly and the patient may receive more radiation than necessary because incorrect exposure may result in a repeat radiograph.

Because x-ray film is sensitive to light, the lamps or safelights used in the darkroom must meet certain requirements. Darkroom lamps are used to provide a minimum of light to allow the operator some illumination. Because exposed screen film is approximately eight times more sensitive to light than unexposed film, safelights must have their light filtered. For blue-sensitive film, an amber (Wratten 6-B) light generally is used. An amber filter will only allow light having wavelengths longer than 550 mm, or beyond the spectral response of blue-sensitive film, to be emitted. A reddish-brown filter is used with green-sensitive film and can also be used with blue-sensitive film. Safelights should be installed at least 3 feet from the area where the film will be handled and processed. Light bulb wattage in the safelight should not exceed the manufacturer's recommendations for the specific type filter.

Safelights are designed for either indirect ceiling illumination or direct illumination. One way to determine whether a safelight is actually safe is to check the safelight illumination, evaluate the results, and take necessary action if an unsafe condition exists. Remember that safelight illumination as well as light leaks into the darkroom area and can cause fog or an undesirable film darkening that decreases the diagnostic value of the radiograph. It is important to periodically check the safelight filter for cracks and light-leaks in the lamp (filter) housing.

Film Identification

Patient identification, date, right or left marker, and other data must be (legally) permanently marked on a radiograph. Two common methods of identification are: (1) attaching lead markers to the cassette before the exposure is made, and (2) a photographic transfer of data. Generally, both methods are used. The lead marker contains the patient's identification number, date, a right or left letter, and the doctor or facility name. The photographic marker usually contains more detailed data such as the patient's address, sex, age, religion, insurance identification, and so on.

In the photographic method of identification, a card containing the patient data is inserted into a camera device. With the white lights off, the exposed radiograph is placed in the camera window, and a very quick light exposure is made, thereby transferring the patient data to the film. Cassettes used with this method of identification must have a lead blocker that protects the area of the film that will later be imprinted with patient data.

Radiographic-Film Storage and Handling

Radiographic film is sensitive to x-rays, heat, light, chemical fumes, moisture, pressure, and any kind of rough handling, such as bending, scratching, crimping. Radiographic film must be properly stored and carefully handled to ensure that damage does not occur.

Film Packaging

Radiographic film is packaged in a moisture-free, sealed bag with cardboard supports. The bag is packaged in a heavy-duty plastic bag within a sealed cardboard shipping carton. The outside of the carton indicates the type of film, quantity, and expiration date. Film is available in quantities of 25, 50, and 100 sheets per carton. Individually wrapped sheets of film can also be purchased; such film is called interleaved or prewrapped film.

Film Storage

Radiographic film should be stored in a cool, dry place. The temperature of the storage area has a direct influence on the length of time unexposed film can be maintained and used (refer to Table 12-1). The best temperature for film storage is

TABLE 12-1   Film Storage Temperature/Time Length Usable Relationships

Maintained Storage Temperature	Approximate Length of Time Film Stays Usable
90–100°F	2–3 days
70°F	2 months
60°F	6 months
50°F	1 year

between 60°F and 70°F and 40% and 60% relative humidity. Stored film should also be protected from x-radiation, fumes, chemicals, and any gas-producing substance. Film boxes should never be subjected to excessive pressure. To avoid pressure marks, warping, and bending, boxes of unexposed film should always be stored upright.

Stored film should be used prior to the expiration date. Stored film boxes should be rotated as new shipments arrive. Rotate the stock so that film with the most recent expiration date is always used first. This avoids having to discard expired film and saves money in film expense.

Once a film box is opened, a film bin (Figure 12-5) provides ideal storage. A film bin has separate compartments to hold different film sizes and is usually installed beneath the film loading area. Film bins may be electrically connected to the overhead lights. In this case, the lights will not turn on if the film bin drawer is open. Also, the darkroom entrance door may be electrically connected to the film bin to prevent accidental light exposure to the film should the door be opened while the bin is open.

Film fog is defined as an undesirable increase in the density of the emulsion, either before or after radiation exposure. The additional film density or fog

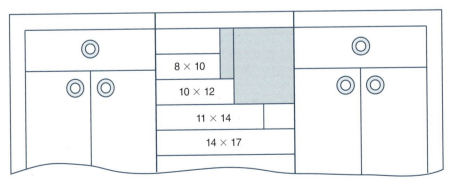

FIGURE 12-5   Film bin. A film bin is generally installed in existing counter space.
Source: Delmar, Cengage Learning.

decreases the quality of the radiographic image by reducing the visibility of the diagnostic information. Some common causes of film fog follow.

- Light—White light, either direct or indirect, can cause film fog.
- Chemical fumes—Certain chemical fumes cause emulsion to become fogged; film may be stored in poorly ventilated areas.
- Temperature—Room temperature should range between 60°F and 70°F.
- Humidity—Films should be stored in a room with 40% to 50% relative humidity.
- Radiation—Film must be stored in an area that is protected from primary and secondary scatter radiation.
- Pressure—Film boxes should never be stacked; they should be stored on edge with the expiration date showing on the end of the box.
- Age—Film should be used by rotating boxes in order of expiration date.

Film Handling

X-ray film must be handled carefully to avoid extraneous marks and images on the radiograph; such marks or images are called artifacts. An artifact can also be defined as an area of increased or decreased film darkening or density. Handle film carefully, avoiding creasing or bending and rapid movement of the film, which can cause static electric discharges to be conveyed to the film (Figure 12-6). Proper loading and unloading of cassettes and direct-exposure film envelopes are essential.

When films are carelessly handled by an individual loading and unloading cassettes, the films may be bent. This damages the emulsion and results in artifacts called crescent or crinkle marks, semicircular in shape. A white crescent-shaped mark results from bending the film before exposure. A black crescent-shaped mark is caused from bending the film after it has been exposed.

Film should also always be handled with clean, oil-free, and dry hands. Film-handling errors are one cause of film artifacts. For further information on film artifacts, refer to the "film processing" section of this chapter.

Maintaining Radiographic Film

Processed radiographs are a permanent, legal patient record and should be stored at 60°F to 70°F temperature and 40% to 50% relative humidity. The storage area should be free of chemical fumes, moisture, and excessive changes in temperature or humidity.

Each facility establishes a particular protocol for film filing and retrieval. It is important that the system provide quick access to the records as needed. Film filing folders should be made of materials that do not contain chemicals that can react with the stored radiographs. There are many ways to file and maintain radiographs.

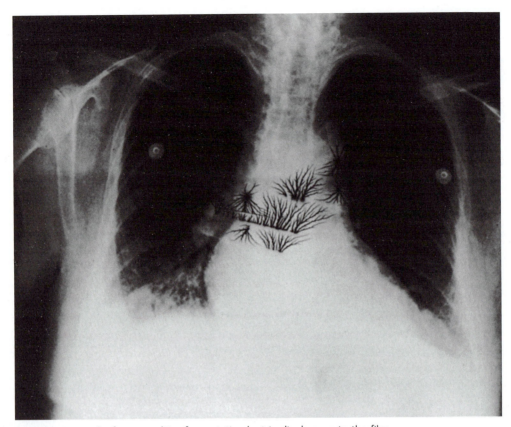

FIGURE 12-6 Artifacts resulting from static electric discharges to the film
Source: Delmar, Cengage Learning.

Each facility will also determine how to handle requests for loans of radiographs. One example would include information on who may request films, whether a written request is required, and if all or only the most recent radiographs are provided. Rather than loan original radiographs, a facility may provide duplicates at a nominal charge. Duplication of radiographs allows the facility to maintain a complete record, yet share the information with others providing medical care to the same patient.

Intensifying Screens

In 1895, German physicist Wilhelm Conrad Roentgen was operating a vacuum tube when he noticed a glow coming from a cardboard coated with a chemical, barium platinocyanide. The vacuum tube was covered so that no light escaped, yet the glow or fluorescence from the cardboard seemed to intensify when it was moved closer to the tube. Roentgen called his discovery "x-radiation" and began to investigate its properties further. In 1901, Roentgen won the first Nobel prize in physics for his discovery. His investigation led not only to the discovery and application of x-radiation but also to the use of chemically coated fluorescent screens in radiography.

Since less than 2% of the x-rays produced are absorbed by the film emulsion, the light emitted by the **intensifying screens** increases the effect on the emulsion, thereby allowing a decrease in x-ray exposure to the patient. In the last decade, the most dramatic reductions in radiation exposure to patients have resulted from the introduction of intensifying screens that have rare-earth phosphors capable of emitting even greater amounts of light.

Intensifying screens look like thin sheets of plastic. They are available in sizes corresponding to film sizes. Screens are mounted inside cassettes. Screens, like radiographic film, consist of layers, each having a specific purpose. Most intensifying screens have four layers: protective coating, phosphor, reflective layer, and base (Figure 12-7).

The protective coating is the outermost layer of the screen and is closest to the film. This coating is transparent and serves to reduce abrasion that would damage the screen surface. It also reduces the accumulation of static electricity. This protective surface may be cleaned without causing damage to the active fluorescent phosphor.

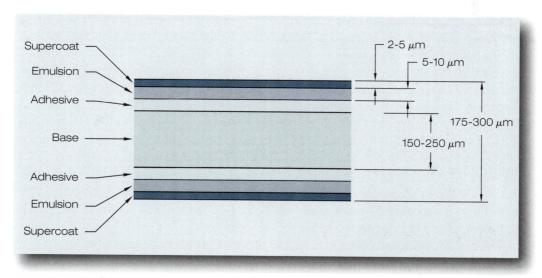

FIGURE 12-7 Cross-sectional view of diagnostic radiographic film
Source: Delmar, Cengage Learning.

The phosphor, or active layer, is responsible for emitting light when struck by x-rays. Another way of expressing this phenomenon is to say that the phosphor is responsible for converting the energy of the x-ray beam into visible light. Phosphors used in screens may be crystalline calcium tungstate, zinc sulfide, barium lead sulfate, or the rare-earths gadolinium, lanthanum, and yttrium. Today, however, calcium tungstate or the rare earths are most commonly in use. Although rare-earth phosphor screens are more costly, they are the phosphor most often used. The major advantage of rare-earth screens over conventional calcium-tungstate screens is speed. Since rare-earth screens are faster, they require less x-ray exposure to the patient. Differences in intensifying screens result from the differences in the phosphor composition, concentration, and crystal size.

For a phosphor to be used in an intensifying screen, it must have the following properties:

1. A high atomic number allowing for greater x-ray interaction with the phosphor
2. A high *conversion efficiency*, or the ability to emit a great amount of light
3. *Spectral matching*, meaning that the light emitted is of a wavelength (color) to match the sensitivity of the x-ray film
4. Should not continue to flow or emit light after the x-ray interaction stops. *Phosphorescence* is the continued emission of light by the phosphor after the exposure has ended. This is often referred to as screen afterglow or screen lag.

The reflective layer of the screen is between the phosphor and the base. The reflective layer keeps the light emitted by the phosphors directed toward the film.

The purpose of the base layer of the screen is to provide support for the phosphor layer. It consists of a tough polyester that is chemically inert, flexible, and resists damage from the radiation.

Intensifying screens have characteristics that are important to the limited radiographer. These characteristics include intensification factor (screen speed) and resolution. The intensification factor measures the speed of the screen. Screen speed is defined simply as the screen's ability to produce density with a given exposure to x-rays. There are three major speed categories of calcium-tungstate screens: medium speed, high speed, and fine detail (slow) speed. Rare-earth screens can be up to twelve hundred times faster than the categories listed for calcium-tungstate screens. Generally, these categories are described by comparing one against the others. Screen speed cannot be accurately measured, so in most discussions, the speeds will be compared in relation to their use and results.

The higher the speed of the screen, the more density will be produced at a given exposure. Use of high-speed screens reduces radiation exposure to the patient. This is possible because a greater intensification (more light) is produced by the high-speed screen, therefore, less exposure is needed to produce an image.

Although medium- and fine-detail-speed screens are available, most limited radiographers will use high-speed screens or rare-earth screens. Medium- and fine-detail-speed screens are used for specialty radiography when increased visibility of anatomic detail is desired. However, the patient may receive more radiation exposure with medium- and fine-detail-speed screens than with fast-speed screens or rare-earth screens.

Resolution is another important characteristic of intensifying screens. It is defined as the ability of a system to consistently produce an image of an object. To demonstrate resolution, one might look through a camera lens. If the object being viewed is out of focus, it has poor resolution. A rule of thumb to remember about screen resolution is that those conditions that increase the intensification factor reduce resolution. This means that high-speed screens with their large-size phosphor crystals will have a lower resolution than fine detail screens. Resolution increases as the phosphor crystals become smaller and the phosphor layer thinner. As previously mentioned, one can increase resolution with fine detail screens; however, the patient radiation exposure increases because these screens require more exposure than do fast-speed or rare-earth screens.

The choice of a film-screen combination, or film-imaging system, can significantly affect the patient's radiation exposure and the diagnostic quality of the radiation. A rule to follow regarding the selection of film and screens is to use the type and speed of film for the particular screen (e.g., high-speed film with a high-speed intensifying screen).

Direct Exposure or Cassette

Two types of film holders are used for radiography examinations: a direct exposure holder or a cassette that contains intensifying screens. Both film-holding devices will be discussed; however, direct exposure film holders are obsolete because of the increase in exposure required. Because cassettes contain a pair of intensifying screens that light up when struck by radiation, the patient's exposure dose is less than is required by a direct exposure holder containing no intensifying screens.

A direct exposure film holder, commonly called a "cardboard," is a lightproof envelope. Direct exposure (nonscreen) film is used with this type of film holder. These holders have a radiographic tube side that must face the tube during the exposure and a back side lined with lead foil to prevent scatter radiation from striking the film. Direct film holders were used for radiography of body parts measuring less than 12 centimeters. The advantage of direct exposure was that it provided good resolution or detail of the image. This resulted from the direct information transfer to the film as compared to the intensification factor of intensifying screens where some detail was lost as a result of the delay in light emitted by the crystal phosphors. Today, however, the potential benefit of direct exposure cannot be justified because of the increase in radiation exposure required as compared to using a cassette.

A cassette is a rigid holder containing intensifying screens. The front surface, or tube side, is made of thin, yet sturdy, plastic. The back of the cassette provides some type of spring closure device to maintain an even pressure on the film when the holder is closed. Attached to the inside are the front and back intensifying screens. A compression material such as felt is installed between each screen and the cassette cover. This material serves to further provide a good film-screen contact when the cassette is closed. Proper film loading and unloading is important in maintaining the surface of the screen as well as the condition of the film.

The outside of a cassette may be cleaned with a disinfectant as frequently as necessary. The intensifying screens, however, require regular inspection and cleaning. Care must be taken to keep the screens dry and to avoid stains and scratches that may cause permanent damage. Common types of soiling are from blood, lipstick, hair dressing, and processing solutions. Foreign objects, such as small pieces of paper, hair, etc., can also find their way into a cassette. Static electricity can cause dust particles to be attracted to the screen. Many commercial screen-cleaning solutions include an antistatic compound to reduce static electricity.

Always remember the important contribution of light energy that intensifying screens make to the formation of the latent image. With this in mind, it is easy to understand that any stain, soil, or matter on the screen surface can interfere with the amount of light reaching the film. An object or stain on a screen surface will appear as an unwanted shadow or artifact on the finished radiograph.

Keeping cassettes closed and properly stored away from moisture will help to avoid damage to the intensifying screens. This also protects the screen's phosphors from light, which can weaken the chemical fluorescence of the phosphor.

A cassette that is closed and latched is assumed to be loaded with unexposed film. If, at any time, a cassette must be closed and latched without film, identify it with a note stating that it is unloaded. This precaution will help to avoid a repeat examination and unnecessary radiation exposure to a patient.

Good darkroom housekeeping to keep the darkroom and film-loading areas clean is essential. Screens should be cleaned according to the manufacturer's instructions, which often recommend a specific commercial cleaning solution. Also, cleaning solutions for calcium-tungstate screens may not be suitable for rare-earth screens because of optical residue that can interfere with the light emission. The frequency at which intensifying screens are cleaned depends upon a number of factors: manufacturer's suggested cleaning schedule, amount of use the screens receive, and overall cleanliness of the darkroom environment and operator.

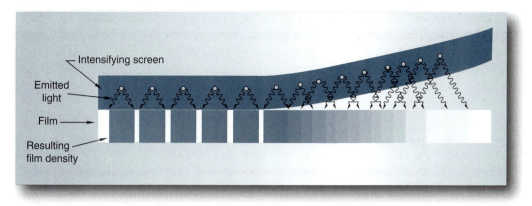

FIGURE 12-8 Poor resolution and increased image density due to loss of film/screen contact
Source: Delmar, Cengage Learning.

Screen-Film Contact

Intensifying screens must be in direct contact with the film across its entire surface. Poor screen-film contact results in a severe loss of recorded detail and a slight decrease in density on the finished radiograph. The compression material (such as felt) and metal backings on the cassette are responsible for proper screen-film contact (Figure 12-8). As a result of constant use or abuse, the compression material, spring latches, or backing may become warped. When this happens, even pressure is not exerted on the screens, which causes poor screen-film contact. Other factors that can contribute to poor screen-film contact are: (1) air trapped between screen and film, (2) foreign matter on the screen surface, and (3) improperly mounted screens. The loss of screen-film contact may be gradual, and for this reason, the contact should be checked on a regular basis.

Film Processing

Chemical processing changes the latent image held in the film emulsion into a manifest image. In the early days of radiography, film processing was done manually, by moving the film from the developer to the fixer tank by hand. Drying of the radiograph was accomplished by the clothesline method of air drying. Needless to say, manual processing was not always a precise procedure and often did not allow for consistent processing results. Today, most medical facilities have automatic film processors; however, a brief section will be included on manual processing because many small medical clinics may still use this method. The basic steps of film processing are similar for automatic and manual processing: development, fixation, wash, and drying processes. The chemicals used in each method are similar, except that the strength concentration is higher for automatic processor chemistry. Also, of course, automatic processing involves higher solution temperatures and shorter processing times.

Overview of Film-Processing Steps

After the cassette is unloaded in the darkroom, the exposed film is ready to be developed. The developer is responsible for converting the exposed silver halide crystals into metallic silver. The fixer actually performs two important functions: it removes the unexposed and undeveloped silver halide crystals from the emulsion and hardens the soft gelatin. The washing process removes fixer solution from the film emulsion. Drying the radiograph prepares it for viewing and later storage.

Processing Solutions

Tables 12-2 and 12-3 list the chemical ingredients of the developer and fixer.

Preparation of Solutions

Preparation of solutions is very important in processing. Chemical solutions should be prepared according to the manufacturer's directions and safety specifications.

TABLE 12-2   Developer Chemistry

Solvent	Water	Dissolves the developer chemicals and causes gelatin in film emulsion to swell
Developing Agents	Phenidone (automatic processing) Elon and hydroquinone (manual processing)	Converts exposed silver halide crystals into metallic silver
Accelerators	Sodium or potassium hydroxide	An alkali added to the developer to increase the chemical activity
Preservatives	Sodium sulfite	Prevents oxidation
Restrainers	Potassium bromide Potassium iodide	Controls activity of reducing agents and prevents chemical fog
Hardener	Glutaraldehyde	**ONLY** used for automatic processing; controls swelling of the emulsion

TABLE 12-3 Fixer Chemistry

Solvent	Water	Dissolves the fixer chemicals
Clearing and Fixing Agents	Ammonium thiosulfate (Hypo)	Dissolves and removes undeveloped silver halide crystals and changes the unexposed areas of the film from milky to clear and translucent
Preservatives	Sodium sulfite	Prevents decomposition of the clearing agents
Hardener	Aluminum chloride or Potassium alum	Shrinks and hardens the emulsion
Acidifier	Acetic acid	Provides an acid pH and neutralizes the alkaline developer
Buffer		Chemicals added to fixing solution to stabilize and balance the acid-alkaline pH of the solutions

Processing chemicals are available in dry and liquid form. It is important to follow the manufacturer's directions for mixing chemicals. Some general precautions include:

1. Dry chemicals should be mixed away from stored film.
2. Liquid chemicals should be mixed with water of the same temperature.
3. All chemicals should be thoroughly stirred while mixing.
4. Follow recommended safety precautions regarding inhaling chemical vapors or dry particles and eye and skin contact when using processing chemicals.

Chemical safety standards have been written by the Occupational Safety and Health Administration (OSHA). Included are standards for personal protection equipment (PPE), which refers to goggles, face shields, or ear protection as needed in typical industrial environments. Additionally defined is hazard communication, known as the "right to know" standard. This requires that communication of information regarding the safe use of chemical products in the workplace be available to employees.

Processing Steps

The four steps to be considered in film processing are developing, fixing, washing, and drying. The developer is an alkaline solution that converts exposed silver halide crystals to metallic silver by a chemical reaction. This reaction is often called a reduction process because the silver ion is said to be reduced to metallic silver.

The developer contains water, which is a solvent for the other chemicals and softens the film's emulsion. Hydroquinone is the main ingredient of developer solution with phenidone and Metol® as secondary agents. Hydroquinone and elon are combined for manual processing and hydroquinone and phenidone for rapid processing. These chemicals, when combined, have many electrons that are easily released to neutralize the positive silver ions in the film emulsion. Hydroquinone is responsible for bringing out the blackest shades on the radiograph, whereas phenidone influences the gray shades. Glutaraldehyde (hardener) is included in the developer for automatic processing. It is added to control emulsion swelling.

Unexposed silver halide crystals have a positive electrostatic charge whereas exposed silver halide crystals have a negative electrostatic charge. Because the electrostatic charge of the developer chemicals is negative, the chemicals cannot penetrate the silver halide crystal *except* in the region of exposure or where there are sensitized specks. In these areas, the developer chemicals penetrate through to the exposed specks and reduce the silver ions to atomic silver (Figures 12-9 and 12-10). Unexposed silver halide crystals are not changed or affected by the developer solution.

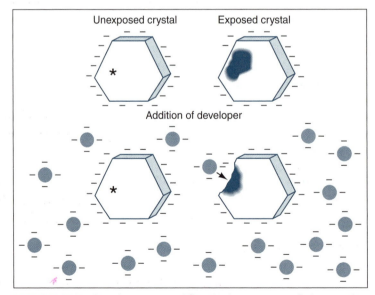

FIGURE 12-9 Development amplifies the latent image. Only crystals that contain a latent image are reduced to metallic silver by the addition of developer. This is known as the Gurney-Mott theory.
Source: Delmar, Cengage Learning.

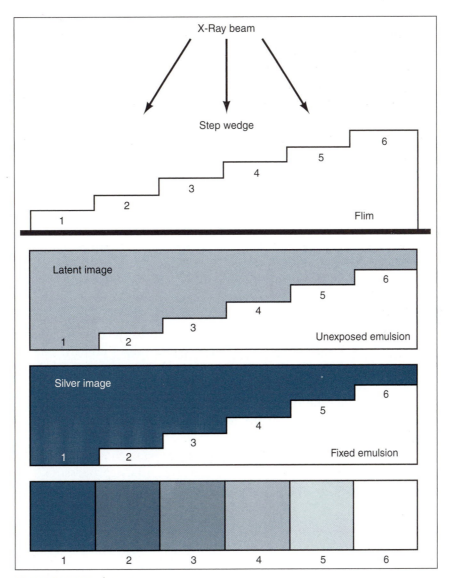

FIGURE 12-10 Latent image process
Source: Delmar, Cengage Learning.

Other ingredients in the developer consist of an activator (such as sodium carbonate), a preservative, and restrainer. The preservative sodium sulfite serves to retard the activity of the reducing agents, thereby decreasing oxidation. Oxidation is undesirable because the chemicals' activity level declines when combined with oxygen. Potassium bromide, a restrainer, limits the action of the developer chemicals to the reduction of only the exposed silver halide crystals. Without proper balance provided by the restrainer, the unexposed silver halide crystals would be attacked. This ingredient is not required when mixing replenishment chemicals because bromide is redeposited into the solution as each film is developed. Because the potassium bromide is used when mixing the initial developer solution, it is commonly called "starting solution" or "starter."

Replenishment of chemicals is very important in providing diagnostic-quality radiographs. Replenishment is used to restore both developer and fixer chemicals to their original strength. As films are processed, they retain a certain amount of chemicals and this depletes the solution level and the chemical strength. In automatic film processing, a pump replenishes the chemicals each time a film is processed; in manual film processing, the amount and rate of replenisher chemical must be performed by the radiographer. In manual processing, replenishment is usually done daily and is based upon the number and size of the films processed.

The fixer is an acidic solution that clears or removes unexposed silver halide crystals from the film emulsion. It also hardens and fixes the film so that it can be maintained as a permanent record. The fixer, like the developer, contains water as a solvent, which serves as a base for the other chemicals. Acetic acid allows the use of potassium alum as a hardening agent but also neutralizes any alkaline developer solution remaining on the film. The clearing agent ammonium thiosulfate (hypo) removes unexposed and undeveloped silver halide crystals from the emulsion. Hardening agents, either aluminum chloride or potassium alum, control the swelling of the emulsion and help to shrink it. Sodium sulfite is included as a chemical preservative to reduce oxidation.

A film must be properly washed to remove processing chemicals. Films must be washed in continuously circulating fresh water. Automatic processors accomplish this by a constant inflow of water.

Automatic Film Processing

Automatic film processing was introduced in the late 1950s. It provided several basic advantages: (1) the operator did not need to have contact with processing chemicals; (2) automatic equipment eliminated long day-to-day hand processing; (3) a finished film could be processed in as little as 90 seconds; and (4) chemicals in automatic processors provided constant control over chemical temperature and chemical strength. Chemicals used in automatic processors are more concentrated than the former manual chemicals, and higher chemical temperature is needed because of shorter development time.

Automatic processing systems include transport, water, recirculation, replenishment, and dryer systems. Each will be discussed briefly.

Transport System. The transport system, consisting of rollers, transport racks, and drive motors, moves the film through the chemical solutions. It also serves to continuously agitate the chemicals, which prevents settling of the solutions. The transport system begins at the feed tray located in the darkroom. As the film is gently pushed on the feed tray, rollers grip the edge and begin moving it through the processor (Figure 12-11). Microswitches located at the entry to the feed tray detect the film size and start the automatic chemical-replenishment pump. The rate at which the film is transported through the processing tanks is very carefully controlled by the roller system. Roller subassembly consists of 1-inch-diameter transport rollers and 3-inch master rollers. Most of the rollers, except for those at the feed tray entry,

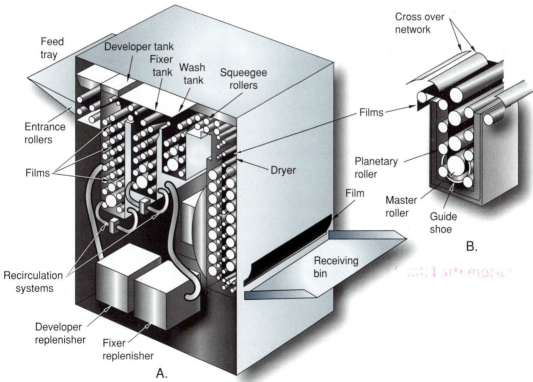

FIGURE 12-11 (A) A modern automatic x-ray film processor. (B) A transport rack and crossover networks in a single tank.
Source: Delmar, Cengage Learning.

are located within a rack. This allows for easy removal to clean and service the assembly. The transport system is powered by a motor whose time is set to the manufacturer's specifications.

Water System. The water system washes the film and helps to stabilize the temperature of the solutions. Incoming water into the processor is maintained by a thermostatic regulating device.

Recirculation System. The recirculation pump blends and mixes the developer and fixer solutions with replenishment solution. This is very important for maintaining the proper temperature and chemical-activity level of the solutions. Constant agitation keeps the solutions mixed and in contact with the film.

Replenishment System. Automatic-processing chemicals are replenished by replenishment pumps each time a film enters the feed tray rollers. Manufacturers recommend replenishment rates based on the number of films processed. This method assumes a common density to each film and bases the quantity of replenishment solution upon a known standard of silver halide conversion to metallic silver. Regular checks are required to assure that the replenishment rates are accurate. This process is considered part of a quality control program.

Dryer System. Automatic-processor drying consists of a blower system that disperses heated air around the film as it moves past.

Limited radiographers should be familiar with automatic-processing components. Each manufacturer provides detailed operating and maintenance manuals, and these should be consulted whenever questions arise. Also, most companies provide representatives who help answer technical film-processing questions.

Artifacts

Film artifacts are undesirable. They consist of a wide range of extraneous marks and areas of increased or decreased density (darkening) that interfere with the diagnostic value of the radiograph. Table 12-4 provides a list of common artifacts. They are caused by physical, mechanical, and chemical means and may be avoided if proper film handling and storage procedures and appropriate film-processing guidelines are observed. Table 12-5 provides a list of common problems and corrections related to handling and processing x-ray film. After films are processed they should be checked for artifacts. If artifacts are visible, the cause or source should be determined and corrected. (See Figures 12-12 through 12-15.)

TABLE 12-4 Artifacts and Sources

Artifact	Source
Brown stain	From old or oxidized developer (too much air has mixed with the solution)
Multicolored stain	From poor rinsing
Yellowish film	From exhausted or weakened fixer solution
Milky-white film	From incomplete washing time
Streaking	From solutions that have not been stirred well or films not agitated well, films not rinsed adequately, poor circulation in automatic processor, and/or withdrawing film after it had started through the entrance assembly of the processor. In manual processing, check the wire hanger clips for chemical residue. Clean with a stiff brush.
Crinkle marks	From kinking the film during handling
Reticulation	Weblike marks that appear in the emulsion when there are extreme differences in the processing solutions.
Hesitation marks	From automatic processor when the film hesitates or stops, causing increased density lines across the film.
Guide Shoe marks	From automatic processor when film guide racks are not lined up properly with the rollers closest to them.

TABLE 12-5 Handling and Processing X-Ray Film: Common Problems and Corrections

Problem	Cause	Correction
Radiograph too dark	1. Overexposure	1. Reduce exposure
	2. Overdevelopment	2. Adjust development time (manual); Check temperatures of water and solutions (automatic)
	3. Concentrated replenishment	3. Adjust replenishment

continues

TABLE 12-5 (continued)

Problem	Cause	Correction
Radiograph too light	1. Underexposure	1. Increase exposure
	2. Underdevelopment	2. Adjust development time (manual); Check temperatures of water and solutions (automatic)
	3. Exhausted replenishment	3. Adjust replenishment
Fog on radiograph	1. Chemical vapor exposure	1. Store film away from hydrogen sulfite, hydrogen peroxide, terpene, mercury
	2. Storage temperatures too high or humidity too high	2. Store film in appropriate place, temperature
	3. Expiration date on film has passed	3. Regularly rotate film stock and use film before expiration date
	4. Safelight exposure	4. Use recommended filter color, bulb wattage, and location of safelight from film-loading bench
	5. X-ray exposure	5. Store film in appropriate place
	6. Pressure	6. Do not apply pressure or stack stored film boxes
Black circular spots	Developer on film before development	Avoid developer splashes on film
White circular spots	Fixer on film before development	Avoid fixer splashes on film
Branched black marks	Static electricity discharge	Use proper film-handling procedures; Avoid clothing that contains excessive static build-up, such as nylon
Crescent-shaped black marks	Bend in the film after exposure	Use proper film-handling procedures
Crescent-shaped white marks	Bend in the film before exposure	Use proper film-handling procedures
Yellow or brown stains	Exhausted developer; exhausted fixer	Replace solution

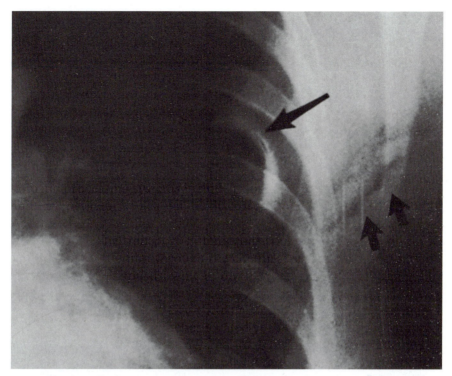

FIGURE 12-12 Both images on this radiograph were caused by mishandling of the film. The single arrow demonstrates a *crinkle mark*, which can occur if the film is bent. The double arrows show an artifact caused by pressure on the surface of the film. Source: Delmar, Cengage Learning.

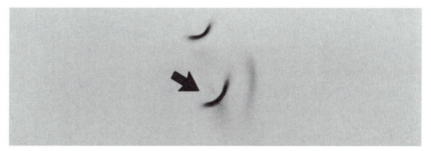

FIGURE 12-13 Kink, crinkle, or half-moon artifact caused by mishandling of the film. A white crinkle mark is caused by bending the film prior to exposure. A black crinkle mark is caused by bending the film after exposure and prior to processing. Source: Delmar, Cengage Learning.

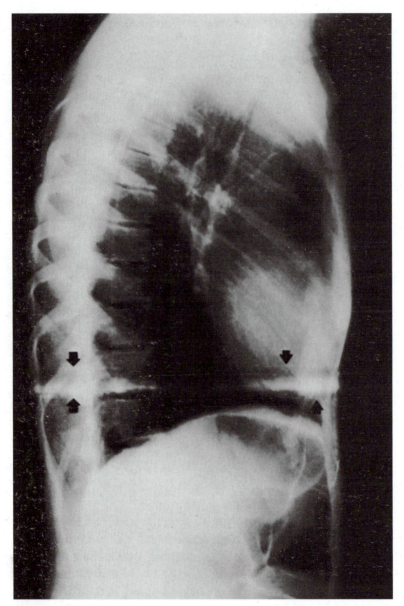

FIGURE 12-14 Pressure artifact resulting from closing the drawer of the film bin on the sheet of film
Source: Delmar, Cengage Learning.

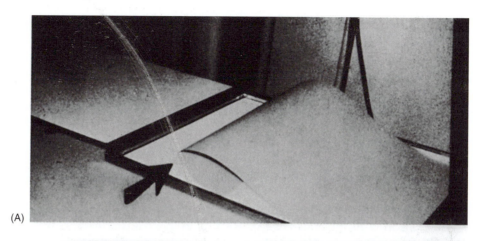

(A)

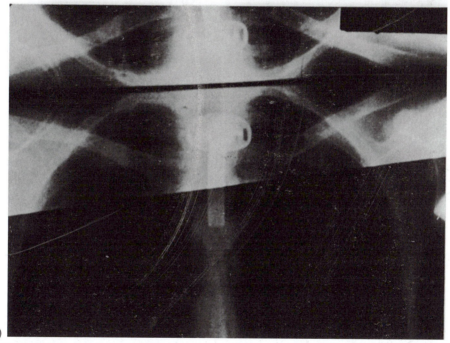

(B)

FIGURE 12-15 (A) A sheet of film may be accidentally loaded into the cassette in a folded position; (B) The artifact in this radiograph resulted from loading the film into the cassette in a folded position.

Source: Delmar, Cengage Learning.

Automatic-Processor Maintenance

Automatic processors, like any electromechanical equipment, must have regular service and repair. Processor maintenance consists of the usual daily, weekly, and monthly care as well as preventive and nonscheduled maintenance. Generally, limited radiographers are not expected to perform preventive or repair maintenance; such procedures are usually performed by skilled service people. Radiographers are, however, expected to perform the usual daily processor care, maintain a designated preventive maintenance schedule and records, and recognize the need for nonscheduled repair. Suggestions for daily processor care follow:

- Clean crossover rollers (use water and a nonabrasive, lint-free cloth).
- Observe all moving parts for wear. Report anything unusual to immediate supervisor.
- Check level of replenishment solutions in storage tanks.
- Drain the wash tank and offset the processor lid at night (this prevents the build up of algae in the tanks).

Preventive maintenance should be regularly scheduled. Each manufacturer will suggest a planned program that should be followed. Consult with company representatives or x-ray sales and service personnel to determine the best schedule to follow.

Nonscheduled maintenance is the most dreaded because it means a mechanical or electrical failure within the processor. The number of these incidents can be reduced with a regular preventive maintenance program. How does one know if something is wrong? Generally, automatic-processor problems will first become evident on the films. Unusual scratches, lines, marks, or improper processing of the films will be noticed. Also, some problems will be noticed first as an unusual operating sound. Limited radiographers are not expected to diagnose such problems, but before making a service call, it is important for the radiographer to note any detail noticed, e.g., nature of the problem, visual appearance of films processed, unusual sounds, or signs of leaks or mechanical failure. It is also a good idea to check all temperature and chemical controls before reporting the problem. Table 12-5 lists common film handling and processing problems and possible corrections.

Sensitometry

Sensitometry is the study of how radiographic film responds to radiation exposure and processing conditions. Sensitometry is used to measure and predict how film density will change as radiation exposure factors and processing conditions change. By monitoring these responses, it provides early detection of equipment

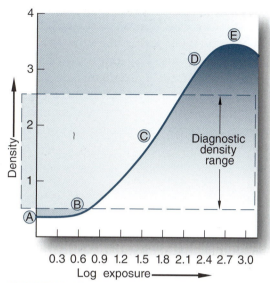

FIGURE 12-16 A typical D log E (characteristic, sensi-tometric, or H&D curve). (A) Base plus fog; (B) toe; (C) straight line portion; (D) shoulder; (E) Dmax
Source: Delmar, Cengage Learning.

malfunctions before they can cause serious operational problems that may result in repeat of patient examinations. Changes in the film characteristics can be easily detected by sensitometry when radiation exposure and processing conditions are constant. Changes in processing conditions may also be identified when film-screen system and radiation exposure factors are constant. Sensitometry measurements include those visibility factors of density, contrast, and fog.

A characteristic curve, sometimes called H & D curve and first used in 1890 for photography analysis by Hurter and Driffield, is used to measure and predict film response to changes. The curve looks like a letter S when plotted on a graph (Figure 12-16). The graph is plotted by exposing a film and plotting the density levels against a logarithm of the various exposure levels.

Sensitometry Methods

There are three methods of performing sensitometry: step-wedge pentrometer and medium exposure, sensitometer exposure, and pre-exposed sensitometry strips. Most limited radiographers will be involved with only the third and easiest method of sensitometric measurement; thus, this is the only method that will be described.

In the procedure for pre-exposed sensitometry test strips, the strips are purchased and are stored in the film bin. When processed, the strips will have areas of increasing density. The processed strips are analyzed in a densitometer, an instrument with a light-sensing device. The amount of light transmitted through each segment on the strip is measured. A characteristic curve should result when this information is recorded and analyzed. Strips are regularly processed and the densities evaluated. This is a very common, widely used method today. Sensitometry application to film processing will be discussed in more detail with radiographic exposures.

Silver Recovery

Silver, a treasured metal, can be recovered from fixer processing chemicals. Silver can also be reclaimed from scrap film and purged radiographic films. Why recover silver? Silver recovery is one way to salvage a scarce natural resource and also provides a small monetary return. The unexposed silver halide is dissolved in the fixer as the radiograph progresses through the film-processing cycle. There are two common methods used to recover silver from the fixer solution: metallic replacement and electrolytic recovery.

Metallic replacement removes silver from the used fixer solution by chemically replacing silver with another metal. As the metal dissolves, the silver moves to the bottom of the container and is removed. Electrolytic recovery uses electrodes placed in the fixer tank. An electric current causes the silver to attach to one of the electrodes (see Figure 12-17A).

Electrolytic recovery is less efficient than metallic recovery and is initially more costly to install. The system requires more careful operational attention. There may be less recovered silver but it may be purer (see Figure 12-17B).

To determine which silver recovery system to use, consult with the processor manufacturer or an x-ray service company.

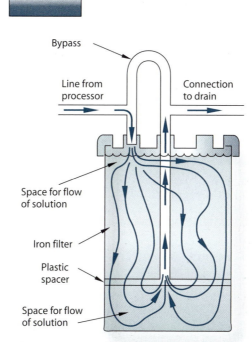

FIGURE 12-17A   A metallic replacement silver recovery unit *(Courtesy of Carestream Health, Inc.)*

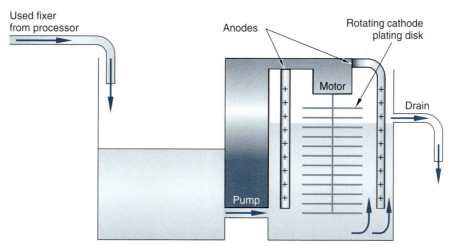

FIGURE 12-17B   An electrolytic silver recovery unit
Source: Delmar, Cengage Learning.

REVIEW QUESTIONS

1. What are the two main parts of radiographic film?
   a. emulsion and gelatin
   b. gelatin and silver halide crystals
   c. film base and gelatin
   d. film base and emulsion

2. A cassette or direct exposure film holder must be:
   a. lighttight
   b. airtight and lightweight
   c. adhesive and airtight
   d. waterproof and fluorescent

3. To reduce excessive radiation exposure to the patient, the following combination should be used:
   a. screen film and cassette
   b. direct exposure film and cassette
   c. direct exposure film and cardboard holder
   d. screen film and cardboard holder

4. The active (phosphor) layer of an intensifying screen:
   a. converts x-ray photons to visible light
   b. makes the screen lightproof
   c. decreases buildup of static electricity
   d. converts x-ray energy into light energy

5. Rare-earth intensifying screens have the following advantage compared to calcium-tungstate intensifying screens:
   a. provide more visible detail
   b. require less radiation and shorter exposure time
   c. permit shorter exposure time but require more radiation
   d. less costly

6. Select the spectral matching combination which would reduce the patient's radiation dose:
   a. high-speed film and high-speed screen
   b. high-speed film and low-speed screen
   c. low-speed film and high-speed screen
   d. low-speed film and low-speed screen

7. Radiographic film is *not* sensitive to:
   a. chemicals
   b. heat
   c. pressure
   d. odors

8. Unexposed silver halide crystals are removed from the film in the
   _____ stage of film processing.
   a. development
   b. wash
   c. final rinse
   d. fixation

9. The following is *not* a component of the fixer:
   a. reducing agent
   b. preserver
   c. hardener
   d. acidifier

10. In an automatic processor, the chemicals are agitated by the _____.
    a. replenishment
    b. water
    c. recirculation pump
    d. dryer

11. If a radiograph is fogged, the radiographic density will:
    a. increase
    b. decrease
    c. no change
    d. none of the above

12. Radiographic film is more easily fogged:
    a. before being loaded into a film holder
    b. after its exposure to x-rays but before processing
    c. after processing
    d. after storage

13. The processing solution with an acid pH is:
    a. developer
    b. fixer
    c. rinse
    d. wash

14. Fogging of the radiograph produces increased:
   a. density
   b. contrast
   c. distortion
   d. recorded detail

REFERENCES

Carlton, R. R., Adler, A. M. (2006). *Principles of Radiographic Imaging: An Art and Science* (4th ed.). Clifton Park, NY: Thomson Delmar Learning.

Eastman Kodak Company. (1980). *The Fundamentals of Radiography* (4th ed.). Rochester, NY: Author.

SUGGESTED READINGS

Cullinan, A. (1987). *Producing quality radiographs*. Philadelphia: J. B. Lippincott Company.

Haus, A. G. (1993). *Film processing in medical imaging*. Madison, WI: Medical Physics Publishing.

Pizzutiello, R. J., & Cullinan, J. (Eds.) (1993). *Introduction to medical radiographic imaging*. Rochester, NY: Eastman Kodak Company.

Quinn, C. B. (2003). *Fuch's radiography exposure, processing and quality control* (6th ed.). Springfield, IL: Charles C. Thomas.

Selman, J. (1995), *The fundamentals of x-ray and radium physics* (7th ed.). Springfield, IL: Charles C. Thomas.

Sweeney, R. J. (1983). *Radiographic artifacts: Their cause and control*. Philadelphia: J. B. Lippincott Company.

CHAPTER 13

BASIC IMAGE QUALITY MANAGEMENT

Key Terms

Evaluation Criteria
Geometric Factors
Image Evaluation
Image Production
Image Quality
Photographic Factors
Radiographic Position

Chapter Outline

Objectives

Upon completion of the chapter, the student will meet the following objectives by verifying knowledge of the facts and principles presented through oral and written communication at a level deemed competent.

⊃ Identify a minimum of four factors that control film quality.
⊃ List some actions that are generally acceptable when adjustments are required on radiographs that are too dark or too light.

⊃ Identify appropriate steps for proper radiographic positioning technique that affect film quality.

⊃ List five basic steps that relate to maintaining proper processing technique.

⊃ Identify and describe an appropriate method for critique of exposure factors for evaluation of radiographic quality.

Introduction

Evaluation of **image quality** is a process of visually assessing the image recorded on a film. When we look at a black and white photograph, we automatically look for detail in a person's face, a building, a landscape, and so forth. If the photograph is too dark, too light, or motion is seen, information is lost.

The radiographer must possess the appropriate knowledge and skills to visualize, inspect, and determine that technical qualities of the radiographic image are satisfactory. This chapter will address photographic qualities related to visual concepts of a recorded radiographic image. Visual inspection of the finished radiographic image under proper illumination (placed on a viewbox) will reveal most black-and-white (photographic) deficiencies related to too much or too little mAs, kVp, or SID.

Evaluation of the radiographic image includes multiple factors that are referred to in sum as *photographic effect* or image quality. These factors have been dealt with fundamentally in Chapter 9 under exposure factors mA, time, mAs, kVp, and SID. Relative to image quality, these exposure factors may be discussed in terms of the following areas: (1) image-quality considerations, (2) preparation of **image production**, and (3) radiographic film processing. The terms radiograph(ic) and image are used interchangeably or in combination in this chapter where appropriate. Digital image control is discussed in Chapter 10.

Image-Quality Considerations

Most people have difficulty seeing what they are not prepared to see. For example, in a stroll through a black-and-white photographic exhibit in a gallery or museum, many viewers react only in terms of whether they like or dislike the subject of a photograph. Others, who have had training in photography or art, additionally react to the shapes, lines, movement, contrast of light and dark, perspective, etc. Details and the quality of the overall effect, rather than the subject, are probably more important to the trained viewer.

In radiography, through educational preparation, the operator must learn about exposure factors and the often delicate balance and interaction between these factors in order to produce film images and then to evaluate the quality of those images. To assess a radiograph, the radiographer's preparation must include knowledge of the following "chain" of factors, their interplay, and their effects on the finished image: the exact mA, time, and kVp; patient's history and present condition; the centimeter measurement of the body part being examined; the processing time and temperature; the characteristics of the film type being processed; and any variation in these factors that may have occurred before or during exposure of the image. Knowing these factors and their interactions is crucial when it becomes necessary to repeat a radiograph. The radiographer who produced the initial image should conduct the second attempt to avoid making the same errors or a different error.

Preparation of Image Production

For quality control when preparing to produce a radiographic image, the operator should employ a systematic approach in order to avoid mistakes. Simple evaluation criteria in the form of a checklist should be followed. Because image quality is affected by improper positioning, these criteria should include steps to avoid poor positioning, which often results in repeating radiographs. Such a checklist should include the following procedures:

1. Carefully read the request for radiographic examination to ensure that you are very clear on the doctor's instructions regarding what radiographic procedure(s) has been ordered. If there is doubt, confirm the radiographic procedure with the doctor.
2. Identify the patient by *asking* his/her name. Do not suggest: "Are you Mr. Smith?" Rather, simply ask "What is your name, Sir?" If the patient cannot respond, check the arm band or follow the appropriate procedure according to office or departmental policy.
3. The patient must be placed appropriately, according to certain basic principles of radiographic positioning.
   a. Proper radiographic positioning may be effective only when applied with sound knowledge of human structure.
   b. Prior to examination, the patient must be given proper instructions regarding the radiographic procedure.
   c. The patient must be made comfortable to avoid the interactive pull of muscle strain that can result in motion.

    d. The patient's entire body must be positioned so that alignment is achieved with the part of the anatomy being examined, to avoid a rotated or twisted effect that may obscure structural information.

    e. After proper body position has been obtained, it is essential that the part being examined be immobilized. Effective mobilization devices that tend to reduce motion are sandbags, tape, or compression bands.
(Although the next three checklist items, f–h, do not all pertain to positioning, each step is crucial to production of an image as a whole.)

    f. A film size that adequately includes only the anatomical part being examined is necessary. The part in focus is placed in the image receptor's (film cassette's) center and a small unexposed border around the image at the film's edges (½″ to 1½″) should be visible. The border indicates exposure limitation.

    g. A very important geometric factor is to place the long axis of the anatomical part being examined parallel to, in the center of and adjacent, to the long axis of the image receptor. This avoids magnification of the structure and/or distortion.

    h. The central ray must be directed perpendicular to the long axis of the image and to the center of the image so that it passes through the center point of the structure.

4. Identify the film inside the image receptor with an appropriate marker (usually lead). Place the marker on top of the receptor in the margins of the film outside the structure. (See 3f.)

5. Measure the part being examined and select the exposure factors—mAs, kVp, and SID (usually standardized, but check to make sure). Measure the part being examined and set kVp unless using automatic exposure.

6. Before making exposure, give the patient final instructions and make a final check of the patient's whole body position. Specifically check the part being radiographed to ensure that the position has not changed.

7. Do not hold your head outside the protection booth to talk to the patient during exposure.

8. Return the patient to the waiting area after completion of all films. It is not wise to leave an unstable patient unattended in the room.

9. Check the film after processing and if image quality is visible, release patient.

The checklist items just cited are largely related to traditional imaging equipment. In today's digital equipment environment, preparation for image production is simpler, that is, the radiographer is responsible for image production according to equipment and processing operations.

Radiographic-Film Processing

You have already learned about what is involved in film processing in Chapter 12. Because film processing, like image production, also involves a chain of events, it is necessary to observe that certain processing elements are constant at all times under any conditions:

1. The time and temperature of the processor must remain at constant levels. Any change in time of processing or degree of temperature will quickly affect the developer solution. If the temperature decreases, the result will be incomplete development (lighter image); if the temperature increases, development of the image will be darker due to chemicals that are too hot.
2. Processor water flow must be constant and maintained at adequate flow pressure.
3. All hoses to the automatic processor and its replenishment tanks must be open, not kinked or clogged, which can cut off chemical flow.
4. The processor must have a schedule for regular maintenance and preventive maintenance.
5. Processor care is generally coordinated with a processor-maintenance person. Day-to-day care of the processor is the responsibility of the radiographer and any others who are involved in equipment care.

Identification of Corrective Factors for Poor Image Quality

There are three image evaluation areas in which the sum of the screen/film image, in terms of photographic effect, may be assessed: (1) photographic factors, (2) geometric factors, and (3) accurate radiographic position.

The finished image will appear either correct or incorrect in the eye of the beholder. If the image is incorrect, then the operator must visually determine if the image is photographically deficient in contrast (kVp) or density (mAs), or if the processing is of poor quality.

When the completed image has been placed on the illuminator (viewbox), the contrast and density (discussed in Chapter 9) of the image should be such that all areas in the anatomy are visible. A rule of thumb is that if the image is so dark (black) that nothing is visible, the mAs should be cut back to one-fourth of what was originally used (e.g., reduce from 40 mAs to 10 mAs) and then determine whether or not the film is adequate for exposure. When the image is dark but some anatomy can be seen by using a bright light or spotlight, reduce the mAs by only one-half (e.g., from 40 mAs to 20 mAs).

Unless appropriate preparation for image production has taken place, i.e., the radiographer understands and has carefully selected mAs, kVp, and SID (usually standard), only guesses can be made—trial and error—to correct radiographic technique (density and contrast) of poor quality in a recorded image.

Except in the case of patient motion, geometric factors are seldom a problem because most are standardized. Errors involving blurring or distortion (shape, size) are generally related to improper positioning, incorrect body alignment, misjudgment of the patient size and shape (body habitus), or inexperience. When an image is assessed for quality, consideration should be given to the accuracy of all of the factors used to produce the image. Most often, when the image is of poor quality, overexposure or, less frequently, underexposure is the problem and is usually correctable by an adjustment of the exposure time. However, not all problems may be so simply corrected. Tables 13-1 and 13-2 provide some basic category information that may be useful for evaluating the quality of radiographic images.

TABLE 13-1   Image Quality Chart Visibility

DENSITY: Overall Image Appears Overexposed or Underexposed Factors to be considered:
mAs: Review the amount of mAs used kVp: Review measurement of the part for amount of kVp used (too much scatter) Processing: Check processor temperature and time (rarely a problem)   Check for chemical contamination (fog) (If the problem is not related to above areas, investigate further.)
CONTRAST: Overall Image Appears Flat and Gray or All Appropriate Structures   Are Not Penetrated Factors to be considered:
kVp: Review the amount of kVp used and part measurement. A flat gray or fogged appearance is usually caused by scattered radiation from excessive kVp. mAs: Review the amount of mAs used. A gray appearance (added density) may be the result of using too much mAs. Processing: Check processor temperature. A gray appearance (added density) may also result from processing at a temperature too high. Check for chemical contamination (fog).

TABLE 13-2 Image Quality Chart–Geometric Factors

IMAGE BLURRING: Image Appears Blurred (Unsharp) on the Processed Radiograph
Factors to be considered:

Patient breathed/moved:
Determine if patient breathed or moved during exposure. If the patient breathed, check the reason and use a faster time, if necessary, to eliminate motion. The most effective recourse against motion is a faster time. Immobilization and sandbag support should also be considered when motion is a problem.

Film-screen contact:
Although poor screen contact is rare today with the excellent construction of cassettes, it still occurs. When it occurs, the screens must be replaced in the cassette. It is unusual for screen contact to be a problem with cassette sizes other than 14″ × 17″.

DISTORTION: Shape/Size of Image Appears Distorted
Factors to be considered:

SID/OFD:
If the part is or must be placed away from the film surface, the SID should be increased to reduce magnification of size caused by the increase in part-image receptor distance. The part should be no more than 1½″–2″ away from the image receptor at 40″ SID or 2½″–3″ away from the image receptor at 60″ SID.

Tube angulation:
Elongation or foreshortening of the part is usually caused by incorrect alignment of the tube or part. Remember, the part to be examined must be parallel to the plane of the image receptor and the tube directed perpendicularly (no angle) through the center point of the anatomy to be viewed. Whenever possible, it is more desirable to rotate the part and keep the anatomy parallel to the image receptor than to angle the tube through the part.

POSITIONING: The Image Appears to Be Incorrectly Positioned
Factors to be considered:

Relationship of anatomy to the image receptor plane and relationship of the CR (central ray) to the anatomy:
Review exactly how the patient was aligned for proper position and how the part to be examined was aligned with the image receptor plane. Poor positioning is a common error and is usually the result of working hurriedly or not checking the position carefully enough. Remember, only one patient can be done at any given time, so there is no need to rush and make mistakes.

Some problems are basic and relatively common in the production of radiographic images. By now you have probably determined that two of the most likely technique errors include overexposure (too much density) and poor positioning. Most overexposure and poor positioning errors generally occur because of the radiographer's lack of attention to details. Table 13-3 identifies a checklist that will acquaint the student with tasks that need to be applied each time a radiographic image is produced.

TABLE 13-3 Checklist for Evaluating Image Quality

Student's Name _____

Exposure Factors: mAs (mA/T) _____ kVp _____ ; AEC _____

Processing: Time _____ Temperature _____

Radiographic Procedure(s) Requested:

Evaluation Criteria	Yes	No	Corrective Action
Anatomy centered on film			
All necessary anatomical borders are visible			
Right/Left/Date marker visible			
Adequate density (mAs)			
Adequate contrast (kVp)			
Magnification/distortion visible			
Adequate detail/definition visible			
Gonad shielding visible (if req.)			
Collimation (clear border edge)			
Artifacts/visible			
Appropriate image receptor placement			

Table 13-3 is intended to be general in design. Most radiography programs develop their own checklist for evaluating image quality. The checklist in the table may be modified to adapt to any program.

REVIEW QUESTIONS

1. To evaluate radiographic quality means to:
   a. visually assess a recorded image
   b. visually inspect a finished radiograph
   c. visualize, inspect, and determine correct image technique
   d. all of the above

2. The limited radiographer's educational preparation must include knowledge of:
   a. mA, time, kVp, SID
   b. patient's history and condition assessment
   c. film processing
   d. all of the above

3. In the preparation of image production, which of the following must be done first?
   a. check room availability
   b. check with doctor
   c. carefully read examination request
   d. identify the patient

4. If an overall image appears overexposed or underexposed, generally the first factor to be considered for corrective action is:
   a. kVp
   b. mAs
   c. mA
   d. processing

5. If an image has a flat or gray appearance, the problem most likely will be related to:
   a. kVp
   b. mAs
   c. processing
   d. time

6. When all anatomy related to a particular image is not visually penetrated, the problem is most likely:
   a. kVp too low
   b. kVp too high
   c. mAs too high
   d. mAs too low

7. A blurred image is most likely the result of:
   a. motion
   b. kVp too low
   c. mAs too low
   d. no immobilization

8. The most common problem related to image size or shape is:
   a. incorrect SID
   b. incorrect kVp
   c. incorrect positioning
   d. incorrect CR

9. If the image appears too long or too short, the _____ is probably not perpendicular to the structure.
   a. image receptor plane
   b. CR
   c. tabletop surface
   d. tube

10. A slight change in the _____ will be seen on the image results almost immediately when film quality is evaluated.
   a. processor water flow
   b. processor time or temperature
   c. processor replenishment rates
   d. processor preventive maintenance

SUGGESTED READINGS

Papp, J. (2006). *Quality management in the imaging sciences* (3rd ed.). St Louis, MO: Mosby Inc.

Quinn, C. B. (1993). *Fuch's Radiographic Exposure, Processing and Quality Control* (5th ed.). Springfield, IL: Charles C. Thomas.

Quinn, C. B. (2007). *Practical radiographic imaging* (Fuch's Radiographic Exposure Processing & Quality Control) (8th ed.). Springfield, IL: Charles C. Thomas.

IMAGING SPECIALTIES

Key Terms

Chapter Outline

Bone Densitometry
Bone Densitometry Equipment
Patient Preparation, History, and Positioning
The Examination
Bone Densitometry Machine Operator Certification

Objectives

Upon completion of the chapter, the student will meet the following objectives by verifying knowledge of the facts and principles presented through oral and written communication at a level deemed competent.

⊃ Define what is meant by the terms: special imaging procedures, diagnostic imaging procedures, and interventional imaging procedures.
⊃ Explain the purpose of administration of contrast agents during imaging procedures.
⊃ Discriminate between vascular and nonvascular interventional imaging procedures.
⊃ Identify applications of computed tomography, magnetic resonance imaging, nuclear medicine, and ultrasound.
⊃ Recall advantages and disadvantages to the application of computed tomography, magnetic resonance imaging, nuclear medicine, and ultrasound.
⊃ Recall facts about molecular imaging, optical imaging, and fusion imaging.
⊃ Differentiate between screening and diagnostic mammography.
⊃ Recall the recommended guidelines for screening mammography and the guidelines for at-risk populations.
⊃ State the purpose of radiation oncology.
⊃ Recall the patient preparation instructions for bone densitometry examinations.

Introduction

This chapter provides an overview of imaging specialties and introduces the most common diagnostic and interventional imaging procedures. Many diagnostic and interventional procedures require the administration of contrast agents. In many states, law prohibits limited radiographers from administering contrast agents, participating in procedures requiring the administration of contrast agents, and performing contrast-imaging procedures. Despite such restrictions, the limited radiographer often communicates with patients and imaging facility staff about scheduling diagnostic and interventional procedures.

According to Standard Three (Patient Education) in *The Limited X-ray Machine Operator Standards* published by the American Society of Radiologic Technologists (ASRT), the limited radiographer provides information about procedures and related health issues according to protocol (2008). To meet the requirements of this standard, the limited radiographer should be knowledgeable of the procedures performed by each of the imaging specialties. The limited radiographer will apply this information when responding to patients' questions and concerns about imaging specialty procedures.

The limited radiographer is encouraged to continue to expand their knowledge about these topics. Additional information on this subject may be obtained from imaging facilities, hospitals, clinics, etc., that perform these procedures.

Diagnostic and Interventional Procedures

Diagnostic and interventional imaging procedures are commonly referred to as "special procedures." A special procedure is best defined as radiography of certain anatomic structures that require the instillation of a contrast agent before they can be visible during imaging procedures. As advancements have occurred in radiography, procedures once referred to as special procedures (e.g., studies of the gastrointestinal tract, urinary system, and the gallbladder) have become routine and are now considered routine diagnostic imaging procedures.

Interventional imaging procedures are used to intervene with the course of certain disease conditions without subjecting the patient to the risks of surgery or other invasive procedures. Interventional imaging procedures includes angioplasty, atherectomy, thrombolysis, and stenting of affected arteries.

Diagnostic and interventional imaging procedures are generally recognized as being either vascular or non-vascular and are performed to diagnose and treat disease conditions. These procedures are performed in facilities that have dedicated room(s) reserved just for these advanced examinations. A dedicated specialized imaging room or rooms may also be designed to support minor surgery procedures and are equipped with cardiac monitoring devices, emergency supplies, and instruments.

Introduction to Contrast Agents

The human body contains a variety of organic and inorganic substances, and the balance of these substances determines how the anatomic part or area will appear on the radiographic image. Many of the routine procedures (e.g., barium enemas, intravenous pylegrams, cholecystography) as well as diagnostic and interventional imaging procedures require the use of a contrast agent.

Internal organs and soft tissue structures do not sufficiently attenuate the x-rays and thus are not generally well-visualized on plain (non-contrast) radiographs. Contrast agents are used in many x-ray examinations to increase or decrease the tissue density (i.e., alter attenuation). By adding a contrast agent to certain organs and vessels, the density of the structure is changed and radiographic visualization is improved.

The tissues and organs of the human body can be categorized into one of four groups: air, fat, muscle, and bone. Anatomic structures containing air are considered to be lower density tissue. Organs and tissues containing air absorb fewer x-ray photons and thus more x-rays reach the film or image receptor (IR) and produce a greater radiographic density. The lungs and sinuses are examples of anatomic structures that contain air.

Fat and muscle are both soft-tissue structures in the body. Muscle attenuates the x-ray beam to a slightly greater degree than fat. For example, on a radiograph of the abdomen, the psoas muscles are usually demonstrated without the use of a contrast agent (Figure 14-1). It is also possible to see a faint outline of the kidneys on an abdomen radiograph because the fat capsule surrounding them increases the structural density and attenuates the x-rays.

Bone tissue has the greatest attenuation factor of the four classifications. Calcium has a high atomic number that effectively attenuates (absorbs) x-rays. Because of this increase in attenuation of x-rays, the bones of the skeleton are readily visualized on the radiographic image.

To review, contrast agents are administered during routine and specialized imaging procedures to enhance the visualization of certain organs and tissues (Figure 14-2).

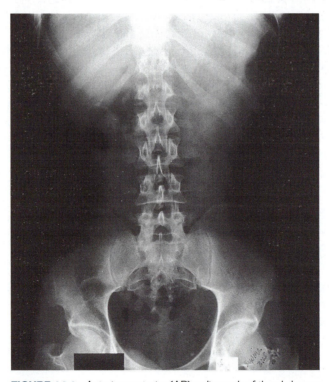

FIGURE 14-1 Anterior-posterior (AP) radiograph of the abdomen
Source: Delmar, Cengage Learning.

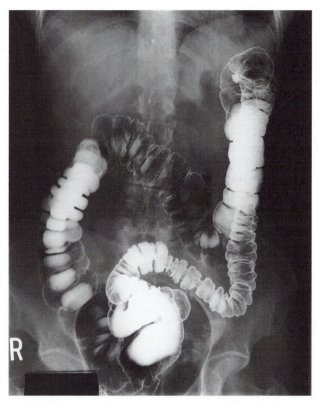

FIGURE 14-2 Examination of the large bowel using
contrast media to enhance visualization
Source: Delmar, Cengage Learning.

Radiographers and physicians performing procedures requiring contrast agents must have sufficient skills to be able to respond to emergency situations that may occur during the examination. Various state laws regulate who may participate in these procedures. The limited radiographer should obtain information about patient preparation and scheduling requirements from facilities used by their clinic or office. Many imaging facilities will provide written patient preparation and scheduling instructions to those referring patients for procedures.

Contrast Agents

Contrast agents may be classified into five groups:

1. Barium sulfate products
2. Aqueous iodine compounds
3. Oily iodine compounds

4. Gases

5. Ionic and nonionic agents

Barium sulfate is an inert inorganic salt of the chemical element barium and is used exclusively for imaging procedures of the gastrointestinal (GI) tract. Barium sulfate is commercially available in many forms, ranging from bulk containers requiring reconstitution with water to individual pre-measured applications. The dilution of the barium sulfate depends on the administration route. Barium sulfate may be prepared for oral and rectal administration.

Aqueous iodinated contrast agents are used when administration of barium sulfate may be too hazardous due to a patient's particular condition of allergies. Adverse reactions to an iodinated contrast agent range from nuisance side effects, such as hives and vomiting, to potentially lethal reactions, such as anaphylaxis and laryngeal edema. The limited radiographer should alert outside imaging facilities if the patient has a history of bronchospasm, laryngeal edema, or anaphylaxis.

Oily iodinated contrast agents may also be called ethiodized oils. Ethiodized oils are preferred in imaging studies in which absorption of contrast into the surrounding tissues or mixing of contrast with body fluids is not desired.

Air and gases are referred to as negative contrast agents because they appear black or very dark as compared to barium sulfate, which appears white, or very white (light). Carbon dioxide is generally the gas of choice because the body absorbs it much faster than other gases.

Ionic and nonionic compounds are used for a variety of procedures. The major difference between ionic and nonionic contrast agents is the atomic structure of the compounds. Common ionic contrast compounds include diatrizoate (trade name Hypaque), iothalamate (trade name Conray), and metrizoate (trade name Isopaque). Examples of nonionic contrast agents include Omnipaque and Amipaque. The nonionic contrast agents are less toxic to the patient and cause fewer anaphylactic shock reactions.

Introduction to Imaging Specialties

Fluoroscopy

Within months of Röentgens' discovery of x-rays, the first fluoroscope was created. The first fluoroscopes were of simple construction until Thomas Edison discovered that calcium tungstate screens could produce a brighter image, thus creating the first commercially available fluoroscope. Early users of these devices had limited knowledge of the potential effects of radiation exposure. These early pioneers often received significant radiation doses and suffered grave side effects.

Fluoroscopy is an imaging modality that uses an x-ray source to obtain real-time images of internal structures of a patient through the use of a fluoroscope (Figure 14-3).

The x-ray tube is located beneath the table. It emits a continuous x-ray beam that passes through the patient and falls onto a continuously fluorescing screen and image intensifier. The images are viewed in real time and a permanent image may be acquired during the procedure. Gastrointestinal imaging studies are generally obtained using fluoroscopy.

"Fluoroscopy carries the same types of risks as other x-ray procedures . . . and the radiation dose that the patient receives varies depending on the individual procedure." The most immediate or acute risk associated with fluoroscopy procedures is radiation-induced "burns" to the skin and underlying tissues ("How innovations," 2007). Most interventional procedures are focused on a relatively small area of skin

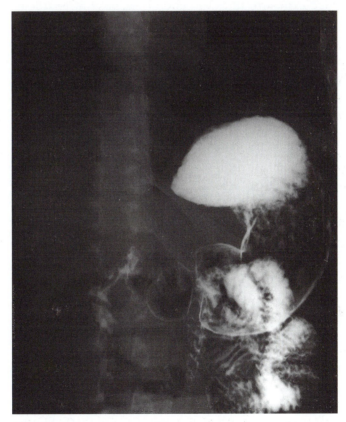

FIGURE 14-3 Abdomen radiograph taken in the upright position
Source: Delmar, Cengage Learning.

for an extended period of time. In these procedures, the skin receives the highest radiation dose of any portion of the patient's body. Such short-term effects of radiation exposure from fluoroscopy include sunburn like injuries and hair loss, or in rare cases, skin necrosis has been reported. Long-term effects include the potential risk of cancer (National Cancer Institute, 2007).

Today, modern fluoroscopic equipment consists of an x-ray tube, image intensifier, and an image system. An image intensifier increases the brightness of the real-time image produced on the fluorescent screen during fluoroscopy. This allows for a reduction in time for the radiologist as well as a reduction of radiation exposure to the patient.

Filtration in fluoroscopy is used to reduce the skin dose received by the patient. A minimum of 2.5 mm of total aluminum filtration permanently installed in the path of the useful beam is required in fluoroscopy units. Current federal standards limit skin entrance exposure rates of general-purpose intensification fluoroscopy units to a maximum of 10 roentgens (R) per minute.

Reduced radiation exposure during fluoroscopy has become possible primarily through digital technology. The use of digital correction functions allows for the production of spot films from previously captured fluoroscopy images instead of creating new images. Also, pulsing fluoroscopy x-ray imaging has allowed a reduction in radiation exposure. Pulsing fluoroscopy employs short radiation pulses. During the radiation-free periods, the last stored digital image is visible until a new and more current image is available. Use of pulsing fluoroscopy as opposed to continuous fluoroscopy results in reduced radiation exposure because beam-on time is shortened. Because fluoroscopy procedures take varying lengths of time, radiation beam-on time management is critical. During the fluoroscopy procedure, the radiologist is in control of beam-on time. The radiologist controls the time by a foot switch, which is designed as a "dead-man" type switch connected to a 5-minute timer.

Fluoroscopic images can be mixed or overlaid with one or more previously stored images. In this case, the dose rate can be significantly lowered and is referred to as digital filtering or recursive filtering. Last image hold is a technique that can be used during the fluoroscopy procedure. The radiologist can study the last image obtained without further radiation exposure. This also can lead to a reduction in total beam-on time and thereby reduce the overall radiation dose.

Frame grabbing can also occur during the fluoroscopy examination. The radiologist can "grab" or extract a chosen image from a series of images without additional beam-on time radiation exposure.

Roadmapping may be used to overlap two images. In this technique, a stored image may be superimposed upon a current image. Also, a current image may be saved and later called up for superimposition. One use for roadmapping is the visualization of blood vessels. An image of a blood vessel filled with contrast can be later superimposed on the same vessel filled with a catheter. By using roadmapping, fluoroscopy beam-on time during interventional studies can be reduced.

Computed Tomography

Computed tomography (CT), originally known as computed axial tomography (CAT or CT scan), is a medical imaging procedure that provides clinical information in the detection and differentiation of disease (American College of Radiography [ACR], 2007). In 1979, Godfrey Newbold Hounsfield and Allan McLeod Cormack were awarded the Nobel Prize in medicine for the invention of CT. Hounsfield conceived the first commercially viable CT scanner in Hayes, England (1967) at Thorn EMI Central Research Laboratories, while Cormack was also independently working on the concept at Tufts University. The first U.S. scanner was installed at the Mayo Clinic.

CT imaging employs tomography where digital geometry processing is used to generate a three-dimensional image of the internals of an object from a large series of two-dimensional x-ray images taken around a single axis of rotation. CT produces a volume of data, which can be manipulated, through a process known as windowing, in order to demonstrate various structures based on their ability to attenuate x-rays.

During a CT examination, the patient lies on a mechanical table that slowly moves through a doughnut-shaped scanner (Figure 14-4). Inside the scanner, an x-ray emitter rotates around the patient in the axial plane. On the opposite side of the patient, 180 degrees from the emitter, electronic x-ray detectors receive the x-ray beam and calculate how much of the beam was transmitted and how much was absorbed by the patient. A computer then calculates the x-ray absorption of each voxel within the slice and assigns it a numeric value. A pixel is a single dot within a two-dimensional image and has unique coordinates along the "X" and "Y" axes of the image. A voxel is a pixel with three dimensions.

Serial CT and helical (or spiral) CT are variations of the standard CT equipment. In serial CT scanning, the emitter/detector whirls 360 degrees around the patient to acquire a slice, the table then moves the patient, and the emitter/detector whirls 360 degrees the other way to acquire the next slice. In helical (spiral) scanning, the emitter/detector array moves around the patient continuously in the same direction, and the table also moves continuously through the scanner while the patient is being imaged.

CT has far greater contrast resolution than plain radiography and is superior in demonstrating abnormal calcifications or fluid/gas patterns in the viscera or peritoneal space. There are many applications of CT including studies of the brain, spine,

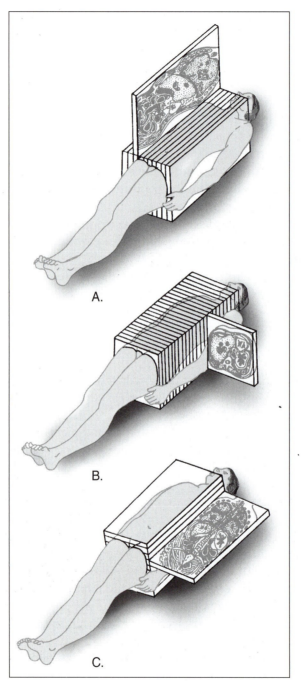

FIGURE 14-4 Computed tomography sections:
(A) sagittal; (B) transverse; and (C) coronal
Source: Delmar, Cengage Learning.

abdomen, pelvis, chest, neck, and paranasal sinuses. CT is also superior at demonstrating solid organs. CT may be performed with or without contrast. Compared to plain radiography, CT is expensive and delivers a relatively high radiation dose to the patient (Figure 14-5).

Multislice CT (MSCT) is another development in imaging technology that provides data acquisition using multiple rows of arrays. MSCT is quicker, provides better image quality, and covers more patient area. MSCT is valuable in three-dimensional imaging and also lends itself to other clinical application, such as CT angiography and virtual endoscopy.

Three concerns with MSCT involve the large number of images produced, causing delays when they are processed; decisions about benefit versus risk in emergency care use; and the cost of MSCT equipment.

After a CT study is acquired, radiographers may crop the images to focus on internal organ structures at the expense of subcutaneous tissues (Uppot, Sahani, Hahn, Gervais, and Mueller, 2008). Abdominal and pelvis CT is a sensitive imaging modality for diagnosis of abdominal disease and is used to investigate acute abdominal pain and in detecting solid organ injury after trauma. CT imaging is also being used increasingly in the guidance of surgical and radiation therapy treatment procedures.

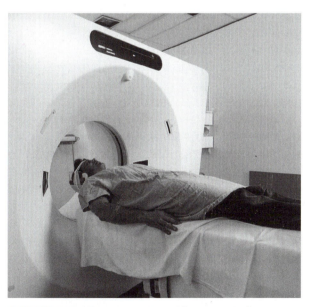

FIGURE 14-5 Patient positioned for computed tomography (CT) of brain
Source: Delmar, Cengage Learning.

Despite all the advantages of CT, the benefits of using CT imaging must be carefully weighed against the risks. "The amount of radiation dose from clinical imaging exams experienced by the U.S. public may have increased more than 600% in the last two decades, most of it due to CT" (National Council on Radiation Protection and Measurements [NCRP], 2007). A preliminary assessment from a National Council on Radiation Protection and Measurements (NCRP) scientific committee found that CT and nuclear medicine exams account for the largest increase in dose, with CT representing 12% of all procedures and 45% of the estimated collective dose. The growth of CT has been greater than 10% per year with 3 million CT scans in 1980 to more than 62 million by 2006 (NCRP, 2007).

The Food and Drug Administration (FDA) states that the principal risk associated with the radiation dose to a person resulting from a CT procedure is the small possibility of developing a radiation-induced cancer some time later in that person's life. However, one must weigh the probability for absorbed radiation dose to induce cancer to the greater benefits of discovering a disease process while at an early treatable stage.

Recognizing the real risks from radiation dose, the equipment design industry has been working to improve certain components of CT equipment. Some of these improvements are listed below.

Pediatric radiation exposure during CT examinations is a very real concern and CT manufacturers, radiologists, and health physicists are continuing to collaborate in the ongoing development of special pediatric CT protocols. These protocols, when used properly, allow lower mAs and kVp values to be used on children.

The Alliance for Radiation Safety in Pediatric Imaging has started a campaign called "Image-Gently™." The Alliance is a consortium of professional societies who are concerned about the radiation exposure children receive when undergoing medical imaging procedures (2008). Currently, thirteen societies representing the fields of radiology, pediatrics, and medical physics and radiation safety are involved. The Alliance recognized the often life-saving value of medical imaging but notes that pediatric imaging may not be tailored to children's smaller bodies, resulting in radiation exposures that are greater than necessary ("How innovations," 2007). This is especially true for CT scans (Alliance for Radiation Safety, 2008). The Alliance estimates that there are approximately 7 million CT studies performed on children every year in the U.S. and the number is increasing approximately 10% per year. CT is widely used among all ages of children, with 33% performed in children under 10 years of age ("How innovations," 2007). CT is the largest contributor to medical radiation dose in the U.S. (Alliance for Radiation Safety, 2008).

The Image Gently campaign recognizes that the radiographer plays a key role on the imaging team and that radiology and CT scanning are critical in diagnosing illness in children. One of the tenants of the campaign is that it is the responsibility of technologists and all members of the health care team to ensure that every imaging study in pediatric patients is thoughtful, appropriate, and indicated for each and every child. It is recognized that imaging departments and technologists are very busy with a varied work load and it is sometimes hard to ensure that action plans are adjusted to use "child-size" protocols. According to the Image Gently Campaign, there are five simple steps that radiographers can engage to improve patient care in everyday practice.

1. Increase awareness for the need to decrease radiation dose to children during CT scanning and to encourage fellow professionals to get involved with the effort.
2. Be committed to making a change in daily practice by working as a team with the radiologist, physicist, referring doctors, and parents to decrease the radiation dose. Sign a pledge, found on The Alliance for Radiation Safety in Pediatric Imaging web site, to join the Image-Gently™ campaign today.
3. Follow the practice standards #1 and #2 on assessment and analysis to ensure an appropriate action plan is established for completing CT examinations.
4. Work with the physicist, radiologist, and department manager to review the adult CT protocols; then use the simple CT protocols found on the Image-Gently to "down-size" the protocols for children. More is not better; adult-size kVp and mAs are not necessary for small bodies.
5. Be involved with the patients. Be the patient's advocate. Ask the questions required to ensure that CT protocols are appropriate for each child and adult patient (Alliance for Radiation Safety, 2007).

Interventional Radiography

Dr. Charles T. Dotter's landmark study in 1964 describing transluminal treatment of atherosclerotic lesions expanded and improved the techniques of angiocardiography and officially launched the growth of interventional radiology procedures (Kinney, 2008).

Diagnostic and interventional radiography procedures may be performed individually or together as part of the treatment plan. Interventional radiography procedures are usually performed in a specialized room and conducted by a radiologist. Fluoroscopy is used to guide and direct the catheters and instruments used during the procedure. Interventional procedures may be classified as vascular or non-vascular procedures. As follows is a brief description of the more common vascular and non-vascular procedures.

Vascular Interventional Imaging Procedures

Embolization is an interventional imaging procedure that employs the use of a catheter to restrict blood flow by creating an embolus in a vessel. Embolization is used to reduce blood flow to a highly vascular area of pathology and to stop active bleeding. Examples of embolization include uterine artery embolization to shrink fibroid growths in the uterus and intracranial endovascular coil used to occlude brain aneurysms.

Angioplasty

Angioplasty is used to treat a vessel that has become occluded or stenosed. Under fluoroscopic guidance, a catheter with a deflated balloon is placed at the vessel stenosis and the balloon inflated. A stent may be inserted to assist in maintaining patency of the vessel (Figure 14-6).

Insertion of venous access devices such as a peripherally inserted central catheter (PICC line), Hickman line, or subcutaneous port may be used for administering chemotherapeutic agents or for large amounts of antibiotics and for providing total parental nutrition and monitoring. Additional vascular interventional imaging

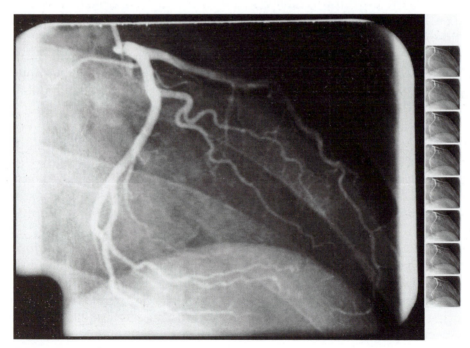

FIGURE 14-6 Coronary arteriography
Source: Delmar, Cengage Learning.

procedures include thrombolysis, infusion therapy, and the extraction of vascular foreign bodies.

Nonvascular Interventional Imaging Procedures

Percutaneous vertebroplasy is an example of a nonvascular interventional procedure that is used to treat patients who have one or more compressed vertebral bodies. Under fluoroscopic guidance, a special type of acrylic cement is injected into the vertebral body to help stabilize the area and reduce pain resulting from the compression.

Additional nonvascular interventional radiography procedures include colonic stenting, nephrostomy, percutaneous biliary drainage (PBD), percutaneous abdominal abscess drainage (PAD), percutaneous needle biopsy, and percutaneous gastrostomy.

Magnetic Resonance Imaging

Felix Bloch of Stanford University and Edward Purcell of Harvard University made the first successful nuclear magnetic resonance experiment to study chemical compounds in 1956. Bloch and Purcell were awarded the Nobel Prize for Physics in 1946. In the early 1980s, the first "human" magnetic resonance imaging scanners became available, producing images of the inside of the body. Current MRI scanners produce highly detailed two-dimensional and three-dimensional images of the human anatomy (Figure 14-7).

Magnetic resonance imaging (MRI) is primarily used in medical imaging to visualize the structure and function of the body. It provides detailed images of the body in any plane and has much greater soft tissue contrast than CT making it especially useful in neurological, musculoskeletal, cardiovascular, and oncological imaging (Merck Manuals, 2009a).

Magnetic resonance imaging (MRI) uses magnets and sequences of radiowaves to generate different types of images. MRI has greater contrast than CT and ultrasonography and, with different pulse sequences, has multiple ways of illustrating contrast between tissues. An advantage of MRI over CT is that MRI data can be obtained in three planes; axial, sagittal, and coronal. CT data acquired in the axial plane can be reformatted to generate the other planes. MRI provides excellent imaging of the soft tissues of the nervous system and is useful in the diagnosis of many types of pathology, including brain and spinal cord tumors and diseases such as multiple sclerosis.

MRI is also used in imaging the soft tissue around joints, providing an alternative to arthrography of the knee, shoulder, and temporomandibular joint. MRI is also being used for imaging procedures involving the intervertebral discs.

The patient is placed in a scanner that generates a very strong magnetic field (Figure 14-8).

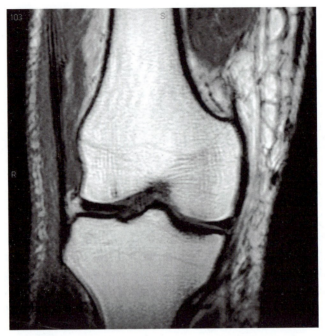

FIGURE 14-7 Magnetic resonance image (MRI) of the knee
Source: Delmar, Cengage Learning.

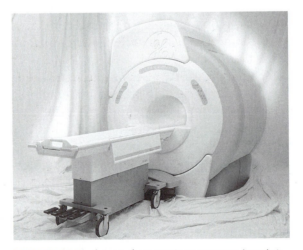

FIGURE 14-8 A typical magnetic resonance imaging unit, with the relationship of the stationary magnet, gradient coil, and RF coil to the patient illustrated (*Courtesy of GE Medical Systems*)

Radiofrequency waves are then pulsed in and once stopped, hydrogen nuclei tend to realign along the magnetic field. Realignment occurs at different rates in different tissue, thus the differential relaxation rates are used to create the MR image. MRI can be performed with or without contrast agents and when these agents are used can cause allergic reactions.

Advantages to MRI are that it is not invasive and the patient does not receive a radiation dose. MRI has some contraindications that are related to the magnetic field itself and to patients who fear being confined in a close space. The effects of the MR magnet on objects within the room and possibly inside the patient's body may be hazardous. Patients with implanted electronic devices such as pacemakers, defibrillators, neurostimulators, and cochlear implants should not be placed in the magnetic field. A directory is available for the technologist to use to determine the safety of specific devices within the MRI suite. Additional conditions that may require assessment prior to MRI, include pregnancy, orthopedic pins and screws, and metal fragments or shrapnel in the soft tissues. Loose metal items are prohibited from the MRI suite since these items may be drawn to the magnet and endanger bystanders and damage the MRI gantry. Other metal objects that cannot be taken into the MRI suite include stretchers, wheelchairs, crutches, and oxygen tanks unless specifically constructed for use with MRI.

Patients with extreme claustrophobia may not be able to withstand the imaging procedure; however, some facilities may have an "open field" scanner to accommodate the claustrophobic patient.

Whole-body imaging MRI is performed on subjects to screen for a range of benign and malignant disease processes. The combination of a variety of multiple time-consuming imaging studies may eventually be replaced by whole-body MRI. Whole-body MRI is an expensive imaging tool that is not intended to replace dedicated MRI examinations. MRI is an accurate alternative to conventional multimodality evaluation for disease staging purposes.

Nuclear Medicine Imaging

Nuclear medicine is referred to as "emission imaging" because photons are emitted from inside the patient and subsequently detected by a gamma camera imaging system (Merck Manuals, 2009c). A radiopharmaceutical agent tagged with a radioactive compound is administered to the patient. As photons are emitted from the radiopharmaceutical agent in the patient, a gamma camera is used to detect the distribution. An image is then created by a computer system. Unlike images produced in plain radiography, ultrasound, CT, and MRI, nuclear medicine studies sacrifice spatial resolution but offer information about organ function (Figure 14-9).

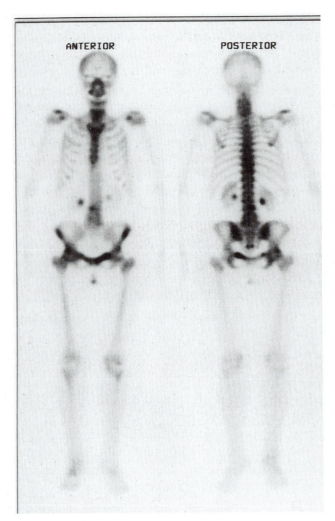

FIGURE 14-9 Whole body radionuclide scan
Source: Delmar, Cengage Learning.

Some common clinical indications for performing nuclear medicine studies include ruling out pulmonary embolism, acute cholecystitis, gastrointestinal bleed, and osteomyelitis.

Molecular Imaging

Molecular imaging is a new discipline that unites molecular biology and *in vivo* imaging (Society for Molecular Imaging, 2009). It enables the visualization of the cellular function and the follow-up of the molecular process of living organisms.

Molecular imaging refers to a varied set of imaging techniques used to observe disease processes. Molecular imaging differs from traditional imaging in that probes, known as biomarkers, are used to help image particular targets or pathways (Society for Molecular Imaging, 2009).

Biomarkers interact chemically with their surroundings and in turn alter the image according to molecular changes occurring within the area of interest. There are many different modalities that can be used for noninvasive molecular imaging. Each has its different advantages and disadvantages and some are more adept at imaging multiple targets than others. The major modalities used in molecular imaging are single photon emission computed tomography (SPECT), positron emission tomography (PET), optical imaging, and magnetic resonance imaging.

Single Photon Emission Computed Tomography

Single photon emission computed tomography (SPECT) is a nuclear medicine tomographic imaging technique using gamma rays (National Cancer Institute, 2009b). It is similar to conventional nuclear medicine planar imaging but provides true three-dimensional images (Figure 14-8). The data is typically provided as cross-sectional slices through the patient but can be reformatted as required.

SPECT procedures require administration of radiopharmaceuticals and the images are acquired by rotating a gamma camera around the patient. Projections are acquired at defined points during the rotation, typically every 3 to 6 degrees.

SPECT can be used to complement any gamma imaging study where a true three-dimensional representation can be helpful, such as in tumor imaging, imaging for infections, thyroid, or bone imaging (National Cancer Institute, 2009b). SPECT is also used in myocardial perfusion imaging and functional brain imaging.

Positron Emission Tomography

Positron emission tomography (PET) is a nuclear medicine imaging technique that produces a three-dimensional image or map of functional processes in the body (National Cancer Institute, 2009a). The system detects pairs of gamma rays emitted indirectly by a positon-emitting radionuclide (tracer), which is administered into the body on a biologically active molecule. Images of the tracer concentration in three-dimensional space within the body are then reconstructed by computer analysis.

Positron emission tomography is important in diagnostic imaging and has proved useful in cancer imaging. PET has 100% sensitivity and 91% specificity for detecting distance metastases (National Cancer Institute, 2009a). It is used in staging and managing cancer diagnosis and treatment.

PET scans are increasingly interpreted alongside CT or MRI scans, the combination (co-registration), giving both anatomic and metabolic information. Because PET imaging is most useful in combination with anatomical imaging, such as CT, modern PET scanners are now available with integrated CT scanners.

Optical Imaging

Optical imaging is an imaging technique that involves inference from the deflection of light emitted from a laser or infrared source to anatomic or chemical properties of material. Diffusive and ballistic optical imaging systems are currently only used in research and development conducted by universities and scientific laboratories (Medline Plus, 2009).

Fusion Imaging

Fusion imaging is also referred to as hybrid imaging. Hybrid imaging combines such modalities as PET/CT and SPECT/CT. Significant advantages of PET/CT include better diagnostic accuracy, treatment planning and response evaluation, and enhanced guided biopsy methods. Fusion imaging is providing previously unattainable levels of precision in detecting numerous conditions such as tumors, Alzheimer's disease, and neural disorders.Combined SPECT with CT scanners are currently being used in clinical research applications to attempt to identify future applications to imaging diagnosis.

Since PET/CT became commercially available in 2000, the number of installations has steadily increased and is expected to keep growing. Multi-skilled imaging technologists will increase as the demand for fusion or hybrid-imaging examinations increases. Currently no training program prepares hybrid technologists; rather technologists become proficient through experience with the technology itself and in preparation for either PET or CT.

Mammography

The American Cancer Society (ACS) predicts that one in eight American women will develop breast cancer sometime in her life (American Cancer Society, 2008). Males are also susceptible to breast cancer; however, breast cancer in males is less prevalent. The risk of breast cancer in women increases with increasing age.

Mammography is a low radiation dose imaging procedure that allows visualization of the breast tissue (Figure 14-10). Mammography is highly accurate, and on average will detect 80 to 90% of breast cancers in women without symptoms. Mammography has a false-negative (missed cancer) rate of at least 10% and about 5 to 10% of women have their mammograms interpreted as abnormal or inconclusive until further tests are done (American Cancer Society, 2008).

High-quality images are necessary for the radiologist to detect discrete and often subtle changes indicative of breast disease. A patient's physical size and shape

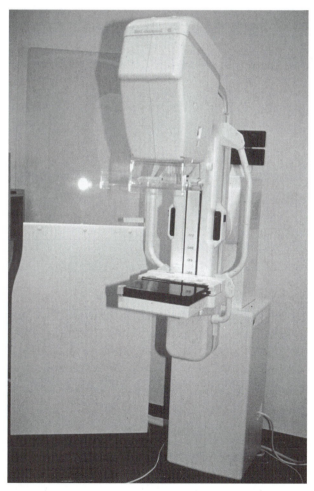

FIGURE 14-10 Mammography unit
Source: Delmar, Cengage Learning.

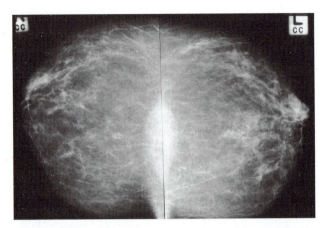

FIGURE 14-11 Mammogram illustrating a fatty breast
Source: Delmar, Cengage Learning.

can result in less than ideal positioning of the breast thus reducing the sensitivity and increasing specificity of the mammography image (Figure 14-11).

In 1992, the federal government enacted the **Mammography Quality Standards Act (MQSA)** in order to ensure that the technical aspects of mammography meet minimum standards. This act also mandated that those performing and interpreting mammograms have mammography training and demonstrate clinical competency.

Screening mammography provides valuable information for the detection of breast cancer and breast diseases. Screening mammography is indicated for asymptomatic women 40 years of age or older. Screening mammography consists of two projections of each breast; a craniocaudal (CC) and a mediolateral oblique (MLO). Diagnostic mammography provides additional information about patients who have signs and/or symptoms of breast disease.

There has been controversy among medical experts about sensitivity of screening mammography in young women. The mammography screening guidelines reflect this fact; however young women who have a family history of breast cancer are advised to begin mammography screening at an earlier age. The ACS guidelines for the early detection of breast cancer include the following:

Age 40 and older

- Annual mammogram;
- Annual clinical breast examination; and,
- Monthly breast self-examination (optional).

Age 20–39

- Clinical breast examination every three years; and, monthly breast self-examination (optional) (American Cancer Society, 2008).

Patients with a strong family history of breast cancer or a history of chest disease treated with radiation may be candidates for earlier screening. For patients with a history of a first-degree relative with breast cancer (mother, sister, aunt, etc.), screening should begin 10 years before the age at which the relative was diagnosed (American Cancer Society, 2008).

A diagnostic mammography is performed under the direct supervision of a qualified physician in mammography and may include mediolateral oblique (MLO), craniocaudal (CC), and/or additional views. Diagnostic mammography is performed when the patient has a history of breast cancer or presents with a breast-related complaint or overt symptoms. Diagnostic mammography consists of the routine screening views with additional projections and positions depending on the nature of the abnormality.

Adjunct diagnostic breast imaging modalities include ultrasound, ductography, and MRI. Ultrasound is typically used to further evaluate masses found on mammography or palpable masses not visualized on mammograms. Ductograms are useful for evaluation of bloody nipple discharge when the mammogram is non-diagnostic. MRI is used for additional evaluation of questionable findings, or for pre-surgical evaluation. Stereotactic breast biopsies are also used to further evaluate suspicious findings.

Digital tomosynthesis is digital tomography that involves x-ray tube movement and multiple low-dose exposures, which blurs out the tissue above and below the plane of interest. This allows for digital data reconstruction in approximately 1-millimeter slices. It is anticipated that digital tomosynthesis will be routinely used in both screening and diagnostic mammography in the next several years.

Ultrasonography

Ultrasonography (US) is an imaging technique used to visualize muscles and internal organs, their size, structures, and possible pathologies or lesions. In the late 1940s, Dr. George Ludwig at the Naval Medical Research Institute in Bethesda, Maryland, was the first to apply US energy to the human body for medical purposes (Merck Manuals, 2009d).

Ultrasound (US) is an imaging technique that uses sound waves that are well above the frequency audible to humans or animals. The procedure is conducted by applying a handheld transducer to the body. The transducer reflects sound waves via a cable to the US scanner and the data rendered on a monitor. A US coupling gel is used to help transmit US waves to and from the transducer. Sound waves encountering a tissue can be attenuated, reflected, or transmitted by tissue (Figure 14-12).

Hyperechoic and hypoechoic are terms used in ultrasound that refer to the brightness of an object relative to other things in the image (Figure 14-13). Air,

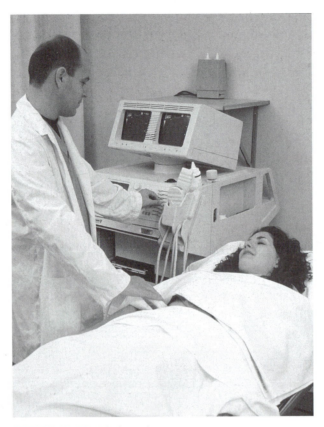

FIGURE 14-12 Modern ultrasonic equipment
Source: Delmar, Cengage Learning.

bone, and soft tissue reflect a great deal of sound and are markedly hyperechoic (Figure 14-10). Fluid-filled structures such as the urinary bladder, cysts, and large blood vessels are generally very hypoechoic.

Two- and three-dimensional echocardiology imaging is a component of ultrasonography. Dimensional cardiology ultrasound applications include stress echo, valvular morphology, myocardial biopsy, septal ablation, defining apical artifacts, and myocardial perfusion.

Breast ultrasound studies are generally performed after mammography imaging to further evaluate a palpable abnormality and to characterize a mammography finding or abnormality. Transabdominal pelvic ultrasound provides an overall view of the pelvis and first-trimester ultrasound is performed when the pregnancy is considered high risk.

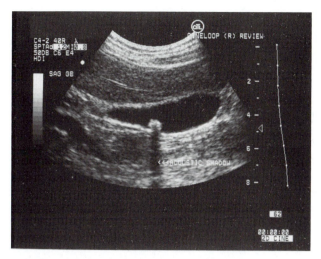

FIGURE 14-13 Ultrasound image of the gallbladder
demonstrating a gallstone
Source: Delmar, Cengage Learning.

Some of the strengths of US are:

- It images muscle and soft tissue very well and is particularly useful for delineating the interfaces between solid and fluid-filled spaces;
- It renders "live" images, where the operator can dynamically select the most useful section for diagnosing and documenting changes, often enabling rapid diagnoses;
- It shows the structure of organs;
- It has no known long-term side effects and rarely causes any discomfort to the patient;
- The equipment is widely available and comparatively flexible;
- Small, easily carried scanners are available and examinations can be performed at the bedside; and,
- The procedure is relatively inexpensive compared to other modes of investigation (e.g., CT, x-ray tomography, and MRI) (Merck Manual, 2009d).

Some of the weaknesses of US imaging are:

- US devices have trouble penetrating bone;
- US perform very poorly when there is a gas between the transducer and the organ of interest, due to the extreme differences in acoustic impedance;
- Even in the absence of bone or air, the depth penetration of US is limited, making it difficult to image structures deep in the body, especially in overweight and obese patients;

- The method is operator-dependent. A high level of skill and experience is needed to acquire diagnostic quality images; and,
- There are no scout images so once an image has been acquired there is no exact way to tell which part of the body was imaged (Merck Manuals, 2009b).

Radiation Oncology

Radiation oncology is commonly referred to as radiation therapy and involves the use of ionizing radiation for the treatment of malignancy and some benign diseases. The discovery of x-ray in 1895 and later the discovery of natural radioactivity in the late 1890s set the stage for the application of radiation as a therapy (Merck Manuals, 2009b).

Today, radiation therapy radiation is used in cancer treatment to control malignant cells and may be used for curative or adjuvant cancer treatment. Total body irradiation (TBI) is a radiotherapy technique used to prepare the body to receive a bone marrow transplant. Radiotherapy has several applications in non-malignant conditions, such as the treatment of trigeminal neuralgia, severe thyroid eye disease, pterygium, pigmented villonodula synovitis, and prevention of keloid scar growth.

Radiation therapy is in itself painless; however most side effects are predictable and expected. Side effects from radiation treatments are usually limited to the area of the patient's body that is under treatment. Side effects are divided into the acute side effects and the medium and long-term effects. Acute side effects of radiation therapy include:

- Damage to the epithelia surfaces. The rates of onset of damage and recovery depend upon the turnover rate of the epithelial cells;
- Swelling and general inflammation of the soft tissue;
- Infertility; if the gonads are directly exposed; and,
- Generalized fatigue.

Medium and long-term side effects are often referred to as latent effects and depend on the tissue that received the treatment. Medium and long-term side effects include:

- Fibrosis;
- Hair loss;
- Dryness (i.e., dry mouth, eyes, skin, and mucosa);
- Fatigue;
- Cancer (Merck Manuals, 2009b).

Surgery, chemotherapy, and radiotherapy are methods used to treat cancer and may be combined with radiation therapy. Radiation therapy may be administered by external beam radiotherapy, brachytherapy, or sealed and unsealed source.

Brachytherapy sealed sources are usually extracted later, while unsealed sources may be administered by injection or ingestion. Radioisotope therapy may also be delivered through a bloodstream infusion or ingestion.

A specialized team of professionals plans and delivers the radiation therapy treatment plan. The team usually includes a radiation oncologist, a doctor who prescribes the treatment and area to be treated, and a medical radiation physicist who advises the oncologist. A medical dosimetrist outlines the plan for obtaining the desired radiation dosage and works closely with the radiation oncologist and medical physicist. The radiation therapist administers the treatments and maintains the patient records.

Bone Densitometry

Bone densitometry is an imaging study that measures bone mineral density (BMD) and is used to determine whether a person may have or be at risk of having **osteopenia** or **osteoporosis** (Health Line, 2009) (Figure 14-14).

There are several methods and types of equipment that measure bone density. Currently, a physician may recommend a bone mineral density (BMD) test when an individual has one of the following conditions:

- long term use of medications such as glucocorticoids or anti-seizure drugs
- overactive thyroid gland (hyperthyrodism) or taking high doses of thyroid hormone medication
- overactive parathyroid gland(hyperparathyrodism)

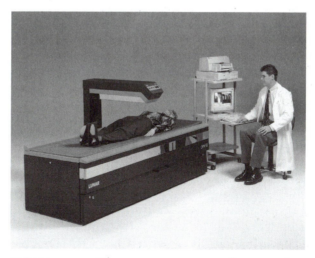

FIGURE 14-14 Densitometry equipment (*Courtesy of Lunar Corporation, Madison, WI*)

- spinal x-ray indicating fracture(s) or bone loss
- fracture resulting from minor injury or strain
- loss of sex hormones at an early age
- chronic disease that can lead to bone loss

Osteoporosis is recognized as one of the most common and serious health problems facing the aging population in the United States (National Institutes of Health, 2002). Additional information about osteoporosis and other bone loss diseases is discussed in Chapter 11, Radiographic Pathology.

After osteoporosis has been diagnosed, a physician prepares a treatment plan designed to help maintain the patient's current bone mass and prevent additional bone loss. Treatment usually involves a long-term program that includes medication, diet, exercise, and regular serial BMD monitoring. It is important that serial BMD measurements used to monitor a patient's response to treatment be precise and accurate in order to detect small changes in BMD.

Bone Densitometry Equipment

In the late 1980s, the **dual energy x-ray absorptiometry (DEXA)** technology was introduced and was applied to the measurement of bone mass. The introduction of new technologies to measure bone mass was critical since ordinary x-ray techniques could not detect less than 30% loss in bone mass. Using bone mass measurement technologies, as little as 1% change in bone mass is detectable (National Institute of Health, 2000; National Osteoporosis Foundation, 2009).

Tests for bone mass density are classified as either central or peripheral tests. A central test is used to quantify BMD in the spine and proximal femur. A peripheral test is used to quantify BMD in the heel, radius, and ulna. Bone densitometry has four major applications in clinical practice: quantification of bone mass or density, assessment of fracture risk, skeletal morphology, and body-composition analysis. Bone mass testing may be performed to confirm:

- suspected bone loss (osteopenia)
- diagnose osteoporosis
- document or follow the effect of a disease process that causes changes in bone mineral content or bone density
- follow response to therapy over time

Current bone measurement devices do not actually measure BMD, rather information is provided about bone mineral content (BMC) and the length or area of bone. The information provided, as a BMD score, is useful when related to a comparative score. The method used to develop the reference data for which the score is compared has a great impact on the estimation of peak bone mass of young normal women and on the estimation of population standard deviations. The FDA sets strict specifications for equipment that is to be used for BMD measurements in the U.S. Although BMD equipment must meet these specifications, the following equipment characteristics are important considerations.

Radiographers and physicians involved in BMD testing must be familiar with testing objectives, diagnosis, and treatment protocols. They must also be proficient in machine operation and calibration. Radiographers who perform BMD testing must have a thorough understanding of basic computer applications. They must also be proficient in using the computer system applications that have been installed on the equipment and recognize the importance of installing manufacturer software upgrades according to instructions. The radiographer is also responsible for archiving and storing the scan image. Usually, machine manufacturers provide initial hands-on staff training in the application and use of the BMD equipment.

Patient Preparation, History, and Positioning

No special preparations are required prior to a bone density examination other than refraining from taking calcium and vitamin supplements the day of the examination. Some special considerations include:

- If there is any possibility of pregnancy, the bone density study should not be done until the pregnancy is ruled out.
- Patients who have had diagnostic testing that included contrast material or radioisotopes (nuclear medicine testing) must wait at least 7 days before undergoing a bone density study.
- There may be weight restrictions on table equipment; for example, certain tables may have a maximum weight limitation such as "capacity is 300 pounds."

Patients may wear their street clothes during the bone density procedure. Metal objects such zippers, belt buckles, and snaps should be removed from the area being scanned. The radiographer should evaluate each patient to determine if they require assistance in sitting or lying down and especially in regaining equilibrium after the examination.

Questionnaires are useful in gathering relevant patient information that may assist in bone density measurement. Most importantly, patient history questionnaires provide consistency so that every patient is asked the same questions. The radiographer should review all available patient records and the physician request to confirm appropriate anatomic site and positioning placement of the region of interest (ROI) prior to beginning the scan examination.

The Examination

Bone density measurements may be made in the vertebral spine, promixal femur, forearm, metacarpals, phalanges, and calcaneus. A physician is responsible for issuing the request for a BMD examination. The radiographer is responsible for ensuring that the measurement is made of the region requested and that patient positioning is correct. When serial BMD examinations are conducted to monitor therapy, evaluate bone-loss, and to follow patients not being treated, but at risk; consistent positioning in subsequent examinations is critical. Many facilities require that the radiographer note in the patient record the evidence of artifacts and any positioning that is unique to the particular patient. The radiographers's competency skill level and knowledge of the procedural applications are important because accuracy and precision in BMD measurements determine ongoing patient monitoring and treatment.

The data obtained from the various types of bone densitometry equipment contains similar information, which can be categorized as follows:

- the skeletal image
- the measured and calculated BMD parameters
- comparisons to the reference database
    percentage % comparisons
    standard score comparisons
- standardized BMD
- age-regression graph
- assignment of diagnostic category based on WHO criteria

Most x-ray densitometry machines provide a paper copy image of the skeletal area being studied. Although these images are not FDA approved for making a structural diagnosis, the technologist should review the image.

In bone densitometry, if a patient's Z-score is +2, this implies that the patient's value is 2 SD above the average value. Likewise, if the patient's Z-score is −2, the implication is that the patient's value is 2 SD below the average value. Because the WHO criteria for a diagnosis of osteoporosis is based on the number of SD's from the average peak bone density of the young adult, the SD comparisons are more widely used in clinical practice.

Physicians use BMD values to predict the patient's likelihood of future fracture risk. Predictions of fracture risk are either global or site-specific fracture risk predictions. A doubling of fracture risk for each SD decline in bone density is used for global fracture predictions. For site-specific fracture predictions, the predicative value depends on the anatomic site where the measurement is obtained. Typically, after a bone densitometry test, a woman will receive one of four diagnoses: normal, osteopenia, osteoporosis, or established osteoporosis with fragility fracture.

- Normal—the skeletal system is as strong as that of a young, normal person.
- Osteopenia—the skeletal bone density is 10% to 25% below peak mass, and the person is at risk for osteoporosis.
- Osteoporosis—the skeletal bone density is 25% or more below peak mass.
- Established osteoporosis with fragility fracture—the skeletal bone density is 25% or more below peak bone mass and the person has had a fracture, typically in the spine, hip or forearm.

Bone Densitometry Machine Operator Certification

Approximately two-thirds of the states have licensing laws governing those who operate equipment that generates x-radiation. The equipment used to measure BMD generates small amounts of ionizing radiation, and as such, their use may be regulated by state law. To comply to a state's radiation control laws, persons who wish to perform BMD tests may be required to provide documentation proving clinical experience in bone densitometry. Also, they may be required to pass an examination covering the following topics: osteoporosis and bone health; equipment operation and quality control; patient preparation and safety; and dual-energy x-ray absorptiometry (DEXA) scanning of the lumbar spine, proximal femur, and the forearm.

Persons who have already attained certification by ARRT, in the supporting categories of radiography, nuclear medicine technology, or radiation therapy, can take the ARRT post-primary bone densitometry machine operator examination. Post-primary candidates must document clinical experience in BMD testing to be eligible for the examination. Refer to Chapter 1, Introduction to Limited Radiography: The Occupation, for a complete outline of the content specifications for the Bone Densitometry Machine Operator examination administered by the ARRT.

For those who do not have the ARRT certification and are not eligible to take the ARRT administered post-primary bone densitometry examination, the International Society of Clinical Densitometry (ISCD) offers both Bone Densitometry training and a certification examination. The ISCD training course, which is offered throughout the U.S., provides a comprehensive training session with separate tracks for physicians and technologists. The ISCD course offers essential education for bone densitometry staff and preparation for ISCD certification examination. For additional information the ISCD may be contacted at www.iscd.org.

Certification in bone densitometry offers personal recognition of bone densitometry skill and demonstration of proficiency in bone densitometry. Continuing education is essential to both technologists and physicians who perform BMD testing since innovations in measurement technology and approaches to prevention and treatment of osteoporosis and other bone loss diseases are occurring at a rapid rate.

REVIEW QUESTIONS

1. Many radiographic imaging studies once referred to as special procedures are now considered routine diagnostic imaging procedures.
   a. True
   b. False

2. Interventional imaging procedures are used to:
   1. intervene with the course of certain disease
   2. replace a thorough medical examination
   3. provide the patient with an alternative treatment method to surgery or other invasive procedures

   Possible Responses
   a. 1 and 2
   b. 1 and 3
   c. 2 and 3
   d. 1, 2, and 3

3. **All** of the following are true regarding the tissue and organs of the human body, **except**:
   a. can be categorized into one of four groups: air, fat, muscle, and bone
   b. air and gas attenuates the x-ray beam to a greater degree than fat or muscle
   c. bone tissue has the greatest attenuation factor of the four classifications
   d. contrast agents are administered during routine and specialized imaging procedures to enhance the visualization of certain organs and tissues

4. The contrast agent used exclusively for imaging procedures of the gastrointestinal tract is:
   a. aqueous iodinated liquids
   b. air and gases
   c. oily iodinated liquids
   d. barium sulfate

5. **All** of the following are true regarding computed tomography (CT) imaging procedures, **except**:
   a. images produced are slice-like multiple image sections
   b. a computer calculates x-ray absorption and converts it to an image
   c. compared to plain radiography, CT delivers a relatively low dose of radiation to the patient
   d. has far greater contrast resolution than plain radiography

6. **All** of the following are examples of vascular interventional imaging procedures, **except**:
   a. percutaneous vertebroplasty
   b. embolization
   c. angioplasty
   d. thrombolysis

7. Indications for magnetic resonance imaging (MRI) include:
   1. non-invasive
   2. the patient does not receive radiation
   3. is useful for patients with implanted electronic devices
   4. provides excellent images of soft tissue

   Possible Responses
   a. 1 and 2
   b. 2 and 4
   c. 3 and 4
   d. 1, 2, and 4

8. Positron emission tomography (PET) is reported to have a sensitivity of _____%.
   a. 100
   b. 91
   c. 75
   d. 50

9. The American Cancer Society predicts that 1 in ___ American women will develop breast cancer sometime in her lifetime.
   a. 25
   b. 15
   c. 8
   d. 5

10. The American College of Radiology recommends that asymptomatic women begin screening mammography at age:
    a. 25
    b. 30
    c. 40
    d. 50

11. Clinical indications for performing nuclear medicine studies include ruling out or diagnosing:
    1. pulmonary embolism
    2. cholecystitis
    3. cardiac infarct
    4. gastrointestinal bleed

    Possible Responses

    a. 1 and 2
    b. 3 and 4
    c. 1, 2, and 4
    d. 2, 3, and 4

12. **All** of the following are markedly hyperchoic, **except**:
    a. urinary bladder
    b. air
    c. bone
    d. soft tissue

13. Radiation therapy administered by internal radiation is referred to as:
    a. sclerotherapy
    b. brachytherapy
    c. teletherapy
    d. thermotherapy

14. According to the National Osteoporosis Foundation, more than _____ million Americans have osteoporosis.
    a. 15
    b. 24
    c. 30
    d. 45

15. The World Health Organization (WHO) study group defined osteoporosis as a systemic skeletal disease characterized by **all** of the following, **except**:
    a. low bone mass
    b. microarchitectural deterioration
    c. decrease susceptibility to fracture
    d. increase in bone fragility

16. **All** of the following factors may contribute to an increased risk of osteoporosis, **except**:
    a. Caucasian or Asian descent
    b. African American or Black ancestry
    c. corticosteroid use
    d. early menopause

17. Ordinary x-ray techniques cannot detect less than _____% loss in bone mass.
    a. 5
    b. 15
    c. 20
    d. 30

18. Current bone measurement devices actually measure bone mineral density.
    a. True
    b. False

19. Peripheral dual energy x-ray absorptiometry is best used for:
    a. serial BMD measurements
    b. a single-event measurement
    c. measurements to follow therapy progress
    d. long-term management of osteoporosis

20. The only measurement technology that provides a three-dimensional or volumetric measurement of bone density is:
    a. peripheral dual energy x-ray absorptiometry
    b. quantitative ultrasound
    c. quantitative computed tomography
    d. dual energy x-ray absorptiometry

REFERENCES

American Cancer Society. (2008). *Breast Cancer Facts and Figures 2008.* Retrieved from http:www.cancer.org

American College of Radiology. (2007). *ACR guidelines and standards, ACR practice guideline for performing and interpreting diagnostic computed tomography (CT).* Retrieved from www.acr.org

American Society of Radiologic Technologists. (2008). *The practice standard for medical imaging and radiation therapy. Limited x-ray machine operator standards.* Retrieved from http://www.asrt.org

Bone mineral density key predictor of fracture. (2004). *Radiology Today.* Retrieved from http://www.radiologytoday.net

Health Line. (2009). Dual-energy X-ray Absorptiometry (DEXA). Retrieved from http://www.healthline.com

How innovations in medical imaging have reduced radiation dosage (executive summary). (2007). Retrieved from http://www.medicalimaging.org

Kinney, T. B. (2008). *Radiologic History Exhibit.* Charles T. Dotter: A Pioneering Interventional Radiologist. Retrieved from http://www.radioeraphics.rsnajnls.org

Medline Plus. (2009). *Envisioning the future.* Retrieved from www.nlm.nih.gov

National Cancer Institute. (2007). *Interventional fluoroscopy: reducing radiation risks for patients and staff.* Retrieved from www.cancer.gov

National Cancer Institute. (2009a). Positron Emission Tomography Scan. Retrieved from http://www.cancer.gov

National Cancer Institute. (2009b). Single-photon Emission Computed Tomography. Retrieved from http://www.cancer.gov

National Council on Radiation Protection and Measurements (NCRP). 2007, April 16. Diagnostic Imaging Online. *Report from NCRP: CT-based radiation exposure in U.S. population soars.* Retrieved from www.diagnosticimaging.com

National Institutes of Health. Osteoporosis and related bone diseases. National Resource Center. (2000). Fast Facts on Osteoporosis. Retrieved from http://www.niams.nih.gov

National Institutes of Health. Osteoporosis and bone related diseases. National Resource Center. (2002). Osteoporosis Overview. Retrieved from www.osteo.org

National Osteoporosis Foundation. (2009). America's Bone Health: The State of Osteoporosis and Low Bone Mass. Retrieved from http://www.nof.org

The Alliance for Radiation Safety in Pediatric Imaging. (2008). *What can I do?* Technologists. Retrieved from http://www.pedrad.org

The Society for Molecular Imaging. Molecular Imaging (2009). Available at http://www.molecular imaging.org

The Merck Manuals Online Medical Library (2009a). Magnetic resonance imaging. Retrieved from http://www.merck.com

The Merck Manuals Online Medical Library (2009b). Radiation Therapy. Retrieved from http://www.merck.com

The Merck Manuals Online Medical Library (2009c). Radionuclide Scanning. From http://www.merck.com

The Merck Manuals Online Medical Library (2009d). Ultrasonography. Retrieved from http:www.merck.com

Uppot, R., Sahani, D., Hahn, P., Gervais, D., Mueller, P. (2008). *Impact of obesity on medical imaging and image-guided intervention.* Retrieved from http://www.medscape.com

World Health Organization. (1994). Assessment of fracture risk and its application to screening for postmenopausal osteoporosis: Report of a WHO study group. *WHO Technical Report Series.* Geneva: WHO.

SUGGESTED READINGS

National Institute of Arthritis and Musculoskeletal and Skin Diseases (2009). (Topics of interest.) Retrieved from http://www.niams.nih.gov

U.S. Department of Health & Human Services. Office of the Surgeon General (2009). Bone Health as Osteoporosis: A Report of the Surgeon General (issued October 14, 2004). Retrieved from http:www.surgeon.general.gov

CHAPTER 15

RADIATION BIOLOGY

Key Terms

Absorption

Absorbed Dose

Acute Radiation Syndrome (ARS)

Absorbed Dose Equivalent (ADE)

Apoptosis

Attenuation

Direct Effect

Dose Fractionation and Protraction

Dose-Response Relationship

Genetic Effects

Indirect Effect

Ionization

Ionizing Radiation

Law of Bergonié and Tribondeau

Linear Energy Transfer (LET)

Meiosis

Mitosis

Radiation Biology

Radiosensitivity

Radiolysis

Relative Biological Effectiveness (RBE)

Somatic Effects

Target Theory

Wilhelm Conrad Röentgen

Chapter Outline

Introduction
Ionization: A Review of the Facts
Cell Anatomy
Radiosensitivity
   Reproductive Cells
   Biologic Factors of Radiosensitivity
Levels of Biological Effects
   Molecular Effects of Radiation
   Cellular Effects of Radiation
   Effects of Radiation on Cell Division
   Organic Effects of Radiation
Absorbed Dose
Absorbed Dose Equivalent
Dose-Response Relationship
Linear Energy Transfer (LET)
Relative Biological Effectiveness (RBE)
Dose Fractionation and Protraction
Direct and Indirect Effect
Radiolysis

Objectives

Upon completion of the chapter, the student will meet the following objectives by verifying knowledge of the facts and principles presented through oral and written communication at a level deemed competent.

➲ Define common radiation biology terminology.
➲ Review the ionization process as it relates to potential biologic damage in humans.
➲ Discuss how attenuation affects both of the following:
  ➲ The patient's absorbed dose of radiation.
  ➲ The radiographic image.
➲ Identify and state function(s) of the basic components of a cell.
➲ Differentiate between meiosis and mitosis.
➲ Select correct statements concerning the Law of Bergonié and Tribondeau.
➲ State biological factors that affect radiosensitivity.
➲ Differentiate between the terms absorbed dose and absorbed dose equivalent.
➲ Recall the theory of linear, non-threshold relationship as it related to the ALARA concept.
➲ Discriminate between the definitions of linear energy transfer and relative biological effectiveness.
➲ Draw an illustration to show what occurs in the direct-hit and indirect-hit theory.
➲ Compare and contrast short-term and long-term radiation-induced biologic effects.
➲ Compare and contrast somatic and genetic effects of radiation.

Introduction

Almost as soon as x-ray was discovered (November 1895) by Wilhelm Conrad Röentgen, biological damage to the skin was observed (Figure 15-1). This biological effect should not be surprising because the rays were virtually unfiltered and of very low energy and penetration. No one considered that there might be any potential health hazard from being exposed to the "invisible light." It was a novelty, a new discovery that people actually exhibited at social events.

Thomas Alva Edison, an American scientist and inventor, brought x-rays to the public's attention through lectures and demonstrations. The first record of injuries from x-ray exposure occurred in Edison's laboratory in 1896. Edison's assistant, Clarence Dally, experienced radiation burns that later resulted in cancer. Dally was

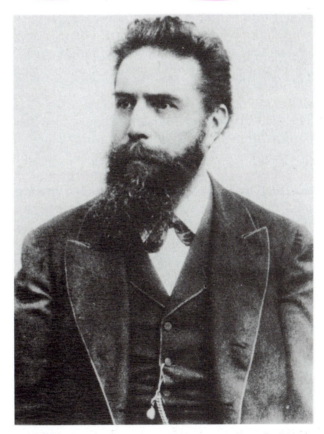

FIGURE 15-1 Wilhelm Conrad Röentgen *(From O. Glasser, Dr. W. C. Roentgen, 2nd Edition, 1958. Courtesy of Charles C. Thomas, Publisher, Springfield, Illinois.)*

the first person to die from radiation exposure (1904, age 39). In 1901, Röentgen was awarded the first Nobel Prize in physics.

The newly discovered light and its effects of skin reactions are known today as erythema x-ray or 'x-ray dermatitis.' Other documented health effects from exposure to the "invisible light" were epilation (hair loss), telangiectasia (dilation of capillaries), and changes in the skin's texture. These early injuries were primarily seen in the clerks who volunteered as radiographers at the London Hospital in Great Britain. Four such clerks, Ernest Harnack, Reginald Blackall, Ernest Wilson, and Harold Suggars, developed signs of skin damage, and by 1903, they all had very obvious radiation injuries. Wilson documented his injuries in a photographic series showing progressive bone damage to his hands. Wilson died of his injuries in 1911 and Harnack ultimately had both arms amputated. Suggars and Blackall continued to work with the "new light" and helped to establish the College of Radiographers. In 1920, the Society of Radiographers was incorporated in the United Kingdom, with the objective of promoting and developing the science and practice of radiography, and also to protect the honor and interests of radiographers. The first examinations were held in 1921, and the first successful candidates from the examination were admitted to membership in March 1921.

Ionizing radiation used during diagnostic imaging studies has been proven to be harmful to any human exposed, whether for diagnostic or therapeutic purposes. Exposure to ionizing radiation is also a serious concern to those who use it in their occupations, such as radiographers, doctors, medical staff, and industrial workers. The extent and nature of the damage is dependent on the type of ionizing radiation, the radiosensitivity of the tissue exposed, and the amount of radiation absorbed. Many factors may influence the type and severity of biologic effect experienced by humans such as a person's genetic makeup, age, and health status. Because many of these influencing factors cannot be controlled, any measures that the radiographer can take to reduce the overall radiation exposure to human tissue is very important.

The radiographer is a key person in the effort to reduce ionizing radiation exposure in the diagnostic imaging setting. By understanding how ionizing radiation produces harmful effects, radiographers can apply radiation protection procedures to reduce exposure to themselves, patients, and staff. Radiographers can further reduce unnecessary radiation exposure by performing each diagnostic imaging study with the utmost attention to detail, thus avoiding retake radiographs, which increase the amount of radiation received.

Radiation biology, a branch of the biological sciences, involves the study of the effects of ionizing radiation on living tissue. This chapter covers the basic concepts of this science by providing a review of the ionization process, introduction to cell biology, mechanisms, and impacts of biologic effects on humans.

Ionization: A Review of the Facts

The effects of radiation on living organisms are a result of ionizations that occur at the atomic level. During ==ionization, an electron is removed from its energy shell, resulting in a positively charged atom.== The free electron can deposit its energy to surrounding tissue. Molecules may be altered, causing cellular damage that may result in abnormal cell function or loss of cell function. If enough cells are damaged, the tissues, organs, and systems may be affected and exhibit symptoms of radiation damage.

A diagnostic x-ray beam passing through living matter will result in ionization in the cells comprising the matter. Because x-ray interaction with matter and ionization are random, some x-rays will pass through matter without interacting, as shown in Figure 15-2. When interaction does occur, x-ray photons will give up their energy to atoms during the interaction, thus altering the atom. When x-ray photons interact with living tissue, the energy is absorbed and is referred to as absorbed dose. ==The greater the absorbed dose, the greater the possibility of biologic effect.== Because there is differential absorption of x-rays in body structures of different densities, x-rays can be used to visualize these body structures (see Figure 15-2).

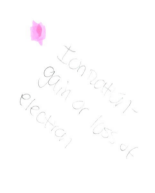

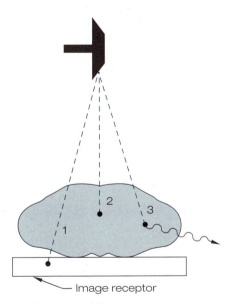

FIGURE 15-2 When x-rays interact with the patient, they will either (1) pass through unaffected, (2) be absorbed, or (3) interact and change direction (scatter). Source: Delmar, Cengage Learning.

For example, x-rays are absorbed preferentially in bone as compared to soft tissue, thus producing the traditional radiographic image. The transference of x-ray energy to the atoms of human tissue is called absorption and the amount of energy absorbed per unit mass is referred to as the absorbed dose (D).

The phenomenon of absorption and the difference in absorption properties of various body structures allow for the production of a diagnostic radiography

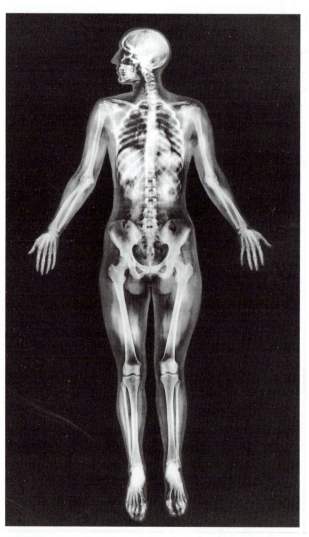

FIGURE 15-3 An antique full-body radiograph (Reprinted with permission of the International Society of Radiographers and Radiological Technicians from the K.C. Clark Archives, Middlesex Hospital, London, England)

or for visualization of these structures during fluoroscopy and other medical imaging procedures. The amount of energy absorbed depends on the atomic number Z (number of protons in the nucleus) of the tissues, mass density of the tissue, and energy of the radiation. For example, bone tissue has a higher atomic number (13.8) than does soft tissue, which has an atomic number of (7.4). In diagnostic kilovoltage ranges of 30–150 kVp, bone tissue will absorb more x-ray energy than soft tissue or fat tissue. As the atomic number of the irradiated tissue increases, the absorbed dose increases (Figure 15-3). Additional information on absorption and absorbed dose will be discussed further in this chapter.

To review, attenuation of the x-ray beam refers to any process that prevents x-ray photons from reaching the patient or the radiographic film. Both absorption and scatter of x-rays (redirection of x-ray photons after interaction with an object) are factors affecting attenuation.

Cell Anatomy

The human body is composed of various types of cells that perform many different functions (Figure 15-4).

The cell is the basic component of all living organisms. Each cell is a single functioning unit, capable of performing the processes essential for life. A single cell reacts to stimuli, ingests and metabolizes nutrients, synthesizes new materials, excretes wastes, and reproduces itself. Cells are involved in an ongoing process of obtaining and converting energy; and any alteration to a cell's usual functions.

Every mature cell is highly specialized, having specific functions to perform. A cell's specialized function is determined by its molecular structure. This delicate balance can be damaged if the cell's structure and/or chemical balance are changed.

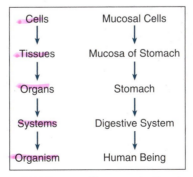

FIGURE 15-4 The organizational structure of a biological organism
Source: Delmar, Cengage Learning.

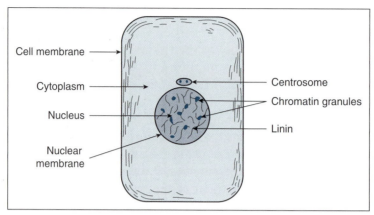

FIGURE 15-5 Diagram of a cell
Source: Delmar, Cengage Learning.

A cell has three basic parts: membrane, cytoplasm, and nucleus, as shown in Figure 15-5. The cell membrane is permeable allowing substances to pass into and out of the cell. The cytoplasm, a watery substance inside the cell, contains many structures referred to as organelles. Organelles are responsible for receiving and converting raw materials into energy.

The nucleus, separated from the cytoplasm by a double-walled membrane, consists of fluid (the nucleoplasm) in which the nucleolus and chromatin material are found. The nucleolus is composed of ribonucleic acid (RNA) and deoxyribonucleic acid (DNA) in the chromatin. The RNA and DNA direct the activities that maintain cell life. Chromosomes that transmit the genetic code of hereditary are composed of DNA.

Cell division or multiplication is controlled by the nucleus (Figure 15-6). Two types of cell division occur: mitosis and meiosis. Genetic cells, such as spermatogonium, undergo meiosis; all other cells in the human body undergo mitosis. In mitosis, the cell divides forming two cells. Mitosis occurs in five phases: interphase, prophase, metaphase, anaphase, and telephase, Figure 15-7.

Meiosis, or reduction division, creates two identical cells produced each containing only one-half (23) of the usual forty-six chromosomes.

One of several events can occur when radiation strikes a cell. These are:

1) Radiation may pass through without damage to the cell;
2) Radiation may damage the cell but the cell partially repairs the damage;
3) Radiation may damage the cell so that the cell fails to repair itself but reproduces in damaged form; and
4) Cell death may occur.

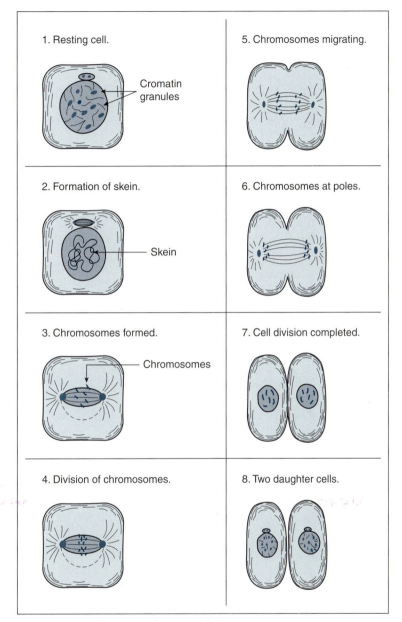

1. Resting cell.

Cromatin granules

2. Formation of skein.

Skein

3. Chromosomes formed.

Chromosomes

4. Division of chromosomes.

5. Chromosomes migrating.

6. Chromosomes at poles.

7. Cell division completed.

8. Two daughter cells.

FIGURE 15-6 Diagrams showing cell division
Source: Delmar, Cengage Learning.

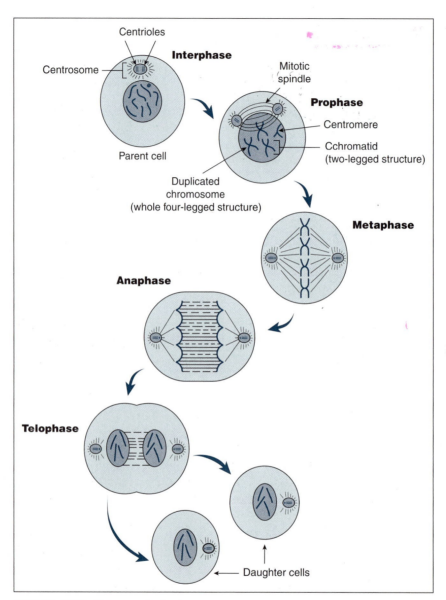

FIGURE 15-7 Diagram of mitosis
Source: Delmar, Cengage Learning.

Radiosensitivity

Each type of cell differs in their **radiosensitivity** to radiation. The **Law of Bergonié and Tribondeau** attempts to explain the basis of cell radiosensitivity. The law states the following: *Stem cells* (handwritten)

1. Immature, nonspecialized cells are most radiosensitive. Mature, specialized cells are most resistant to radiation damage.
2. Cells with a high metabolic level are radiosensitive.
3. Cells that are rapidly growing and dividing are radiosensitive.
4. Immature tissues and organs are radiosensitive.

Ionizing radiation exposure to the bone marrow causes a decrease in the number of immature stem cells produced and ultimately a reduction in the number of mature blood cells in the blood stream. Erythrocytes are precursors of red blood cells and are sensitive to ionizing radiation, as are all immature cells that are in an undifferentiated (nonspecialized) state of maturation. The most highly sensitive blood cell is the lymphocyte, a subgroup of the white blood cells. Lymphocytes have a short life span of only 24 hours during which time they produce antibodies that defend the body against invading pathogens. A radiation dose as low as 0.25 Gy (25 rad) is sufficient to depress the number of lymphocytes in the peripheral blood circulation, making them the most radiosensitive blood cells in the human body. A whole body dose of ionizing radiation (0.5 Gy to 1 Gy or 50 to 100 rad) will cause the lymphocyte count to decrease to zero within a few days.

The neutrophil, an infection fighting cell, may also be decreased in number by a dose of ionizing radiation (0.5 Gy or 50 rad). The number of granulocytes, cells that also fight infection, and thrombocytes, platelets that initiate blood clotting and prevent hemorrhage, also may be reduced in number as a result of radiation exposure.

In the early years of diagnostic medical x-ray use, the periodic blood count was used as a measure of radiographer's exposure to ionizing radiation. However, a blood count is a relatively insensitive test that cannot measure radiation exposures less than 10 cGy (10 rad) and not useful in the diagnostic radiology levels. As such, the blood count is not an accurate measure of radiation exposure received by those working in radiation occupations. Today in medical radiography, limited radiographers and staff wear radiation monitoring badges or similar devices, which more accurately record radiation exposure. These devices are discussed in detail in Chapter 16, Radiation Protection.

Epithelial tissue lines and covers body tissues and is found in the lining of blood and lymphatic vessels, intestines, respiratory tract, and the pulmonary alveoli. This tissue contains cells with no blood vessels and regenerates through mitosis. Epithelial cells are constantly in the process of regeneration, making them highly radiosensitive.

Muscle and nervous system tissue are composed of cells that are highly differentiated and specialized in their functions, making them less radiosensitive as compared to either epithelial tissue or lymphocytes. However, developing nerve cells in the embryo-fetus are more radiosensitive than mature nerve cells of the adult. Epidemiological studies conducted on the Japanese atomic bomb survivors provide evidence of a "window of maximal sensitivity" extending from 8 to 15 weeks after gestation. During this time, neuron organogenesis occurs and there is a high degree of radiosensitivity. Irradiation during this period causes central nervous system anomalies, microencephaly, and mental retardation.

Reproductive Cells

The human reproductive cells (germ cells), spermatogonia and the ova, are relatively radiosensitive. The male and female reproductive cells react differently to ionizing radiation because of the process of development from immature to mature status. In the male testes, both immature and mature spermatogonia exist. As with any cells that are mature and highly specialized, their radiosensitivity decreases. So the concern is more with the immature spermatogenia that may receive doses as low as 0.1 Gy (10 rad) or more. Any amount of radiation exposure to the immature cell may cause genetic mutations in future offspring. Radiation doses of this magnitude are not common in routine diagnostic radiology procedures; however, radiation protection procedures including shielding of the testes should be used whenever possible. Gonad shielding procedures will be discussed in detail in Chapter 16, Radiation Protection.

The female reproductive (germinal cell) ovum, unlike the male spermatogenia (sperm), does not constantly divide. During the female reproductive lifetime (from approximately age 12 to 50), one of the two ovaries expel a mature ovum for fertilization by the male sperm. In a lifetime, approximately 400 to 500 mature ova are expelled and these are less radiosensitive than the immature ova still in the ovaries. The concern in irradiating women of childbearing age is twofold: first to reduce the amount of ionizing radiation that the immature ova receives and secondly to prevent radiation exposure to a newly fertilized ovum or embryo. Reducing ionizing radiation exposure to the ovaries of women in the childbearing age can reduce the potential risk of genetic mutations in future offspring.

Reducing ionizing radiation exposure to a newly fertilized ovum, embryo, or fetus also may reduce the potential adverse genetic and somatic effects to the offspring. Thus, shielding of the reproductive organs is important for women of childbearing age.

Biologic Factors of Radiosensitivity

Individual biological variables must also be considered when discussing cell radiosensitivity. These variables are based on the biological variations of individual organisms.

Radiosensitivity is highest before birth and until maturity. In diagnostic radiography, according to the Law of Bergonié and Tribondeau, the most radiosensitive state of human growth and development is the embryonic and fetal period. During this period, there are a great number of immature, nonspecialized cells, which are more susceptible to radiation damage when compared to the adult stage. This does not mean that the mature adult is resistant to potential biologic damage from radiation exposure; rather the Law of Bergonié and Tribondeau provides a ranking or hierarchy of cell radiosensitivity. This hierarchy is given for the growth stages of human development and ranks cells in order from the least radiosensitive to the most radioresistant. Consistent application of radiation-protection measures is very important for protection of the developing embryo and fetus, all children, and all women and men who may have a likelihood of reproducing.

Human cells are capable of recovering from radiation damage. The repair mechanism is dependent upon many biological and environmental factors.

Levels of Biological Effects

The biological effects of radiation occur at three levels: molecular, cellular, and organic.

Molecular Effects of Radiation

Damage to the human body caused by ionizing radiation begins at the molecular level. Several theories attempt to explain how biological damage occurs. These are the direct-hit theory and the indirect-hit theory. The two theories refer to the way radiation interacts with a cell. These theories will be discussed in detail later in this chapter.

Cellular Effects of Radiation

Instant death of a large number of cells occurs when a radiation dose of about 1000 Gy (100,000 rads) is absorbed in a period of a few minutes. Cell death occurs due to gross disruption of normal cellular form and structure such as the breakup of DNA macromolecules and coagulation of proteins. Such radiation exposures exceed those delivered during diagnostic medical imaging procedures and even in some therapeutic radiation treatments.

Reproductive death occurs when a cell receives radiation exposure in the range of 1 to 10 Gy (100 to 1000 rad). The cell does not actually die but loses its ability to procreate; thus it does not genetically pass on any radiation-induced mutations.

Apoptosis, a nonmitotic, or nondivision, form of cell death, occurs when cells die without attempting division during the interphase. Apoptosis occurs spontaneously in both normal and abnormal tissue. In humans, apoptosis is related to cell death and considered part of the cycle of development and maintenance of the organism. For example, skin cells constantly die, shed, and are replaced. Radiosensitivity of particular cells governs the amount of radiation dose required to cause apoptosis.

The organ or tissue weighting factor attempts to equate the various risks of cancer and genetic effects to the tissues or organs exposed to radiation (see Table 15-1).

Various tissues and organs are not equal in radiosensitivity, thus a tissue weighting factor is used in the current effective dose limiting system that is discussed in detail in Chapter 16, Radiation Protection.

Effects of Radiation on Cell Division

Ionizing radiation may retard or permanently inhibit cell division. Mitotic, or genetic, death of a cell occurs when a cell dies after one or more cell divisions. As little as 0.01 Gy (1 rad) can cause the cell to delay division on its regular interval. The

TABLE 15-1 Organ or Tissue Weighting Factors

Organ or Tissue	Weighting Factor
Gonads	0.20
Breast	0.05
Thyroid	0.05
Skin	0.01

Data from National Council on Radiation Protection and Measurements (NCRP): *Report #116, Limitation of exposure to ionizing radiation*, Bethesda, Md., 1993, NCRP.

[handwritten notes: most dangeous for RTs. High dose whole body short time]

[handwritten notes: ways we measure Radiation — Absorbed dose — Bone marrow dose — Gonadal dose — entrance skin exposure]

cell may also experience permanent or temporary interference of function but still maintain its ability to divide, thus replicating any cell mutations.

Organic Effects of Radiation

The cellular effects of radiation can result in organic damage, causing problems such as cataracts and leukemia. The degree of damage generally depends upon the following: quantity of ionizing radiation, ionization ability of the radiation, body part exposed, amount of body area exposed.

Absorbed Dose

Several physical factors should be considered in the determination of radiosensitivity: 1) absorbed dose, 2) absorbed dose equivalent, 3) dose response relationship, 4) linear energy transfer, 5) relative biologic effectiveness, 6) **dose fractionation and protraction**, and 7) an individual person's unique biologic factors.

As previously discussed, the human body consists of many different types of matter each having their own atomic structure. It is these differences that allow for the creation of a diagnostic radiograph. The amount of x-ray energy absorbed per unit mass is called absorbed dose, and the calculable potential for biologic damage is directly related to absorbed dose. The rad was developed as a unit of absorbed energy or dose and pertains to any material. This unit is not restricted to air and can be measured in other absorbing materials.

The maximum exposure received by the patient is not at the area of interest but at the skin entrance to the body. This is known as the entrance skin exposure and although medical radiation physicists often discuss organ and gonadal doses, the entrance skin exposure is the most common expression to approximate patient exposure.

Radiation exposure to the patient can be estimated by recording mR/mAs when the x-ray system is calibrated. This is calculated by recording a reading for any average exposure and then dividing the reading in mR by the total mAs used. In developing x-ray imaging technique charts for diagnostic radiography procedures, the various combinations of milliaperage, time, and kilovoltage have a direct effect on the absorbed dose of the patient. For example, as the x-ray kilovoltage decreases, and the electromagnetic wavelength produced increases (becomes longer), thus the absorbed dose to the tissue increases. The procedure for this process is discussed in detail in Chapter 9, Fundamentals of Radiographic Exposure.

Absorbed Dose Equivalent

Absorbed dose equivalent (ADE) is a method used to calculate the effective absorbed dose for all types of ionizing radiation. It is known that not all types of radiation are equal in their ability to cause biologic damage to living tissue. For example, 25-rad of fast neutrons would result in greater biologic damage than 225-rad of x-ray. The ADE method of calculating considers the differences in radiation damage by using a modifying or quality factor (QF). The formula used to calculate the absorbed dose equivalent is ADE (absorbed dose equivalent) = AD (absorbed dose) X QF (quality factor).

Gamma rays, beta particles (high-speed electrons), and x-rays have a quality factor value of 1 because they produce nearly the same biological effects in body tissue for equal absorbed doses.

Dose-Response Relationship

A radiation dose-response relationship refers to a point or level of radiation exposure (dose) at which a response or reaction first occurs (Figure 15-8).

The relationship between radiation and some biologic response is a linear, non threshold relationship. This means that any amount of ionizing radiation, no matter how small, may cause biologic effects (response). The linear, nonthresh-

no amount of radiation is safe. (non-threshold)

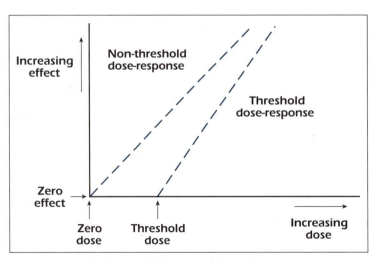

FIGURE 15-8 A theoretical depiction of the radiation dose-response relationship
Source: Delmar, Cengage Learning.

old relationship model indicates that there is no amount of radiation exposure that is safe. It is assumed that all ionizing-radiation exposure presents the potential to cause biologic effect. Therefore, any such exposure to radiation requires the consistent use and application of measures to protect the patient and those performing the radiographic examination.

Linear Energy Transfer (LET)

Linear energy transfer (LET) is a unit of measurement that relates to the quantity of absorbed dose and is an important concept in radiation biology. The amount of ionization that occurs in tissue is directly related to how much radiation energy is absorbed. The extent of biologic damage is directly related to the degree of ionization that occurs. Ionization resulting from various types of electromagnetic radiation is not equal. For example, particulate radiation, such as alpha particles, loses energy quickly as the particles interact with tissue. Because of the quick loss of energy and the resultant ionizations (in the tissues), particulate radiation, such as alpha particles, are referred to as high-LET radiation. High-LET radiation has the potential to cause a greater amount of ionization in tissue. Alpha radiation has a LET of 20 whereas x-rays have a LET of 1.

To review, x-rays and gamma rays are examples of low-LET radiation whereas alpha particles are considered high-LET radiations.

Relative Biological Effectiveness (RBE)

Biologic damage resulting from radiation interaction with tissue increases as the LET of radiation increases. Many scientists have attempted to quantify different types of radiation as to their biological effectiveness in relation to absorbed dose quantities. This, however, has proven difficult; therefore, the relative biological effectiveness (RBE) is not practical for delineating radiation protection dose levels. The quality factor (QF), as previously discussed, is basically a measure of RBE and is used in calculation of the absorbed dose equivalents.

Dose Fractionation and Protraction

If the quantity of radiation (dose) is delivered over a long period of time, the biological effect of the same dose will be less than if it were delivered quickly (short period of time). As the time of delivery of a quantity of radiation is increased, a higher dose will be required to produce the same biological effect. The delivery of radiation may be accomplished in two ways, protracted or fractionated.

A protracted dose is one that is delivered continuously but at a lower dose rate. A fractionated dose is one that is delivered at the same dose rate but divided into equal fractional quantities of radiation. Dose fractionation is used in radiation therapy since it allows time for tissue repair and recovery between the radiation treatments.

Direct and Indirect Effect

There are two means of damaging a cell by radiation: direct and indirect effect (Figure 15-9). Remember cells are composed mainly of water and biologic macromolecules such as deoxyribonucleic acid (genetically active part of the genes that transmits the hereditary code to offspring). The **direct effect** occurs when x-ray photons directly interact with a "target" or master (critical) DNA molecule (Figure 15-9).

In the **indirect effect**, a photon strikes a noncritical molecule, usually water, and the noncritical molecule then transfers the ionization energy to the critical

Indirect effect is also called Radiolysis

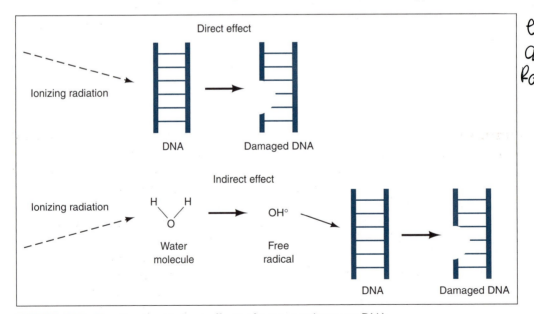

FIGURE 15-9 The direct and indirect effects of ionizing radiation on DNA
Source: Delmar, Cengage Learning.

DNA molecule. Because the human body is composed of approximately 80% water, it is believed that the greatest percentage of ionizations will occur as interactions between photons and water molecules (indirect effect). When a water molecule is ionized, it separates into free radicals. Free radicals are very chemically reactive forms of ions. Free radicals have excess energy and are capable of traveling through the cell and interacting with molecules located at some distance from their place of origin. A free radical is a configuration of one or more atoms having an unpaired electron, but no net electrical charge. This object is highly reactive because the unpaired electron will pair up with another electron even if it has to break a chemical bone to pair up. Molecules containing an unpaired electron in their outer shell are chemically unstable and very reactive. They can produce undesirable chemical reactions and cause biologic damage by transferring their excess energy to other molecules. A free radical can react quickly with other molecules because it has an electron in the outer-energy shell that does not have a partner (another electron to balance the charge). Because free radicals have an unpaired electron, they are very reactive and can impart some of their excess energy to other molecules. It is this transfer of energy by free radicals that causes biological damage (indirect effect). Free radicals are capable of traveling through the cell and causing biological damage at distances away from their origin. This type of radiation damage is referred to as the indirect-hit theory because the damage to the DNA molecules takes place indirectly.

Radiolysis (Indirect)

Radiolysis occurs when a water molecule is ionized resulting in free ions capable of recombining with other free radicals to form new molecules (Figure 15-10).

The free radicals result from the radiolysis, or the breakdown of the molecule has the potential to recombine to form a new water molecule or to combine with other radicals to form new molecules. It is believed that most of the effects of radiation on living organisms are a result of radiolysis or the indirect action caused when an x-ray photon interacts with a noncritical molecule.

The concept of a sensitive target or key molecule is called the target theory. The target theory states that there is a certain critical target molecule in a cell that must be inactivated in order to damage or cause cell death. Scientists believe that the DNA of a cell represents this target and is the area of the cell vital to cell life and replication (Figure 15-11).

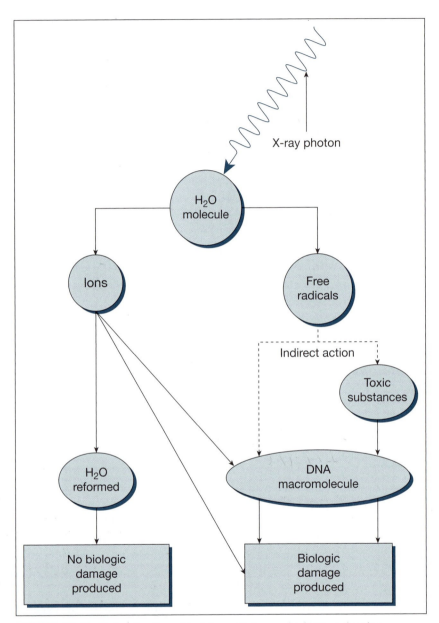

FIGURE 15-10 Indirect action of ionizing radiation on biologic molecules
Source: Delmar, Cengage Learning.

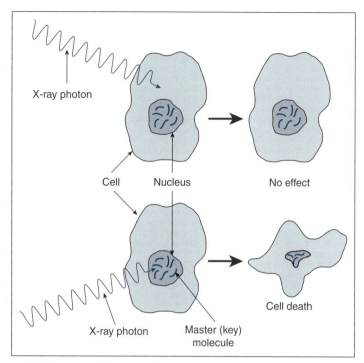

FIGURE 15-11 The target theory
Source: Delmar, Cengage Learning.

Short term show up within 30 days

Short-Term and Long-Term Effects of Radiation

Biologic effects may be classified as either short-term or long-term effects. Biologic effects from radiation fit into one or the other classification, depending upon the length of time it takes for the effect to become evident or demonstrable. As previously discussed, several factors—such as type of radiation, amount of absorbed dose, and body area receiving the exposure—determine the type and intensity of the effect.

Short-term or early effects of exposure to radiation have classically been determined from studies of uranium miners, radium dial painters, survivors of the atomic bombs detonated in Japan during World War II, and survivors of nuclear power plant and nuclear industry accidents.

Short-term effects are found in the acute radiation syndrome, which includes but is not limited to gonadal dysfunction, epilation (hair loss), depression of the white blood cells, and even death. Clinical signs and symptoms of short-term effects include nausea, vomiting, diarrhea, anemia, leukopenia, hemorrhage, fever, infection, and shock (Figure 15-12).

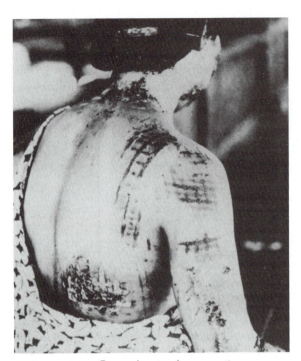

FIGURE 15-12 Dry and moist desquamation *(Reproduced with permission from Statkiewicz-Sherer M. A. [2007] Radiation Protection in Medical Radiography [5th Edition], Oxford: Elsevier/Mosby.)*

takes long time for it to show up

Long-term or late effects of radiation may result from small doses of radiation received over a number of years. Long-term effects may also be demonstrated in individuals who have been exposed to a single dose of radiation and are considered to be in a latent period. Epidemiolgic studies of radiation survivors include the following long-term effects.

Local Tissue Effects

An example of this effect is when the skin undergoes changes in its texture, elasticity, and appearance. It appears dry, chapped, and prematurely aged. Exposed skin may also exhibit an increase in skin lesions, both benign and malignant (Figure 15-13).

These changes are both dose- and time-related to the type and quantity of the radiation received.

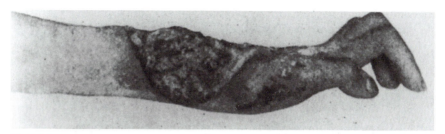

FIGURE 15-13 Carcinoma of the distal arm and hand developing after an x-ray burn (1904) *(From Eisenberg, R. L., Radiology: An illustrated history. (1992). St. Louis, MO: Mosby-Year Book.)*

Effects of Ionizing Radiation on Chromosomes

When radiation exposure causes changes in the DNA molecule, discrete modifications occur. After irradiation and during cell division, some radiation-induced chromosome breaks may be viewed microscopically. Such alterations manifest during the metaphase and anaphase of the cell division cycle, when the length of the chromosomes are visible. Both somatic cells and reproductive cells are subject to chromosome breaks induced by radiation.

Damaged chromosomes appear as fragments that have the ability to adhere to other fragments (Figure 15-14). Chromosome damage may be exhibited as abnormal pairings, translocation, and other phenomena that can result in cell damage and dysfunction. Chromosome aberrations and chromatid aberrations are the two types of anomalies observed during metaphase. Abnormalities may also occur during interphase.

To review: ionizing radiation interacts randomly with matter. As a result of these interactions, a variety of changes in the chromosomes have been identified. These are:

- A single-strand break in one chromosome
- A single-strand break in one chromatid
- A single-strand break in separate chromosomes
- A strand break in separate chromatids
- More than one break in the same chromosome
- More than one break in the same chromatid
- Chromosome stickiness, or clumping together

Structural changes may result in one of the following consequences to the cell: restitution, deletion, and broken-end rearrangement. When fragment breaks rejoin with no visible damage, restitution is said to occur. Healing by restitution is believed

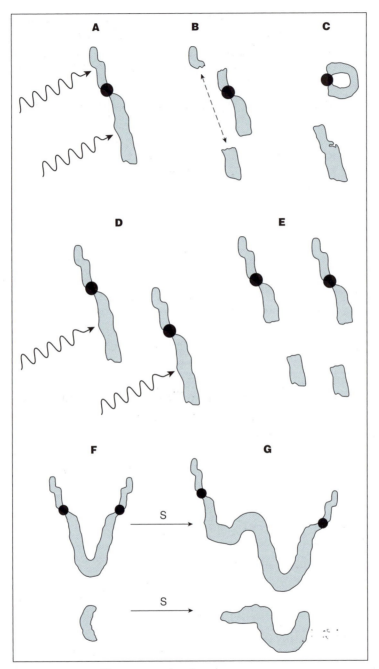

FIGURE 15-14 Chromosome breakage
Source: Delmar, Cengage Learning.

to be the process by which 95% of single-chromosome breaks mend. When part of the chromosome or chromatid is lost at the next cell division, creating an aberration known as an acentric fragment, deletion is said to have occurred. A distorted or grossly misshaped chromosome is referred to as a broken-end rearrangement. A broken-end rearrangement may also occur without visible damage although the genetic material has been rearranged. This type of change generally results in mutation and alteration of the heritable characteristics of the cell.

Cells have a repair mechanism that provides for some recovery and repopulate to occur. Scientific research has shown that repeated radiation exposure has a cumulative effect on cellular damage. Approximately 10% of radiation-induced cell damage is irreparable but the extent of damage determines the potential for recovery.

Cataracts

Radiation-induced cataracts were reported as early as the 1940s. The radiosensitivity of the lens of the eye has been demonstrated to be age-dependent. This means that the older the individual, the more susceptible one is a to radiation-induced cataract.

Life Span Shortening

It is suggested that as a result of chromosomal mutations the fitness and life span of an individual acutely exposed will be compromised and/or shortened. For this reason, the amount of radiation delivered in radiographic imaging procedures should always be as low as reasonably possible to obtain the necessary diagnostic information, and radiation-protection measures should always be used.

Somatic and Genetic Effects

The effects of radiation on living organisms are further classified as **somatic** or **genetic.** Somatic effects occur to the individual who has been exposed to ionizing radiation, whereas the genetic effects may not be apparent in the exposed individual but passed on to future generations through genetically damaged chromosomes. (fetus)

Somatic effects occurring to the living organism may be classified as either early or later somatic effects, depending upon the length of time from the moment of radiation exposure to the first appearance of symptoms.

Acute Radiation Syndrome (ARS)

Acute radiation syndrome (ARS), or radiation illness, occurs after humans receive large doses of ionizing radiation to the entire body within a short time period. Data collected from studies on atomic bomb survivors at Hiroshima and Nagasaki, those accidentally exposed to atomic bomb tests on Marshall Island, and most recently (1986) survivors of the Chernobyl nuclear power plant disaster has been helpful in understanding ARC. Early or acute effects are those that appear within minutes, hours, days, or weeks after the initial radiation exposure. Examples of early or acute effects are loss of bone marrow function (hematopoietic syndrome), gastrointestinal syndrome, and central nervous syndrome.

Acute radiation syndrome (ARS) is a collection of symptoms associated with high-level radiation exposure, which presents in four major stages: prodromal, latent period, manifest illness, and recovery or death. The prodromal stage occurs within hours after a whole-body absorbed dose of 1 Gy (100 rad) or more. Nausea, vomiting, diarrhea, fatigue, and leukopenia characterize this stage. The severity of these symptoms is radiation dose dependent. The prodromal stage may be from hours to a few days. The latent period follows the prodromal stage. During the latent period recovery or lethal effects become evident. The latent period is followed by the manifest illness phase. During the manifest illness period, symptoms that affect the hematopoietic, gastrointestinal, and cerebrovascular systems become evident. *(red + white blood cells) (causes nausea)* *(stroke, coma, seizure)*

The hematopoietic system is responsible for the manufacture of the corpuscular elements of the blood and is the most radiosensitive organ system in humans. The hematopoietic form of acute radiation syndrome (ARS) occurs when human beings receive whole-body doses of ionizing radiation ranging from 1 to 10 Gy (100 to 1000 rad). This quantity of radiation exposure produces a decrease in the number of bone marrow stem cells, which decreases bone marrow function and ultimately causing susceptibility to infection and hemorrhage.

The cerebrovascular syndrome involves radiation doses of 50 Gy (5000 rad) or more. Symptoms of this syndrome include excessive nervousness, confusion, severe nausea, vomiting, diarrhea, loss of vision, and a burning sensation of the skin and loss of consciousness. *Stroke & seizures* Failure of the central nervous and cardiovascular systems may result in death. The term LD 50/30 refers to the whole-body dose of radiation that can be lethal to 50% of the exposed population within 30 days. If intensive medical intervention is afforded to the person exposed to high doses of radiation, a factor of LD 50/60 may apply. This means that 50% of the exposed population will survive for 60 days due to the medical interventions.

Death may occur 6 to 8 weeks after humans receive a whole-body ionizing radiation exposure exceeding 2 Gy (200 rad). As the whole-body dose of ionizing radiation increases from 2 to 10 Gy (200 to 1000 rad), the time to death decreases.

Late Somatic Effects

Late somatic effects are those that appear after a period of months or years after the initial exposure. Late somatic effects may result from an initial high dose of radiation that caused early acute symptoms, and ultimately repair or recovery, or chronic low-level doses of radiation received over a long time period. Carcinogenesis is the most important late somatic effect and is difficult to verify statistically because it cannot be distinguished from cancers normally expected in populations (Table 15-2).

Cancer is the most important late somatic effect caused by exposure to ionizing radiation. Cells that survive the initial irradiation, and then retain a memory of that event, are responsible for producing late effects. Somatic cells provide an example wherein the probability of the induction of malignancy increases with dose, but the severity of the cancer is not dose dependent (Table 15-3).

TABLE 15-2   Major Types of Late Somatic Effects

Stochastic Effects	Nonstochastic Effects
Carcinogenesis	Cataractogenesis
Embryologic Effects	Nonspecific life span shortening

TABLE 15-3   Short- and Long-Term Effects of Radiation

Short-Term Effects	Long-Term Effects
Result from a great amount of radiation delivered over a short period of time	Small doses of radiation delivered over a long period of time
Acute Radiation Syndrome (ARS)	Recovery from short-term effects
(Three radiation syndromes)	Increased cancers
	Life span shortening
	Increase in genetic mutations

Summary of Human Exposure to Ionizing Radiation

Different types of cells have different degrees of radiosensitivity. The most radiosensitive cells include the blood-forming cells and the reproductive cells. Ionizing radiation can result in biological damage to the human body at the molecular, cellular, and organic levels. The damage can be either genetic or somatic. Genetic effects damage the offspring of an individual exposed to radiation; whereas somatic effects damage only the individual exposed.

Generally, short-term somatic effects known as acute radiation syndrome (ARS) are of three types: central nervous system syndrome, gastrointestinal syndrome, and hematopoietic syndrome. Long-term somatic effects, which appear long after exposure, consist of cataractogenesis, life span shortening, carcinogenesis, and embryological effects.

1. Biologic effects are dose-dependent (the greater the amount, the greater the effect).
2. Effects of a given exposure vary from person to person. Predicting exactly how individuals will respond is nearly impossible except at lethal-dose levels.
3. A great amount of radiation delivered over seconds, minutes, or hours is called an acute radiation exposure. Acute doses to the whole body are more dangerous than acute exposure to a specific body part.
4. There is controversy about the long-term effects of low doses of radiation; however, chronic low doses of radiation have been associated with a higher incidence of cancer.

REVIEW QUESTIONS

1. The extent and nature of damage from radiation exposure is dependent upon:
    1. type of ionizing radiation
    2. radiosensitivity of the tissue exposed
    3. amount of radiation absorbed

Possible Responses

   a. 1 only
   b. 1 and 2
   c. 2 and 3
   d. 1, 2, and 3

2. The key person in the effort to reduce ionizing radiation exposure in the diagnostic imaging setting is the:
   a. radiologist
   b. radiographer
   c. referring doctor
   d. medical radiation physicist

3. The amount of energy absorbed per unit mass is referred to as:
   a. absorption
   b. absorbed dose
   c. attenuation
   d. alteration

4. A cell has **all** of the following basic parts, **except**:
   a. membrane
   b. nucleoplasm
   c. cytoplasm
   d. nucleus

5. Genetic cells divide by a process called mitosis.
   a. True
   b. False

6. The Law of Bergonié and Tribondeau refers to:
   a. living-tissue sensitivity to radiation
   b. the way radiation intensity varies with the distance
   c. the fact that 100 mA at 1/10th second equals 10 mAs, and 300 mA at 1/30th of a second equals 10 mAs
   d. the interaction of various types of radiation with atoms

7. Cell sensitivity is determined by:
   1. degree of cell specialization
   2. how rapidly the cell grows and divides
   3. the state of maturity of the cell

   Possible Responses
   a. 1 and 2
   b. 1 and 3
   c. 2 and 3
   d. 1, 2, and 3

8. The most highly sensitive blood cell is the:
   a. lymphocyte
   b. erythrocyte
   c. neutrophil
   d. thrombocyte

9. Instant death of a large number of cells occurs when a radiation dose of about ___ rads is absorved in a period of a few minutes.
   a. 100
   b. 1,000
   c. 10,000
   d. 100,000

10. The quality factor assigned to x-ray is:
    a. 1
    b. 10
    c. 100
    d. 1,000

11. **All** of the following refer to dose-response relationship, **except**:
    a. a level of exposure at which a response first occurs
    b. a relationship between radiation and some biologic response
    c. is the same type of relationship as the Law of Reciprocity
    d. refers to the Law of Bergonié and Tribondeau

12. An example of a high LET radiation is:
    a. gamma
    b. x-rays
    c. alpha
    d. cosmic

13. Some long-term effects of radiation exposure are:
    1. cataracts
    2. life span shortening
    3. epilation

    Possible Responses
    a. 1 and 2
    b. 1 and 3
    c. 2 and 3
    d. 1, 2, and 3

14. **All** of the following are **true** regarding long-term effects of radiation, **except**:
    a. results from a great amount of radiation delivered over a short period of time
    b. may result after recovery from short-term effects
    c. results in increased cancers and genetic mutation
    d. results in life span shortening

15. The most important late somatic effect caused by exposure to ionizing radiation is:
    a. diabetes
    b. skin reddening
    c. cancer
    d. genetic effects

REFERENCES

American College of Radiology. (2006). *ACR guidelines and standards, ACR practice guideline for general radiography*. pp. 17–20. Retrieved from www.acr/org

Brusin, J. A. (2007, May/June). Radiation protection. *Radiologic Technology 78*(5), 378–91.

Bushong, S. C. (2008). *Radiologic science for technologists: Physics, biology and protection* (9th ed.). St. Louis, MO: Mosby Elsevier.

Campeau, F., & Fleitz, J. (1999). *Limited radiography* (2nd ed.). Albany, NY: Delmar, Cengage Learning.

Carlton, R. R., & Adler, A. M. (2006). *Principles of radiographic imaging: An art and a science* (3rd ed.). Albany, NY: Delmar Thomson Learning.

Cohen, B. L. (1991). Radiation standards and hazards. IEEE. *Transformation Education 34*, 261–265.

Diagnostic Imaging Online. (2007, April 24). *Imaging equipment vendors tout innovations to reduce radiation exposure*. Retrieved from www.diagnosticimaging.com

Furlow, B. (2004, May/June). Biological effects of diagnostic imaging. *Radiologic Technology 5*(5), 355–363.

Health Physics Society. (2001, February 6). *Answer to question #641 submitted to "ask the experts"* (Category: Radiation workers-pregnant workers). Retrieved from www:hps.org

Idaho State University. (2000). *Radiation and risk. Radiation information networks*. Retrieved from www.physics.isu.edu

International Commission of Radiation on Radiation Protection (ICRP). (2007a). *Pregnancy and medical radiation* (Report No. 84). Retrieved from www.iscp.org

International Commission of Radiation Units and Measurements. (2007b). *Radiation quantities and units*. (Report 33). Retrieved from www.2000.irpa.net

Mathisen, L. (2007, April 16). Tragedy times two: Late effects of children who undergo radiation therapy. *RT Image. 20*(16), 17–19.

McClafferty, C. (2001). *The head bone's connected to the neck bone.* New York: Farrar, Straus and Giroux.

McGill University. (2007). *Radiation dose limit.* Retrieved from www.mcgill.ca

Mossman, K. L., Goldman, M., Masse, F., Mills, W. A., Schiager, K. J., & Vetter, R. L. (1996, March). *Radiation risk in perspective.* Health Physics Society Position Statement. Retrieved from www.physics.isu.edu

National Cancer Institute. (2005). *Interventional fluoroscopy: reducing radiation risks for patients and staff.* Retrieved from www.cancer.gov

National Council on Radiation Protection. (2004, December). *Recent application of the NCRP public dose limit recommendations for ionizing radiation* (NCRP statement No. 10). Retrieved from www.ncrponline.org

National Council on Radiation Protection and Measurements. (NCRP). (1977). *Medical exposure of pregnant and potentially pregnant women* (Report No. 54). Washington, DC: NCRP.

National Council on Radiation Protection and Measurements. (1981). *Radiation protection in pediatric radiology* (Report 68). Washington, DC: NCRP.

National Council on Radiation Protection and Measurements (NCRP). (1987). *Ionizing radiation exposure of the population of the United States.* (Report No. 93). Bethesda, MD: NCRP.

National Council on Radiation Protection and Measurements. (2007a). Diagnostic Imaging Online. *Report from NCRP: CT-based radiation exposure in U.S. population soars.* Retrieved May 7, 2007 from www.diagnosticimaging.com

National Council on Radiation Protection and Measurements (NCRP). (2007b). *Radiation exposure during pregnancy demands well-informed patient management.* Retrieved from www.diagnosticimaging.com

National Council on Radiation Protection and Measurements (NCRP). (2007c). *Limitations of exposure to ionizing radiation.* (Report 116). Retrieved from www.ncrponline.org

National Electrical Manufacturer's Association (2006, December). *How innovations in medical imaging have reduced radiation dosage (executive summary).* Retrieved from www.medicalimaging.org

National Electrical Manufacturer's Association (2006 December). *How medical imaging has transformed health care in the U.S. (executive summary).* Retrieved from www.medicalimaging.org

National Research Council, Commission of Life Sciences, Committee on Biological Effects of Ionizing Radiation *(BIER V),* Board of Radiation Effects Research. (1989). *Health effects of exposure to low levels of ionizing radiations,* Washington, DC: National Academy Press.

North Carolina University Health and Safety, Radiation Safety Division. (2007). *Radiation safety and alara.* Retrieved from www.ncsu.edu.

Patton, K. T. (2000). *Structure and function of the body* (11th ed.). St. Louis, MO: Mosby, Inc.

Rasussaki, M. T. *Pediatric Radiation Protection (abstract).* Retrieved from www.springerlink.com

Schleipman, A. R. (2005, January/February). Occupational radiation exposure: Population studies. *Radiologic Technology, 76*(3), 185–191.

Seeram, E. (2001). *Rad Tech's Guide to Radiation Protection*, Malden, MA: Blackwell Science.

Sherer, M. A., Visconti, P., & Ritenour, E. R. (2006). *Radiation Protection in Medical Radiography* (5th ed.). St. Louis, MO: Mosby.

Sprawls, P. (1995). The Physical Principles of Medical Imaging. Interaction of Radiation with Matter. Retrieved from http://www.sprawls.org

The Merck Manuals Online Medical Library. (2009). Radiography. Retrieved from http://www.merck.com

Thomas, A. M. K., & Isherwood I. (Eds.). (1995). *The invisible light; The Röentgen centenary: 100 years of medical radiology.* Oxford: Blackwell Science.

United States Food and Drug Administration, Centers for Devices and Radiological Health. (1994, September 30). *FDA public health advisory: Avoidance of serious x-ray induced skin injuries to patients during fluoroscopic-guided procedures.* Rockville, MD: FDA.

U.S. Department of Labor Occupational Safety & Health Administration. (2007). *Ionizing radiation health effects.* Retrieved from www.osha.gov

U.S. Environmental Protection Agency. (2007a). *Estimating risk (Understanding radiation).* Retrieved from www.epa.gov

U.S. Environmental Protection Agency. (2007b). *Health effects (Understanding radiation).* Retrieved May 14, 2007 from www.epa.gov

U.S. Environmental Protection Agency. (2007c). *History of radiation protection.* Retrieved June 6, 2007 from www.epa.gov

U.S. Environmental Protection Agency. (2007d). *Ionizing & non-ionizing radiation.* Retrieved from www.epa.gov

Whalen, J. P., Balter, S. (1984). Radiation Risks in Medical Imaging. Chicago: Year Book Medical Publishers, Inc.

Willis, E., & Slovis, T. L. *Editorials: The alara concept in pediatric CR and DR: dose reduction in pediatric radiographic exams—A white paper conference executive summary.* Retrieved from www.radiology.rsnajnls.org

CHAPTER **16**

RADIATION PROTECTION

Key Terms

Added Filtration

Air Gap Technique

ALARA

American College of Radiology (ACR)

Aperature Diaphragm

Cardinal Principles

Collimation

Cone

Early Somatic Effects

Effective Dose Limiting System

Film Badge

Inherent Filtration

Gonadal Shielding

Grid

Late Somatic Effects

Maximum Permissible Dose (MPD)

NCRP Report No. 116

NCRP Report No. 54

Nonstochastic Effects

Nuclear Regulatory Commission (NRC)

Occupancy Factor (T)

Pocket Ionization Chamber

Chapter Outline

Introduction

Effective Dose Limiting Sysytem

Radiation-Protection Procedures

The Patient

Primary-Beam Limitation

Radiation-Protection Procedures for the Operator

Cardinal Principles

Structural Protective Shielding

Primary Structural Protective Shielding

Secondary Protective Structural Shielding

Protective Apparel

Radiation Exposure and Pregnancy

The Pregnant Patient

The Pregnant Radiographer

Radiation Exposure and the Pediatric Patient

Radiation Detection and Monitoring

Personnel Monitoring Devices

Optically Stimulated Luminescence (OSL) Dosimeter

Film Badges

Thermoluminescent Dosimeters

Survey Instruments for Area Monitoring

Positive Beam Limitation (PBL) System

Primary Structural Protective Shielding

Repeat Examination

Secondary Protective Structural Shielding

Stochastic Effects

Ten-Day Rule

Thermoluminescent Dosimeter (TLD)

Workload (W)

Objectives

Upon completion of the chapter, the student will meet the following objectives by verifying knowledge of the facts and principles presented through oral and written communication at a level deemed competent.

⊃ Recall the ALARA concept and give a minimum of two examples of ALARA activities.

⊃ Define the term, "effective dose limiting system" and state the exposure recommendations for the following categories: occupational, public, embryo-fetus, and education and training.

⊃ Differentiate between stochastic and nonstochastic effects.

⊃ Explain the importance of patient communication, patient preparation, and motion control in reducing unnecessary radiation exposure and retake examinations.

⊃ Select advantages and disadvantages to various beam-limiting devices (cone, aperture diaphragm, collimator, and positive beam limitation system).

⊃ Select the correct response care. Given examples of proper and improper primary beam limitation.

⊃ Explain the purpose and importance of tube filtration and differentiate between inherent and added filtration.

⊃ Select correct responses in regard to film screen combinations, grids, air-gap technique, and gonadal shielding as these relate to radiation protection.

⊃ Recall correct facts about radiation protection and the pregnant patient and pregnant staff.

⊃ Given common situations, select the correct response regarding primary and secondary structural shielding, gonadal shields, and protective apparel (gloves, aprons, etc.).

⊃ Recall basic facts about radiation detection and monitoring devices.

⊃ List methods that can be used to limit radiation exposure in the pediatric patient.

Introduction

The use of radiological imaging procedures in the diagnosis of disease and injury is often considered to be a standard part of the medical evaluation process. Yet few people realize that the physician must consider several factors before requesting a radiographic examination.

Each time a radiographic examination is indicated, the physician must consider the potential diagnostic benefits to be gained from the radiographic examination versus the potential biologic harm to the patient resulting from radiation exposure. This decision is often called the benefit-versus-risk principle and must be considered each time a radiologic examination is requested. Once the decision to perform a radiographic procedure has been made by the physician, it is the radiographer's responsibility to perform the examination and to follow all recognized radiation-protection guidelines. These guidelines consist of cardinal principles and procedures intended to reduce unnecessary radiation exposure to the patient and radiation operator. The main goal of all radiation-protection activities is to keep all radiation exposure *as low as reasonably achievable* (ALARA). This chapter introduces current radiation-protection philosophy, the ALARA concept, effective dose limiting system, and radiation-protection procedures for the patient and radiation operator.

Effective Dose Limiting System

Guidelines limiting the amount of radiation received by the general public and those individuals who use radiation in their work (occupational dose) have been established by several international and governmental agencies (Table 16-1).

The agencies named in Table 16-1 determine effective dose limits and make recommendations that the **Nuclear Regulatory Commission (NRC)**, a national agency, has the responsibility to enforce. There are five regional NRC offices that serve various geographic areas of the United States. Regional NRC offices accept collect telephone calls from employees who wish to register concerns or complaints about conditions or matters within radiologic facilities.

Traditionally, radiation-exposure limits have been expressed as the **maximum permissible dose (MPD)** of radiation to which the radiation-occupation worker or the general public can be exposed. Over the years, as knowledge of the injurious effects of radiation has increased, the MPD has been decreased (Table 16-2).

However, the MPD is no longer used as the criterion of radiation exposure in radiation protection. Risk may be defined as the likelihood of injury, ailment, or death resulting from an activity. For those in the medical radiology fields, risk is viewed as the possibility of developing cancer or genetic defect after radiation exposure.

TABLE 16-1   Groups Responsible for Establishing Effective-Absorbed-Dose-Equivalent Limits

(ICRP)	International Commission on Radiological Protection
(NAS-BEIR)	National Academy of Sciences Advisory Committee on the Biological Effects of Ionizing Radiation
(NCRP)	National Council on Radiation Protection and Measurement
(UNSCEAR)	United Nations Scientific Committee on the Effects of Atomic Radiation

TABLE 16-2   Historical Overview of Radiation Exposure Dose Trends

Year	Approximate Daily Dose	
1902	100 mSv	10 rem
1925	2.0 mSv	0.2 rem
1928	1.5 mSv	0.15 rem
1936	1.0 mSv	0.1 rem recommended by the United States Advisory Committee on X-Ray and Radium Protection
1959	0.2 mSv	0.02 rem recommended by the National Council on Radiation Protection and Measurements

Risk is also assigned to various occupations as the government has worker protection standards for each industry. The occupational risk associated with radiation exposure is similar to the occupational risk in other industries that are generally considered safe.

The **effective dose limiting system** is based on the premise that any organ in the human body is vulnerable to damage from exposure to ionizing radiation. Although there is a difference in the radiosensitivity of various organs and tissues, every organ and tissue is at some risk because of the stochastic probability of somatic and genetic radiation induced effects. Stochastic effects are those that occur in a random way and the severity of the effects are not dose dependent. Cancer and genetic mutations are examples of stochastic effects. Nonstochastic effects are somatic effects that are directly related to the dose of ionizing radiation received. Nonstochastic effects may be classified as either **early** or **late somatic effects**. Refer to Chapter 15, Radiation Biology, for a discussion of early and late somatic effects of ionizing radiation exposure.

As previously discussed in Chapter 15, in an attempt to equate the various risks of cancer and genetic effects to the tissues or organs exposed to ionizing radiation, a tissue weighting factor is used.

Because of scientific controversy regarding the risk of cancer from low-level radiation exposure, the trend by U.S. radiation regulatory agencies has been to propose more stringent radiation protection standards. The NCRP has published these recommended standards in **NCRP Report No. 116**, which supersedes those contained in NCRP Report No. 91, and No. 39 (see Table 16-3).

The age of the radiation worker is also a factor in exposure limitations. Previously, no one under 18 years of age was allowed to work with ionizing radiation. The NCRP Report No. 116 states that for educational and training purposes, radiation workers less than eighteen years old be limited to an annual dose limit of 1 mSv (0.1 rem). In addition to annual dose limitations, a cumulative or lifetime dose

TABLE 16-3   Effective Dose Limit Recommendations   ON Final

Occupational Exposures		
Effective dose limits		
Annual	50 mSv	(5 rem)
Cumulative	10 mSv × age	(1 rem × age)
Dose equivalent annual limits for tissues and organs		
Lens of eye	150 mSv	(15 rem)
Skin, hands, and feet	500 mSv	(50 rem)
Public Exposures (Annual)		
Effective dose limit		
Continuous or frequent exposure	1 mSv	(0.1 rem)
Infrequent exposure	5 mSv	(0.5 rem)
Equivalent dose limits for tissues and organs		
Lens of eye	15 mSv	(1.5 rem)
Skin, hands, and feet	50 mSv	(5 rem)
Embryo-Fetus Exposures (Monthly)		
Equivalent does limit	0.5 mSv	(0.05 rem)
Educational and Training Exposures (Annual)		
Effective dose limit	1 mSv	(0.1 rem)
Dose equivalent limit for tissues and organs		
Lens of eye	15 mSv	(1.5 rem)
Skin, hands, and feet	50 mSv	(5 rem)

Adapted from NCRP Report No. 116: *Limitations of Exposure to Ionizing Radiation*, Table 19.1

limitation must be observed. This limit is determined by the age of the radiation worker. The total allowable cumulative exposure is the age (in years) of the worker times 10 mSv (1 rem). For example, a 30-year-old radiographer is allowed a cumulative exposure of 30×10 mSv or 300 mSv (30 rem).

Guidelines for dose limitations for the general public are less than those for radiation workers. The effective dose limit for continuous or frequent exposures is 1 mSv (0.1 rem) and for infrequent exposure 5 mSv (0.5 rem).

Embryo-fetal exposures are also considered separately. The total dose-limit for the embryo-fetus is 5 mSv (0.5 rem) and the dose-limit in a month is 0.5 mSv (0.05 rem).

Radiation-Protection Procedures

The Patient

The main goal of any radiation-protection procedure is to reduce unnecessary radiation according to the ALARA concept. Reducing unnecessary or excessive radiation exposure is a responsibility shared by everyone involved with radiologic examinations, including the doctor, radiation operator, and all support staff. There are four major areas that relate to reducing radiation exposure: patient preparation, primary-beam limitation, gonadal shielding, and technical factors.

Patient Communication. The first time when radiation-protection guidelines may be applied is when the examination is requested by the attending physician. It is the attending doctor's responsibility to explain why the radiologic examination is necessary, to answer patient questions, and to respond to any concerns about the nature of the examination. Poor communication between the doctor and the patient, the doctor and the radiographer, and/or the radiographer and the patient may result in a repeat examination or even in the wrong patient being radiographed. Communication then becomes an important factor in reducing unnecessary or excessive radiation exposure. Patients have the right to know about the examination; and if inadequately informed, they may have questions or fears regarding the nature, purpose, or even value of the examination. Patients who do not understand what is going to happen or what is expected may even be reluctant to cooperate.

What responsibility does the radiographer have in regard to explaining the radiographic examination to the patient? It is the radiographer's responsibility to give the patient clear, concise instructions and to communicate in such a way that patients understand what is expected of them in order to complete the examination. If at any time the patient refuses to undergo the examination, the radiographer should seek supervisory assistance and never insist that the patient submit to any procedure against his/her will.

One way to ensure that each patient is informed regarding his/her radiographic examination is to take adequate time to explain the procedure so that the patient understands. The radiographer should always answer patient questions within ethical limitations, and if asked a question that cannot be answered, the radiographer should seek supervisory assistance. Remember, patients have the right to be completely informed about their medical care and to have their questions answered.

Patient Preparation.   Radiation protection also extends to patient preparation. Many repeat examinations occur as a result of inadequate patient preparation. It is important to ask the patient to remove all radiopaque objects from the area to be radiographed, such as necklaces, zippers, hair pins, and even long, braided hair. Remember that a repeat examination results in a repeat or double-radiation exposure to the patient.

During patient preparation and initial introductions, it is also important to give instructions regarding breath and motion control.

If positioning or immobilization devices are to be used, explain to the patient why they are needed and how they will be used. Talk to the patient before, during, and after the examination and let the patient be of assistance whenever possible.

Careful attention to radiographic positioning also helps reduce the number of retake radiographs and thus reduces unnecessary radiation exposure. Radiographers should never attempt a radiographic procedure if they are uncertain as to the correct procedure. If in doubt or just inexperienced, the radiographer should *STOP* and *ASK FOR HELP.*

Whenever a radiograph must be repeated, patient radiation dose increases because of additional radiation exposure. The ultimate goal of any radiographic procedure is the production of a high-quality radiograph. A radiographic examination is retaken whenever the diagnostic quality does not provide image quality. The reasons for retake examinations range from simple forgetfulness of the radiographer to complex technical errors. The most common causes include improper positioning of the part or patient, inaccurate calculations of the exposure settings resulting in over or under exposure of the radiographic image, patient motion during the exposure, and improper film processing techniques. The observant radiographer can correct many of these errors and prevent retaking the examination. Prior to retaking the examination, the radiographer should consult with the supervising physician to determine whether the radiographic image can provide the needed diagnostic information. Remember, radiographs should only be retaken if the diagnostic integrity has been so compromised as to render the image useless. For additional information on evaluating image quality refer to Chapter 13, Basic Image Quality Management.

Primary-Beam Limitation

Primary-beam limitation means using a device such as an aperture diaphragm, cone, or collimator to limit the useful or primary radiation beam to the area of clinical interest, thereby decreasing the area of body tissue irradiated. This in turn reduces the amount of secondary scattered radiation and also limits unnecessary exposure to the nearby tissue. A beam restrictor, however, is only as effective as the operator who uses the device. Therefore, it is important that radiographers understand the basic operation of each type of beam restrictor and the operator's role in using the device.

The **aperture diaphragm** is a simple beam-limitation device consisting of a flat piece of lead with a hole in the middle. The size and shape of the hole determine the size and shape of the radiographic beam.

An aperture diaphragm is constructed so that it fits directly below the x-ray tube window. One disadvantage of an aperture diaphragm is that each is designed to be used with a specific film size at a given distance. Because of this feature, it is not easily adaptable to various film sizes or distances. The variable-aperture diaphragm device overcomes this disadvantage because it has a variable opening that can be adjusted for use with various film sizes and source-to-image distances.

Other simple beam-limitation devices are the **cone** (a circular metal tube with a flared end) and the cylinder (a long tube having the same diameter at base and tip), as shown in Figure 16-1. These devices—available in a variety of lengths and diameters—can be inserted and interchanged under the x-ray tube window to accommodate various film sizes and source-to-image distances.

Collimators. A collimator, often referred to as a variable collimator, is an efficient beam-limitation device. Attached to the radiographic tube housing, the collimator looks like a square box with a clear plastic window. It contains two sets of adjustable lead shutters mounted at different levels, a light source, and a mirror to deflect the light source. The lead shutters can be adjusted so as to limit the primary radiation beam to the area of clinical interest as shown in Figure 16-2.

Proper **collimation** of the primary radiation beam will result in an unexposed margin around the edge of the radiograph. Never allow the primary radiation beam to expose an area beyond the area of clinical interest. The examples in Figure 16-3 illustrate proper and improper collimation technique.

The collimator is equipped with a light source that simulates the radiation exposure area. The collimator light is used as a guide in positioning, alignment, central ray placement, and collimation. If the light source becomes misaligned with the actual area of radiation exposure, errors in positioning, alignment, central ray placement, or collimation may occur. Daily use, a bump, or jarring of the collimator housing may result in misalignment. The radiographer should include

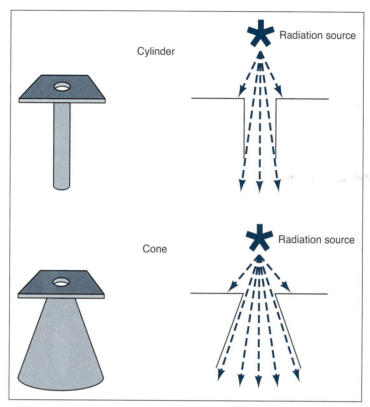

FIGURE 16-1 Beam limitation devices
Source: Delmar, Cengage Learning.

a collimator-light-source-accuracy check as part of a scheduled routine equipment-maintenance check. Whenever in doubt about the collimator-light-source accuracy, perform a light-source-accuracy check.

The efficiency of any beam-restricting device depends upon its regular and proper use by the radiographer. The positive beam limitation (PBL) system was designed in response to the concern about the operator forgetting to limit the beam. The PBL system actually restricts the primary beam to the film size used in the bucky tray. The PBL system consists of electronic sensors installed in the bucky tray holder. When a film holder is locked into the bucky tray, the electronic sensors transmit the film size information to the collimator, which automatically adjusts the primary beam to the size of the film holder (Figure 16-4).

An additional benefit of restricting the primary beam is improved radiographic quality. A properly collimated primary radiation beam produces less secondary scattered radiation, thus reducing possible film fog or increased film darkening.

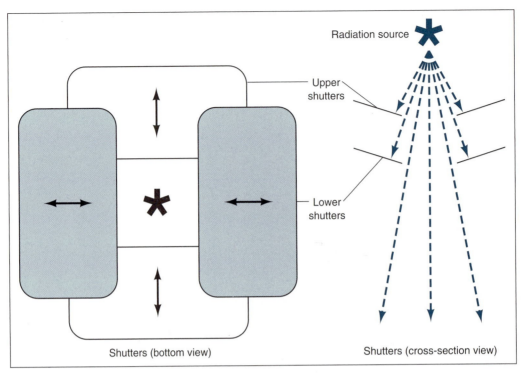

FIGURE 16-2   Two views of shutters
Source: Delmar, Cengage Learning.

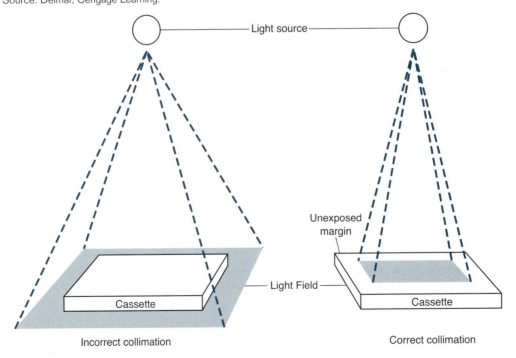

FIGURE 16-3   Proper use of collimation
Source: Delmar, Cengage Learning.

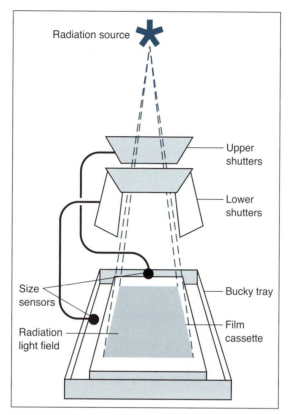

FIGURE 16-4 Positive beam limitation (PBL) device
Source: Delmar, Cengage Learning.

Filtration. Filtration of the primary radiation beam is another method used to protect the patient from unnecessary radiation exposure. Radiographic filters serve two major functions by removing low-energy, long-wavelength photons from the primary beam. These functions are to 1) protect the patients' skin and superficial tissue and 2) improve the quality of the radiation beam. By removing the longer wavelengths, the beam is more homogeneous in wavelength. This filtering is referred to as attenuation of the beam. Ultimately, as primary radiation is restricted and filtered, there is less radiation to scatter.

There are two types of radiographic filtration: inherent filtration and added filtration. Inherent filtration consists of the tube's glass envelope, insulating oil, and the glass window. Inherent filtration is expressed in equivalent aluminum thickness and should be at least 0.5 mm of aluminum. Aluminum is the metal of choice because it effectively removes long wavelengths, is inexpensive, and is sturdy.

Added filtration is any filtration added to the existing inherent filtration. These filters, usually consisting of aluminum sheets, may be added outside the tube housing. The inherent filtration plus added filtration represent the required amount of total filtration. The amount of total radiographic-tube filtration is dependent upon the kilovoltage ranges of the equipment, e.g., 50–70 kVp = 1.5 mm aluminum; above 70 kVp = 2.5 mm aluminum.

Film Screen Combinations. Patient radiation dose is affected by the choice of film-screen combination. The dose to the patient will be lessened when a high-speed film-screen combination is used. The speed of the imaging system describes the way in which the intensifying screen enhances the action of the x-rays and the way the film responds. Use of a rare-earth imaging system rather than calcium tungstate screens will reduce the patient's radiation dose. This is possible because rare-earth screens are from two to ten times as fast as calcium tungstate screens and emit more light and therefore less initial x-ray exposure.

Grids. The primary purpose of a **grid**, whether stationary or moving, is to minimize scattered radiation, which degrades the radiographic image. A grid is placed between the patient and the film and serves to improve radiographic image quality, thus contributing to the reduction of retake radiographs and therefore reducing additional radiation exposure to the patient.

Air-Gap Technique. Air-gap technique may be used when a grid is needed but not available. A distance or "natural" air gap is introduced between the patient and the film holder. This distance allows the scattered photons emerging from the patient to diverge and never reach the film.

Gonadal Shielding. Gonadal shielding protects the patients' gonads from direct primary exposure by placing shielding material between the x-ray beam and the patients' gonads. Gonadal shielding should be used in addition to primary beam restriction and never as a substitute for it.

Gonad shielding should be provided for all persons having reproductive potential, including adults of reproductive age and children. The anatomic location of the testes allows for adequate shielding while not obscuring needed clinical information. The ovaries, however, located near the vertebral spine, ureters, and small and large intestines, do not permit adequate shielding without obscuring a great deal of anatomy nearby.

The two kinds of gonadal shields are *shadow shields* and *contact shields*. Shadow shields are so named because of the shadow cast by the shields. These shields are suspended from the beam-limiting system. They can be positioned to hang over the patients' gonads and are positioned with the assistance of a light localizer. Contact shields may be flat, uncontoured, lead-impregnated material placed on or taped to the patient to cover the gonads, or they may be shaped and contoured to enclose the male reproductive organs (Figure 16-5).

Flat contact shields are most effective for anterior-posterior or posterior-anterior projections when the patient is recumbent. Flat contact shields can be easily used for male and female patients; whereas the shaped contact shield is designed exclusively for use with male patients.

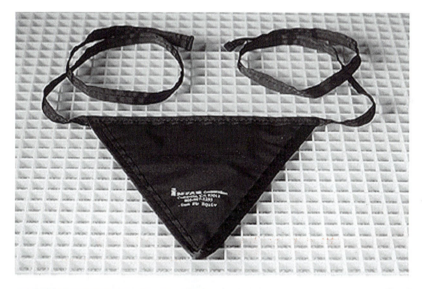

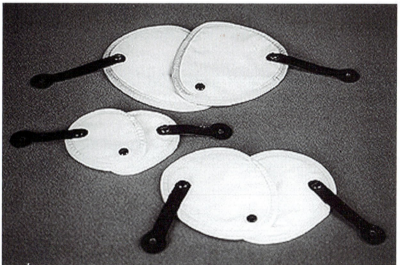

FIGURE 16-5 Examples of gonadal shields *(Courtesy of GE Medical Systems)*

Shaped contact shields are used with disposable supporters. The cup-shaped shield permits enclosure of the scrotum and penis and remains in place with the patient in an upright or recumbent position.

Gonadal shields should meet the following specifications based on the kVp range used:

0.25 mm lead equivalent for 100 kVp or less

0.5 mm lead equivalent for 100–150 kVp

1.0 mm lead equivalent for 150 kVp and above

The decision to use gonadal shielding must be considered with each individual patient's situation and the radiographic request. However, the following criteria provide guidelines for deciding when gonadal shielding should be used:

1. Use gonadal shielding on all patients who have a reasonable likelihood of reproducing.
2. Use gonadal shielding on all children.
3. Use gonadal shielding if the gonads lie within the primary beam or within 5 cm (2½ in) of the primary beam's edge.
4. Use gonadal shielding if the shielding will not obscure (cover) necessary diagnostic information on the radiograph.

Gonadal shields can develop cracks and pinpoint holes with constant use or if improperly stored. Gonadal shields should be stored flat without folds when not in use and should be regularly checked for cracks or pinpoint holes, which can allow radiation leaks to the patient.

Technical Factor Selection.   Selection of the correct combination of technical factors has a direct impact on the amount of radiation received by the patient. Table 16-4 lists technical factors and their roles in radiation protection.

TABLE 16-4   Technical Factors/Roles

Factor	Effect
Exposure selection of high kVp	Reduces radiation doseand low mAs
Proper film processing	Reduces repeat examinations
Use of a grid	Improves radiographic quality
Use of intensifying screen	Reduces amount of radiation exposure required Reduces patient radiation dose
Reduction of repeat examinations	Reduces radiation dose

Radiation-Protection Procedures for the Operator

Cardinal Principles

There are three cardinal principles of radiation protection: time, distance, and shielding (TDS) (Figure 16-6). If used together, the principles of TDS can minimize radiation exposure to the patient and radiographer. These three cardinal principles were developed for nuclear-energy employees who have the potential to be exposed to high levels of radiation in their workplace. The radiographer, of course, is not expected to be employed in a high-level radiation area, such as a nuclear energy plant, but the cardinal principles have practical application to medical radiography.

Time. Radiation exposure is proportional to the amount of time spent in the radiation. A five-minute exposure to radiation would result in a radiation dose five times as great as a one-minute exposure to radiation. This has several implications that can be related to the radiographer and the patient. The radiographer has a responsibility to:

1. Reduce the amount of time exposed to radiation. Do not stay in a radiography room during the exposure unless standing behind a protective barrier.

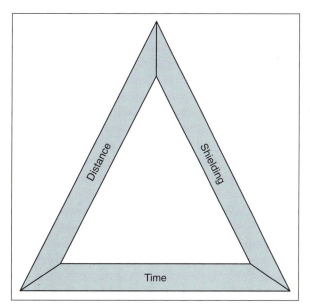

FIGURE 16-6 Three cardinal principles of radiation protection
Source: Delmar, Cengage Learning.

2. Reduce the amount of time that the patient is exposed to radiation. Reduce retake examinations and subsequently reduce time and radiation exposure.

3. Use a fast exposure-time factor whenever possible. A fast exposure time can reduce radiographic motion unsharpness due to patient movement.

Distance. Distance between the radiographer and the radiation source is the most effective way to reduce radiation exposure and the most easily applied principle of radiation protection. The inverse square law which applies to point sources of radiation can be used to demonstrate the effect of distance on radiation intensity (Figure 16-7). Radiation from an x-ray tube is considered to be a point source. Radiation intensity from a point source varies inversely as the square of the distance from the source.

X-rays are similar to light in that the farther you move away from the source, the dimmer the light becomes or the less intense the x-rays become. Figure 16-7

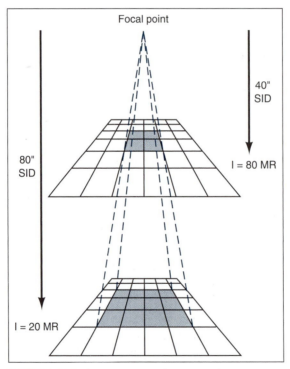

FIGURE 16-7 Inverse square law
Source: Delmar, Cengage Learning.

demonstrates that doubling the distance in an x-ray exposure will spread the radiation over four (4) times the original area size; therefore, the radiation will have only one-fourth its original intensity. Distance is a very important safety guideline because operator protection increases as the distance from the radiation source increases. For example, as the distance doubles from the radiation source, the radiographer gains four times more protection because the radiation intensity is decreased by one-fourth its original intensity.

In clinical situations where mobile radiographic equipment is used, special protection considerations apply. If structural or mobile protective shielding is not available, the radiographer should wear a protective lead apron and gloves. The exposure switch cord should be at least 6 feet (72 inches) long to permit the operator to gain maximum of a 72-inch distance from the radiation source (inverse square law application). The radiographer should also position his/her body at a right angle (90 degrees) to the object creating scatter radiation. Use of the cardinal principles of time, distance, and shielding should be applied to maximize radiation-protection measures to the operator and patient.

The distance principle as applied to patient protection means that every radiographic examination should be performed with the x-ray tube positioned at the proper SID from the patient or part being examined.

Shielding.   Shielding is the third cardinal principle of radiation protection. As x-ray photons travel through the air or through an absorber (such as living tissue), the quantity and energy of the x-ray photons decrease. The degree to which the quantity and energy of the x-ray photons is decreased depends upon several factors: 1) original quantity and energy of the x-ray beam; 2) type of absorber material; and 3) thickness of the absorber material. If x-ray photons travel through enough absorbing material, eventually their energy will be lost to the material and no x-rays will emerge through to the other side.

Protective shields are usually constructed of lead or a concrete wall barrier. This serves as an absorber of the radiation and should be situated so that it intercepts the primary radiation and any radiation that has scattered.

The radiographer should stand behind a lead shield or wall barrier when making the radiographic exposure. The radiographer should not peek around the shield or wall to watch the patient but should watch the patient through the protective glass window installed in the shield or wall (Figure 16-8). Also, x-ray exposures should be made only when the radiographic room doors are closed. This practice provides a substantial degree of protection for patients and staff who may be walking past the radiographic room.

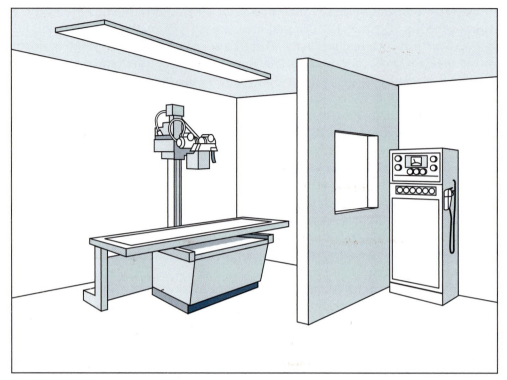

FIGURE 16-8 Arrangement of a control console of an x-ray machine with protective leaded wall and window *(Courtesy of GE Medical Systems)*

Structural Protective Shielding

A radiographic room must be designed to ensure that placement of the equipment is proper and the structural protective shielding meets recommended protective guidelines. Structural protective barriers are designed with certain materials and are of sufficient thickness to reduce radiation exposure to the desired levels. In constructing a radiographic room, the designer has several factors to consider.

A qualified medical radiation physicist must survey the prospective room design and then determines the exact requirements for the shielding. Whether the prospective x-ray room is already in existence or is part of a new construction, appropriate thickness of lead structural shielding will be installed according to the medical radiation physicist's specifications, which are usually mandated by state and/or federal laws. The medical radiation physicist will recommend and provide recommendations for primary and secondary protective barriers.

Some of the factors that the medical radiation physicist must consider are briefly discussed.

The workload (W) of the diagnostic x-ray unit is defined as the radiation output weighted time during the week that the x-ray unit is actually delivering radiation. The actual radiation-on-time factor is used in determining barrier-shielding requirements. Another factor that the medical radiation physicist considers is the use factor (U). Because primary or secondary radiation is not directed or received by every wall or structure in a x-ray room, the use factor allows for consideration of beam-on time during the week for calculating barrier shielding requirements. Rooms adjacent to the x-ray room are also classified as either a controlled or uncontrolled area. A controlled area is an area adjacent to the x-ray room that is used only by personnel who may receive occupational radiation exposures. A nearby hall or corridor that is frequented by the general public is classified as an uncontrolled area.

The occupancy factor (T) is used to modify the structural-shielding requirement for a particular barrier by taking into account the fraction of the workweek that the space beyond the barrier is occupied. Additionally, information about the design of structural shielding for fixed diagnostic x-ray rooms may be found in NCRP Report No. 49: Structural Shielding Design and Evaluation for Medical Use of X-Rays and Gamma Rays of Energies Up to 10 MeV.

Three categories of radiation sources can be generated in an x-ray room. These are classified as *primary radiation, scatter radiation,* and *leakage radiation.* Scatter and leakage radiation is also collectively called *secondary radiation.* Structural protective barriers are named according to their protective nature based on the categories of radiation generated: primary barriers or secondary barriers.

Primary Structural Protective Shielding

Provides protection from the primary x-ray beam. Primary radiation emerges directly from the x-ray tube collimator and moves without deflection toward a wall, door, etc. A wall in the path of the primary radiation requires the most protective shielding. For equipment capable of operating up to 150 kVp, primary structural protective shielding should consist of 1/16th inch lead and be as high as 7 feet from the x-ray room floor. Primary structural protective shielding is located perpendicular to the primary x-ray beam.

Secondary Protective Structural Shielding

Secondary radiation occurs when the primary x-ray beam is deflected or redirected by the object being irradiated. Radiation leakage around the x-ray tube and scatter radiation generated by the patient and other objects receiving radiation comprise secondary radiation.

Secondary protective structural shielding should consist of 1/32nd inch of lead, extend to the ceiling, and be located parallel to the primary beam. Secondary protective shielding is also installed in the control console shield and structural barrier window through which the radiographer can observe the patient. The window is required to contain 1.5 mm lead equivalent.

Protective Apparel

Protective apparel is used for the patient and radiographer whenever additional protection is desired or necessary. Protective apparel consists of lead-impregnated vinyl gloves and apron (Figure 16-9). When operating in the kVp range of 100, the lead gloves and apron should be at least 0.25 mm lead equivalency; however, lead aprons are typically lined with 0.5 mm lead or its equivalency.

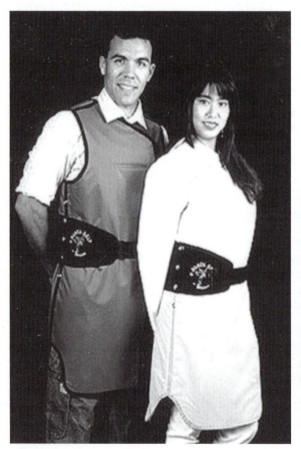
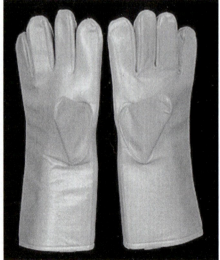

FIGURE 16-9 Use of lead apron and gloves for personnel protection *(Courtesy of GE Medical Systems)*

Handle lead aprons, gloves, and gonad shields with care. Protective apparel should be properly stored when not in use to prevent cracks from developing in the lead. Do not store the items by folding since cracks could result from the bending of the protective lead insert. Cracks could permit radiation to leak through.

The lead apron and gloves should be checked for cracks once every three months.

Radiation Exposure and Pregnancy

Of special concern is radiation exposure during pregnancy. Recent studies published in the Biological Effects of Ionizing Report V (BEIR V) suggest that the fetus may be particularly radiosensitive during the period of 8 to 15 weeks post-conception. It is during this period when certain tissues and organs are developing and are at greatest risk from radiation. Observing all radiation protection guidelines to reduce radiation exposure is extremely important to any pregnant individual, including pregnant (or potentially pregnant) patients and pregnant personnel. The National Council on Radiation Protection (NCRP) guidelines currently recommend that the monthly equivalent dose limit (excluding medical exposure) for the embryo not exceed 0.05 rem (0.5 mSv) once the pregnancy becomes known.

NCRP Report No. 54, Medical Exposure of Pregnant and Potentially Pregnant Women, discusses the risks associated with fetal exposure. The risk is considered to be negligible at 5 rad or less when compared to other risks of pregnancy. At radiation doses above 15 rad, the risk of fetal malformations is significantly increased above control levels. The exposure of the fetus to radiation from diagnostic procedures would rarely be cause, by itself, for terminating a pregnancy.

The Pregnant Patient

It is important to remember that it is the physician's responsibility to evaluate the patient and to determine if the benefits outweigh the risks associated with radiation exposure during the diagnostic procedure. This evaluation is easily made when the possibility of pregnancy can be ruled out. A guideline known as the ten-day rule was recommended by a number of agencies to avert this problem. The guideline stated that pelvic or abdominal x-ray examinations of women of child-bearing age be done only in the first ten days following the onset of menstruation as it would be improbable that a woman would be pregnant during these ten days. The ten-day rule is now considered obsolete and had always been difficult to implement in actual practice. To assist doctors in requesting diagnostic x-ray procedures of women in the childbearing ages, the American College of Radiology (ACR) recommended that a female patient's medical history including a possible pregnancy be reviewed prior to scheduling abdominal and pelvic x-ray examinations.

When a physician does not consider a diagnostic x-ray procedure urgent, it may be regarded as an elective examination and can be scheduled at a time to accommodate patient needs and safety. In NCRP Report No. 102, a recommendation was made to facilitate scheduling of elective examinations. This recommendation states that elective abdominal examinations in the childbearing years should be performed during the first few days following the onset of menses to minimize the possibility of radiation of an embryo.

If the physician determines that it is in the best interests of a pregnant or potentially pregnant patient to undergo a diagnostic x-ray examination, the radiographer's responsibility is to minimize radiation exposure to the patient's lower abdomen and pelvic region. Radiation-protection procedures for the pregnant and potentially pregnant patient conform to the as low as reasonably achievable (ALARA) concept.

The radiographer should also concentrate efforts on producing a diagnostic-quality radiograph the first time (avoid retake examinations) while providing for patient comfort and safety. This can be accomplished by performing all recommended radiation-protection procedures and by providing the pregnant patient with a lead apron or shield placed over the uterus or totally surrounding the pelvis (Figure 16-10).

The potential pregnancy status of all female patients of childbearing ages should always be determined. In many medical facilities, female patients of childbearing ages are asked to provide the date of their last menstrual period (LMP). Pregnancy alert posters are a convenient way to visually inform women to disclose information about a suspected or known pregnancy.

Although the major responsibility for patient radiation-safety rests with the physician and radiographer, the current trend in consumer awareness and involvement focuses some responsibility on the patient. This responsibility involves the patient

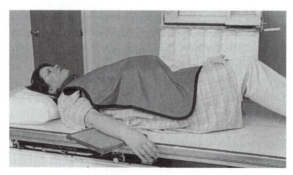

FIGURE 16-10 Use of lead apron when the patient is pregnant *(Reproduced with permission from Statkiewicz-Sherer, M. A. [2007] Radiation Protection in Medical Radiography [5th Edition]. Oxford: Elsevier/Mosby.)*

being aware, asking questions about medical care, and adopting a personal philosophy of not requesting diagnostic radiographic procedures when alternative diagnostic measures are suggested by the attending physician.

The Pregnant Radiographer

A radiographer who becomes pregnant while employed in that capacity should discuss her pregnancy with her supervisor and attending physician. It is the radiographer's responsibility to voluntarily notify the supervisor when she becomes pregnant. The radiographer should review all radiation protection guidelines with the supervisor to ensure that all precautions are being followed to limit radiation to the fetus. The annual occupational effective dose limits for the radiation worker no longer apply and are reduced to reflect the effective dose limits for the embryo/fetus, which is 5 mSV (0.5 rem) for the total period of the pregnancy and 0.5 mSV (0.05 rem) for any given month.

The pregnant radiographer should be reminded that the first trimester (first three months) is the most critical period of fetal development. It is recommended that pregnant radiographers observe all radiation protection measures and closely monitor radiation exposure to ensure that it is kept to a minimum.

Optional protective measures that a pregnant radiographer may use include wearing a protective apron of at least 0.5 mm lead in addition to standing behind the protective barrier and wearing a "Baby" or fetal film badge. The "Baby" film badge may be worn in addition to the operator film badge. The badge worn near the hip or pelvic area should be labeled "Baby" or fetal so that a separate record can be maintained.

If a pregnant radiographer applies the usual recommended radiation safety procedures and uses the optional protective measures mentioned, it is nearly impossible for a radiographer to be exposed to the embryo/fetal exposure near the equivalent dose limit of 0.05 rem (0.5 mSv) per month. The pregnant radiographer should not fear losing her job because of the pregnancy. Discrimination laws prohibit an employer from terminating an employee or putting the employee on a lay-off status due to pregnancy. Pregnancy policies generally apply to both employees as well as to student radiographers during clinical practicum.

Radiation Exposure and the Pediatric Patient

Children command special attention and consideration when undergoing diagnostic x-ray examinations. As no radiation dose is considered "absolutely" safe and experts theorize that all radiation exposure levels possess the potential to cause biologic damage, infants and children should not receive unnecessary radiation exposure.

The same radiation protection procedures used to reduce radiation for adults may also be used to reduce radiation exposure to pediatric patients. There are a few areas however that are unique to the pediatric patient, these being radiation exposure factors and motion control techniques.

Children are not small adults and require lower values of kilovoltage peak (kVP) and mAs compared to adults. Underexposure as well as overexposures and loss of visibility of recorded detail due to motion are the major causes of repeat radiographic examinations, thus increasing the radiation exposure to the pediatric patient. Tips for adapting exposure factors for children based on exposure factors for adults are discussed in Chapter 9, Fundamentals of Radiographic Exposure.

Motion control in pediatric procedures is critical to producing a diagnostic radiograph. Adapting the exposure control factors to allow for the use of very short exposure times is one method used to help control motion in pediatric radiography. Use of a very short exposure time coupled with effective immobilization devices available to hold the pediatric patient securely and safely in the required position is the gold standard in pediatric imaging. For additional information, refer to Chapter 8, Basic Positioning and Patients with Special Needs where the use and application of pediatric immobilization devices are discussed.

Collimation and gonadal shielding are also very important in pediatric radiography. Collimation is most effective when the radiation field size is limited to the area or part being examined. When using the automatic collimation system the dimensions of the radiation field size may require additional manual adjustment to accommodate the smaller size of the pediatric patient. In pediatric radiography, consistent application of gonadal shielding and proper collimation of the primary beam are very important. Because of the small size of the pediatric patient, it may be difficult to precisely place the gonadal shield on the gonadal tissue. Every attempt should be made to use a gonadal shield on the pediatric patient as long as the shield does not obscure necessary anatomic structures on the radiograph. For additional information, refer to discussion on gonadal shielding in this chapter.

In an ideal situation, mechanical immobilization devices would be sufficient to assist the patient. Infants, young children, elderly, and the critically ill or injured patient may not be capable of maintaining the required radiographic position, holding still without movement during the exposure, or safely staying secured on the radiographic table. In these circumstances, someone must remain with the patient during the radiographic exposure. Radiographers should never stand in the primary beam to restrain a patient during a radiographic exposure. The person chosen should also not be pregnant or be concerned about the possibility of an undetected pregnancy. The nonoccupationally exposed person chosen to assist in holding the patient during a radiographic exposure should be provided with appropriate protective apparel. The most common available protective devices are lead aprons and gloves, and leaded glasses and thyroid shields. Protective aprons and gloves are usually made of lead impregnated vinyl within the range of 0.25 to 1.0 mm of lead equivalency. For x-ray exposures with a peak energy of 100 kVp, the protective aprons must possess a minimum of 0.5 mm lead equivalent. Additionally the radiographer should instruct the person as to how to assist in holding the patient and should also position the person so as to minimize their exposure to the primary radiation beam.

Radiation Detection and Monitoring

Accurate radiation detection and measurement is necessary if occupational exposure levels are to be kept below the maximum-permissible-dose levels. Personnel and area monitoring are the most commonly used procedures used to determine occupational exposure.

Personnel Monitoring Devices

Personnel monitoring provides important information regarding the amount of radiation exposure received by an operator. The information gathered from personnel monitoring must then be reviewed to determine if it is within the maximum-permissible-dose guidelines. After the review, corrective actions may be required to reduce or eliminate the radiation exposure. It should be recognized that personnel radiation monitoring is just that—a monitor that records the amount of radiation received and is an indication of the radiographer's working habits and working conditions. One should never assume one is safe just because monitoring is occurring. Nor should it be assumed that because no exposure has ever been recorded, no exposure has ever been or ever will be received. Also, personnel monitoring devices record only the exposure received in the area in which they are worn. The device should be attached to the front of the clothing so it records the radiation received by the radiographer's body trunk. During fluoroscopic procedures when the operator wears a protective lead apron, an additional monitoring device may be worn outside of the protective apron at the collar level to record exposure to the radiosensitive organs of the head, neck, and lens of the eye.

There are several kinds of personnel-radiation-monitoring devices: optically stimulated dosimeter, film badges, thermoluminescent dosimeters, and pocket ionization chambers. Usually, the nature of the occupation and the type of ionizing radiation will determine the choice of personnel monitoring device. A summary of personnel monitoring devices is presented in Table 16-5.

TABLE 16-5   Summary of Personnel Monitoring Devices

Device	Advantages	Disadvantages
Film Badge	• Economical, low-cost • Durable container • Permanent record of personnel exposure • Detects both small and large exposures • Filters allow determination regarding direction of exposure and cause of exposure (scatter/primary) • Control badge provided • Reliable with x-ray and gamma radiation and differentiates between	• Only effective if worn and eared for according to monitoring company directions • Records exposure only in area where badge is worn • Film packet can be fogged by excessive temperature or humidity
TLD Device	• Accurately records dose • Not sensitive to excessive temperature or humidity • May be worn up to three months	• Initial high cost • No permanent record of readings • Not effective if not worn • Person performing readout must follow recommended procedures
Dosimeter Pocket	• Easy to wear • Sensitive and accurately records dose • Immediate readout in self-reading chambers	• Expensive • No permanent record of readings • Chamber should be read and recharged daily • Not effective if not worn
Optically Stimulated Luminescence (OSL) Dosimeter	• Records exposures as low as 1 millirem (MR) • Precision as low as 1 MR	• Only effective if worn and cared for according to monitoring company direction

Optically Stimulated Luminescence (OSL) Dosimeter

One of the most widely used radiation monitoring devices used today is the optically stimulated luminescence (OSL) dosimeter.

When radiation strikes a thin strip of aluminum contained in the device, the quantity is recorded. One of the advanatages of an OSL dosimeter is that radiation exposures as low as 1 millirem can be captured. It also has a precision factor of ±1 millirem. Another advantage is that a read-out can be made on the OSL dosimeter without loss of the stored information.

Film Badges *Radiation Badge*

Film badges are frequently used as a personnel monitoring device. They are economical and considered relatively accurate in recording low doses of radiation if instructions regarding care and use are followed.

A film badge consists of three parts: a film packet, metal filters, and a plastic holder with a clip attachment (Figure 16-11). The plastic holder is made of a low-atomic-number material so that low-energy radiation may reach the film packet. Metal filters of aluminum or copper are contained in the plastic holder and allow for measurement of the radiation energy reaching the film packet. After processing, the degree of film-darkening beneath the filters provides a basis for estimating the radiation exposure. A densitometer is used to measure film density and is then compared to the exposure value of a control film of similar density on a characteristic

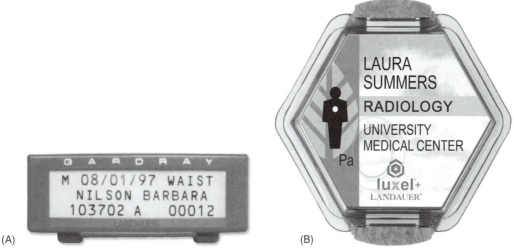

(A)　　　　　　　　　　　　　　　　　　　　　　(B)

FIGURE 16-11　(A) A typical film badge and (B) optically stimulated luminescence (OSL) dosimeter (*Courtesy of Landauer, Inc., Glenwood, IL*)

curve. In addition to the amount of radiation received, the information provided by film-badge films also includes: 1) direction of the radiation exposure (from front to back or from back to front) and 2) whether exposure was from excessive scattered radiation or a single primary beam exposure.

The radiographic-film packet consists of radiation dosimetry film and is similar in size and shape to dental film. Enclosed in a light-free envelope, the radiographic film has sensitivity to doses ranging from 0.1 mSv (10 millirems) to 5 Sv (500 rems). The light-free envelope has a lead foil back that absorbs scatter radiation from behind the device.

Film-badge film packets must be returned to the monitoring company at specific intervals (usually once a month) for processing. The monitoring company provides a control film packet with each shipment of film packets. The control film packet serves as a control for comparing the worn film packets after they have been returned for processing. The control film packet must be stored in a radiation-free area within the medical facility.

Monitoring companies provide a written report containing the results for each film packet and the control packet. These film-badge reports should be reviewed by the facility's radiation safety officer or supervisor to determine compliance with effective-bed-dose-limit guidelines and corrective action taken as necessary. The badge reports should be permanently maintained with personnel records (Figure 16-12).

Although film badges have the advantage of being economical and not easily damaged if dropped, the disadvantages must be considered. The film packet is sensitive to extreme temperature and humidity levels and is not accurate over long periods of recording time, generally not longer than one month.

Thermoluminescent Dosimeters

A **thermoluminescent dosimeter** (TLD) badge is similar in appearance to the film badge; however, it contains a different type of monitoring system. Special crystals in the TLD undergo physical property changes when struck by ionizing radiation. When heated, the crystals emit energy in the form of visible light, equal to the amount of radiation exposure absorbed. A TLD analyzer is then used to heat and measure the amount of radiation received. TLD monitoring devices have several advantages that film badges do not have. They give more accurate recording of low radiation doses; they are less sensitive to extreme temperatures or humidity; and they can be used for up to three months. Disadvantages include initial high cost and no permanent record of the radiation reading since the readout process destroys the stored information.

The most sensitive, yet infrequently used, personnel monitoring device in diagnostic radiology is the **pocket ionization chamber**. The pocket dosimeter

LANDAUER®

Landauer, Inc. 2 Science Road Glenwood, Illinois 60425-1586
Telephone: (708) 755-7000 Facsimile: (708) 755-7016
www.landauerinc.com

SAMPLE ORGANIZATION
RADIATION SAFETY OFFICER
2 SCIENCE ROAD
GLENWOOD, IL 60425

RADIATION DOSIMETRY REPORT

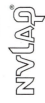

ACCOUNT NO.	SERIES CODE	ANALYTICAL WORK ORDER	REPORT DATE	DOSIMETER RECEIVED	REPORT TIME IN WORK DAYS	PAGE NO
103702	RAD	992150087	6/13/07	06/09/07	4	1

PARTICIPANT NUMBER / ID NUMBER	NAME / BIRTH DATE	SEX	DOSIMETER	USE	RADIATION QUALITY	DOSE EQUIVALENT (MREM) FOR PERIODS SHOWN BELOW — DEEP DDE	EYE LDE	SHALLOW SDE	YEAR TO DATE DOSE EQUIVALENT (MREM) — DEEP DDE	EYE LDE	SHALLOW SDE	LIFETIME DOSE EQUIVALENT (MREM) — DEEP DDE	EYE LDE	SHALLOW SDE	RECORDS FOR YEAR	INCEPTION DATE (MM/YY)
FOR MONITORING PERIOD:						05/01/07 - 05/31/07			2007							
0000H CONTROL	CONTROL		J	CNTRL		M	M	M							5	07/97
	CONTROL		P	CNTRL		M	M	M								07/97
	CONTROL		U	CNTRL				M								07/97
00189	ADAMS, HEATHER 08/31/1968	F	P	WHBODY		M	M	M	9	10	12	29	31	42	5	07/01
336235619																
00191	ADDISON, JOHN 10/04/1968	M	J	WHBODY	PN	90	90	90	100	100	100	200	200	200	5	07/01
471563287					P	60	60	60	70	70	70	170	170	170		
					NF	30	30	30	30	30	30	30	30	30		
00202	HARRIS, KATHY 06/09/1960	F	P	WHBODY		M	M	M	M	M	M	M	M	M	5	02/02
587582144			U	RFINGR				M			30			30		02/02
00005	MEYER, STEVE 07/15/1964	M	P	COLLAR	PL	119	119	113	33	185	174	1387	2308	2320	5	08/97
982778955			P	WAIST	P	10	11	11								08/97
				ASSIGN		19	119	113								
				NOTE		ASSIGNED DOSE BASED ON EDE 1 CALCULATION										
			U	RFINGR				140			690			2180		08/97
00203	STEVENS, LEE 08/25/1951	M	P	WHBODY		ABSENT						M	M	M	4	07/02
335478977			U	RFINGR		ABSENT								M		07/02
00204	WALKER, JANE 03/21/1947	F	P	WHBODY		3	3	3	12	11	11	22	21	21	5	11/02
416995421																
00188	WEBSTER, ROBERT 05/15/1972	M	P	WHBODY		40	40	40	200	200	200	240	240	240	5	07/01
355381469				NOTE		CALCULATED										

QUALITY CONTROL RELEASE: LMR

1 - PR 6774 - PT131 - N1

M: MINIMAL REPORTING SERVICE OF 1 MREM
ELECTRONIC MEDIA TO FOLLOW THIS REPORT

NVLAP LAB CODE 100518-0 **

-21587

FIGURE 16-12 Radiation dosimetry report/front-only page (*Courtesy of Landauer, Inc., Glenwood, IL*)

resembles a fountain pen and contains an ionization chamber, which may be either a self-reading type or a non-self-reading chamber (that requires the use of a special electrometer accessory for a readout).

One advantage of the pocket ionization chamber is that the self-reading type can provide an immediate exposure readout. This is an important and critical feature often required by those who work in high-radiation-exposure occupations. These chambers are expensive and require careful attention to the manufacturer's directions during the readout.

Survey Instruments for Area Monitoring

Radiation survey instruments are used to detect the presence or absence of radiation in a particular area. Generally, radiographers will not be required to use survey instruments to determine radiation exposure; however, it is important to recognize the function of these instruments. The Geiger-Müller (G-M) detector, ionization chamber-type survey meter, and the proportional counter are gas-filled radiation survey instruments used to detect radiation and its exposure quantity. The Victoreen condenser R-meter used to calibrate radiography equipment is also a gas-filled ionization chamber. Survey instruments are commonly used by radiation physicists, equipment inspectors, x-ray service staff, and others who are employed in nuclear occupations where environmental radiation exposure may occur.

REVIEW QUESTIONS

1. The main goal of all radiation protection procedures is to:
   a. reduce radiation exposure to zero
   b. allow exposures up to the maximal limits
   c. limit exposures to non-occupational persons
   d. keep all radiation exposures as low as reasonably achievable

2. The ___ system is based on the premise that any organ in the human body is vulnerable to damage from exposure to ionizing radiation.
   a. skin entrance dosage
   b. minimum exposure guidelines
   c. maximum permissible dose
   d. effective dose limiting

3. Stochastic effects are those that:
   1. are predictable
   2. occur in a random way
   3. are dose dependent
   4. are not dose dependent

   Possible Responses
   a. 1 and 2
   b. 2 and 4
   c. 1, 2, and 3
   d. 2, 3, and 4

4. In regard to occupational exposures, the annual effective dose limit is ___ rem.
   a. 20
   b. 15
   c. 10
   d. 5

5. According to the effective dose limit recommendations, the embryo-fetus equivalent dose monthly limit should not exceed ___ rem.
   a. 5
   b. 2.5
   c. 0.1
   d. 0.05

6. According to the effective dose limit recommendations, the education and training annual limit should not exceed ___ rem.
   a. 5
   b. 2.5
   c. 0.1
   d. 0.05

7. **All** of the following are methods of limiting the primary beam to the area of clinical interest, **except**:
   a. cone
   b. aperture diaphragm
   c. collimator
   d. filter

8. The purpose of tube filtration of the primary x-ray beam includes:
   1. increase radiographic density
   2. improve the quality of the radiation beam
   3. protect the patients' skin and superficial tissue
   4. reduce scatter radiation

   Possible Responses

   a. 1 and 2
   b. 2 and 3
   c. 3 and 4
   d. 1, 3, and 4

9. Inherent filtration in the x-ray tube consists of **all** of the following, **except**:
   a. glass envelope
   b. insulation oil
   c. glass window
   d. added aluminum filters

10. In kVp ranges between 100 and 150, gonadal shields should contain ___ mm lead equivalent.
    a. 0.25
    b. 0.5
    c. 1.0
    d. 1.5

11. The cardinal principles of radiation protection include time, distance, and shielding.
    a. True
    b. False

12. In regard to radiation exposure:
    1. increasing distance increases radiation exposure
    2. decreasing exposure time decreases radiation exposure
    3. increasing shielding decreases radiation exposure

    Possible Responses

    a. 1 only
    b. 1 and 3
    c. 2 and 3
    d. 1, 2, and 3

13. On mobile radiography equipment, the exposure switch cord should be at least ___ feet long to permit the operator to be an appropriate distance from the radiation source.
    a. 2
    b. 4
    c. 6
    d. 8

14. During mobile radiography, the radiographer should position his/her body ___ degrees to the object creating scatter radiation.
    a. 180
    b. 90
    c. 60
    d. 30

15. In regard to structural shielding, a controlled are is used:
    a. only by personnel who may receive occupational radiation exposure
    b. for a holding area for contagious patients
    c. as a reception room for older patients
    d. only by visiting pharmaceutical representatives

16. Secondary radiation consists of:
    a. primary radiation
    b. remnant radiation
    c. scatter and leakage radiation
    d. characteristic radiation

17. For x-ray equipment capable of operating up to 150 kVp, the protective primary structural shielding should consist of ___ inch of lead.
    a. 1/32nd
    b. 1/16th
    c. 1/8th
    d. 1/4th

18. For x-ray equipment capable of operating up to 150 kVp, the secondary protective structural shielding should consist of ___ inch of lead.
    a. 1/32nd
    b. 1/16th
    c. 1/8th
    d. 1/4th

19. The report titled Biologic Effects of Ionizing Radiation V (BIER V) suggests that the fetus may be particularly radiosensitive during the period of __ to __ weeks post-conception.
    a. 1–2
    b. 8–15
    c. 12–24
    d. 36–40

20. Some of the advantages of using a film badge for personnel monitoring include:
    1. low cost
    2. reliability
    3. it is not sensitive to excessive humidity or temperature

    Possible Responses

    a. 1 and 2
    b. 1 and 3
    c. 2 and 3
    d. 1, 2, and 3

21. Some advantages of using a thermoluminescent dosimeter for personnel monitoring include:
    1. low cost
    2. accuracy
    3. it is not sensitive to excessive humidity or temperature
    4. may be worn up to 3 months

    Possible Responses

    a. 1 and 3
    b. 2 and 3
    c. 3 and 4
    d. 2, 3, and 4

REFERENCES

American College of Radiology. (2006). *ACR guidelines and standards, ACR practice guideline for general radiography.* pp. 17–20. Retrieved from www.acr.org

American College of Radiology. (2006). *ACR guidelines and standards, ACR practice guideline for performing and interpreting diagnostic computed tomography (CT).* Retrieved from www.acr.org

Brusin, J. A. (2007, May/June). Radiation protection. *Radiologic Technology 78*(5), 378–91.

Bushong, S. C. (2008). *Radiologic science for technologists: Physics, biology and protection* (9th ed.). St. Louis, MO: Mosby Elsevier.

Campeau, F., & Fleitz, J. (1999). *Limited radiography* (2nd ed.). Albany: Delmar.

Carlton, R. R., & Adler, A. M. (2006). *Principles of radiographic imaging: An art and a science* (3rd ed.). Albany, NY: Delmar Thomson Learning.

Cohen, B. L. (1991). Radiation standards and hazards. IEEE. *Transformation Education 34*, 261–265.

Diagnostic Imaging Online. (2007, April 24). *Imaging equipment vendors tout innovations to reduce radiation exposure.* Retrieved from www.diagnosticimaging.com

Encyclopedia Britannica. (2009). Film badge dosimeter. Retrieved from http://www .britannica.com

Encyclopedia Britannical. (2009). Thermoluminescent dosimeter. Retrieved from http:// www.britannica.com

Furlow, B. (2004, May/June). Biological effects of diagnostic imaging. *Radiologic Technology 5*(5), 335–363.

Health Physics Society. (2001, February 6). *Answer to question #641 submitted to "ask the experts"* (Category: Radiation workers-pregnant workers). Retrieved from www.hps.org

Idaho State University. (2000). *Radiation and risk. Radiation information networks.* Retrieved from www.physics.isu.edu

International Commission of Radiation on Radiation Protection (ICRP). (2007a). *Pregnancy and medical radiation* (Report No. 84). Retrieved from www.iscp.org

International Commission of Radiation Units and Measurements. (2007b). *Radiation quantities and units.* (Report 33). Retrieved from www.2000.irpa.net

Johns Hopkins Safety Manual. (2007). *Personnel monitoring.* Retrieved from www.hopkinsmedicine.org

Mathisen, L. (2007, April 16). Tragedy times two: Late effects of children who undergo radiation therapy. *RT Image. 20*(16), 17–19.

McClafferty, C. (2001). *The head bone's connected to the neck bone.* New York: Farrar, Straus and Giroux.

McGill University. (2007). *Radiation dose limit.* Retrieved from www.mcgill.ca

Mossman, K. L., Goldman, M., Masse, F., Mills, W. A., Schiager, K. J., & Vetter, R. L. (1996, March). *Radiation risk in perspective.* Health Physics Society Position Statement. Retrieved from www.physics.isu.edu

National Cancer Institute. (2005). *Interventional fluoroscopy: reducing radiation risks for patients and staff.* Retrieved from www.cancer.gov

National Council on Radiation Protection and Measurements (NCRP), (1987). *Ionizing radiation exposure of the population of the United States.* (Report No.93). Bethesda, MD: NCRP.

National Council on Radiation Protection and Measurements (NCRP). (2007b). *Radiation exposure during pregnancy demands well-informed patient management.* Retrieved from www.diagnosticimaging.com

National Council on Radiation Protection and Measurements (NCRP). (2007c) *Limitations of exposure to ionizing radiation.* (Report 116). Retrieved from www. ncrponline.org

National Council on Radiation Protection and Measurements, (NCRP). (1977). *Medical exposure of pregnant and potentially pregnant women* (Report No. 54). Washington, DC: NCRP.

National Council on Radiation Protection and Measurements. (1981). *Radiation protection in pediatric radiology* (Report 68). Washington, DC: NCRP.

National Council on Radiation Protection and Measurements. Diagnostic Imaging Online. (2007, April 16). *Report from NCRP: CT-based radiation exposure in U.S. population soars.* Retrieved from www.diagnosticimaging.com

National Council on Radiation Protection. (2004, December). *Recent application of the NCRP public dose limit recommendations for ionizing radiation* (NCRP statement No. 10). Retrieved from www.ncrponline.org

National Electrical Manufacturers Association (2006, December). *How medical imaging has transformed health care in the U.S. (executive summary)*. Retrieved from www.medicalimaging.org

National Electrical Manufacturers Association (2006, December). *How innovations in medical imaging have reduced radiation dosage (executive summary)*. Retrieved from www.medicalimaging.org.

National Research Council, Commission of Life Sciences, Committee on Biological Effects of Ionizing Radiation (BIER V), Board of Radiation Effects Research. (1989). *Health effects of exposure to low levels of ionizing radiations.* Washington, DC: National Academy Press.

North Carolina University Health and Safety, Radiation Safety Division. (2007). *Radiation safety and alara*. Retrieved from www.ncsu.edu.

Patton, K. T. (2000). *Structure and function of the body* (11th ed). St. Louis, MO: Mosby, Inc.

Raussaki, M. T. (2004). *Pediatric Radiation Protection (abstract)*. Retrieved from www.springerlink.com

Schleipman, A. R. (2005, January/February). Occupational radiation exposure: Population studies. *Radiologic Technology* 76(3), 185–191.

Schueler, B. (2003). *Personnel protection during fluoroscopic procedures*. Rochester, MN: Mayo Clinic, Retrieved from www.aapm.org

Seeram, E. (2001). *Rad tech's guide to radiation protection*. Malden, MA: Blackwell Science.

Sherer, M. A., Visconti. P. & Ritenour, E. R. (2006). *Radiation Protection in Medical Radiography* (5th ed.). St. Louis, MO: Mosby.

Sprawls, P. The Physical Principles of Medical Imaging. (1995). Interaction of radiation with matter. Retrieved from http://www.sprawls.org

The Merck Manuals Online Medical Library. (2009). Radiography. Retrieved from http://www.merck.com

Thomas, A., & Sherwood, I. (Eds.). (1995). *The invisible light; The Röentgen centenary: 100 years of medical radiology*. Oxford: Blackwell Science.

United States Food and Drug Administration, Centers for Devices and Radiological Health. (1994, September 30). *FDA public health advisory: Avoidance of serious x-ray induced skin injuries to patients during fluoroscopic-guided procedures*. Rockville, MD: FDA.

U.S. Department of Labor Occupational Safety & Health Administration. (2007). *Ionizing radiation health effects*. Retrieved from www.osha.gov

U.S. Environmental Protection Agency. (2007a). *Estimating risk (Understanding radiation)*. Retrieved from www.epa.gov

U.S. Environmental Protection Agency. (2007b). *Health effects (Understanding radiation)*. Retrieved from www.epa.gov

U.S. Environmental Protection Agency. (2007c). *History of radiation protection*. Retrieved from www.epa.gov

U.S. Environmental Protection Agency. (2007d). *Ionizing & non-ionizing radiation*. Retrieved from www.epa.gov

Whalen, J. P., & Balter, S. (1984). Radiation Risks in Medical Imaging. Chicago, IL: Year Book Medical Publishers, Inc.

Willis, E. & Slovis, T. L. (2005). *Editorials: The alara concept in pediatric CR and DR: Does reduction in pediatric radiographic exams – A white paper conference executive summary*. Retrieved from www.radiology.rsnajnls.org

SUGGESTED READINGS

GE Healthcare. (2006). *Education: X-ray dose*. Retrieved from www.gehealthcare.com

Idaho State University: Radiation Information Network's (2006). *Radiation and risk*. Retrieved from www.physics.isu.edu

Idaho State University: Radiation Information Network's. (2006). *Radiation and us*. Retrieved from www.physics.isu.edu

Jefferson Lab. (2007). *Radiation biological effects*. Retrieved from www.jlab.org

National Commission on Radiation Protection (NCRP). (1987). *NCRP Report 91: Recommendation on limits for exposure to ionizing radiation*. Bethesda, MD. p. 72.

Princeton University. (2007). *Open source radiation safety training. Module 3: Biological effects*. Retrieved from www.princeton.edu

Tolekikids, G. (2007, February). Am I in danger? How far away should you stand during an x-ray exam? *ARST Scanner, 39*(5).

U.S. Environmental Protection Agency. (2007). *Calculate your radiation dose*. Retrieved from www.epa.gov

U.S. Environmental Projection Agency. (2007). *Understanding radiation, estimating risk*. Retrieved from www.epa.gov

U.S. Environmental Protection Agency. (2007). *Understanding radiation*. Retrieved from www.epa.gov

BIBLIOGRAPHY

Bushong, Stewart C. (1997). *Radiologic science for technologists: Physics, biology, and protection*, (6th ed.). St. Louis, MO: Mosby-Year Book.

National Council on Radiation Protection and Measurements, (NCRP). (1977). *Medical exposure of pregnant and potentially pregnant women* (Report No. 54). Washington, DC: NCRP.

National Council on Radiation Protection and Measurements, (NCRP). (1987) *Recommendations on limits for exposure to ionizing radiation*, (Report #91). Bethesda, MD: NCRP Publications.

Statkiewicz-Sherer, Mary Alice, Paul J. Visconti, and E. Russell Ritenour. (1997). *Radiation protection in medical radiography*, (3rd ed.). St. Louis, MO: Mosby-Year Book.

A

Absorbed dose the amount of radiation energy absorbed in tissue; measured in grays

Absorbed dose equivalent (ADE) a method used to calculate the effective absorbed dose for all types of ionizing radiation

Absorption the transference of x-ray energy to the atoms of human tissue

Acromegaly a progressive metabolic disorder caused by excessive secretion of growth hormone from the pituitary gland

Actual focal spot the actual size of the focal spot on the anode (on which the electron stream impacts)

Acute diseases diseases that have a fast onset and last a short period of time

Acute radiation syndrome (ARS) also called radiation illness, occurs after humans receive large doses of ionizing radiation to the entire body within a short time period

Added filtration sheets of metal placed in the path of the primary x-ray beam to make it a more penetrating beam

Administrative regulations written by boards or agencies that have been established by legislative bodies for areas where certain kinds of expertise are required to develop specific regulations

Air gap technique a technique to reduce scatter of radiation by increasing the distance between the patient and the surface of the film; used when a grid is unavailable

Airborne pathogens organisms that cause disease that are transmitted through the environment by dust or droplet contamination

Airbronchograms air-filled bronchi seen as radiolucent, branching bands within pulmonary densities

ALARA (As Low As Reasonably Achievable) means making every reasonable effort to maintain exposures to ionizing radiation as far below the dose limits as is practical

Alpha particles product of radioactive decay composed of two protons and two neutrons; a helium nucleus

Alternating current electrical current that periodically alternates its direction back and forth

American College of Radiology a key medical organization composed of diagnostic radiologists, radiation oncologists, interventional radiologists, nuclear medicine physicians, and medical physicists

American Registry of Radiologic Technologists (ARRT) the largest certifying body in the radiological profession; promotes high standards of patient care by recognizing qualified individuals in medical imaging, interventional procedures, and radiation therapy

American Society of Radiologic Technologists (ASRT) the world's largest and oldest membership association for medical imaging technologists and radiation therapists; provides members with educational opportunities, promotes radiologic technology as a career, and monitors state and federal legislation that affects the profession

Americans with Disabilities Act (ADA) enacted in 1990, a law intended to protect persons with disabilities

Ampere the S.I. base unit of electrical current; also expressed as 1 coulomb/second

Analog-to-Digital Converter (ADC) changes analog signal to digital image of patient part being examined

Anasarca swelling of the subcutaneous tissues throughout the body due to fluid accumulation

Anatomic position the position used to describe the relationship of body parts to each other, known as the standing (erect) position with the body facing forward, the feet together, and the arms down by each side with the palms of the hands facing forward

Angioplasty procedure used to treat a vessel that has become occluded or stenosed

Anode the positively charged side of an electrical circuit; the target side of an x-ray tube

Anterior a positioning terminology, refers to the body position facing the film

Aperture diaphragm a simple beam-limitation device consisting of a flat piece of lead with a hole in the middle

Aplasia the failure of a body part or organ or the congenital absence of an organ or tissue

Apoptosis a nonmitotic or nondivision form of cell death, which occurs when cells die without attempting division during the interphase

Artifacts extraneous marks and images on the radiograph

Ascites refers to fluid accumulation within the peritoneal cavity

Asepsis the absence of all disease-producing microorganisms

Assault any willful attempt or threat to inflict injury upon the person of another

Asthenic a body type that is extremely slender and generally frail in appearance and usually weak

Asymptomatic patient a patient without symptoms of disease or illness

Atherectomy a nonsurgical procedure to open blocked coronary arteries or vein grafts by using a device on the end of a catheter to cut or shave away atherosclerotic plaque

Atom the smallest particle that an element can be reduced to while still maintaining its chemical identity

Atomic mass number the number of protons and neutrons in a nucleus

Atomic number the number of protons in a nucleus

Atrophy a wasting or decrease in the size of tissues, organs, or the entire body

Attenuate a decrease in energy of a wave or a beam of particles, occurring as the distance from the source increases as a result of absorption, scattering, spreading in three dimensions

Attenuation any process that prevents x-ray photons from reaching the patient or the radiographic film

Automatic exposure control (AEC) x-ray exposure timing determined by a radiation sensitive detector

Automatic film processing a process that eliminates manual handling of film in addition to decreasing the time of film processing and providing constant control over chemical temperature and chemical strength

Automatic program radiography (APR) an exposure or technique chart that uses microcomputers to determine kVp and mAs (time)

Autonomy freedom to govern one's self or self-governance

Autotransformer a transformer consisting of two windings on a single core; used in x-ray machines to change the line voltage

Avulsion the tearing away of a body part as of a fragment of bone from the bone shaft

Background radiation the normal amount of radiation exposure expected from unavoidable natural and artificial sources

Bacteria one-celled organisms, both pathogenic and nonpathogenic, which are identified and classified according to their morphology (shape) and structure

Barton's fracture an intra-articular fracture of the distal radius that involves the styloid and articular surface of the distal radius

Battery any unlawful touching of another that is without justification or excuse

Beam filtration use of filters added to the radiation beam to eliminate non-useful, soft, low-energy (long wavelengths) radiation

Beam restriction control of the field size of an x-ray beam

Beneficence in health care, a duty to others to provide or improve conditions that promote physical and emotional well being

Benign the quality of being localized; usually attributed to tumors and other abnormal growths

Bennett's fracture an injury to the thumb that occurs when a direct blow is received on the hand with the metacarpophalangeal (MCP) joint of the thumb partially flexed

Beta particles a product of radioactive decay physically identical to an electron

Binding energy the amount of energy needed to remove an electron from its orbital shell

Bioethics see Biomedical ethics

Biomedical ethics, or bioethics involves the knowledge and application of modern medical technologies

Bit depth number of bits per pixel

Blood pressure (BP) the force of the flow of blood exerted against the walls of the blood vessels

Body habitus physical appearance of the body or body build

Body plane one of the three primary planes used to identify the body in different sections

Bone densitometry an imaging study that measures bone mineral density (BMD) and is used to determine whether a person may have or be at risk of having osteopenia or osteoporosis

Bone Densitometry Equipment Operators one of the ARRT examinations available to states for licensing purposes

Boxer's fracture an injury of the neck of the metacarpal that results from direct trauma to the hand with axial loading or compression

Bremsstrahlung radiation radiation comprising photons that occurs as a result of electrons interacting with atoms of the target material

Bursitis a condition of inflammation of the bursa sacs that protect the shoulder

Calipers a caliper is a measuring device, used in radiography to measure the volume of tissue thickness of a body part

Cardinal principles the key principles of radiation protection: time, distance, and shielding (TDS)

Caring the responsibility and attention towards health, well-being, and safety of clients demonstrated when medical professionals (e.g., limited radiographer) listen, provide information, help, communicate, show respect, touch, and protect

Carpal tunnel syndrome a condition in which the median nerve in the wrist is compressed

Cathode the negatively charged side of an electrical circuit; the side of an x-ray tube where electrons are produced

Central ray the center of the x-ray beam

Certification a one-time process of initially recognizing individuals who have satisfied certain standards within a profession

Chain of command order in which authority and power in an organization is wielded and delegated from top management to every employee at every level of the organization

Characteristic interactions interactions of incoming electron with an inner-shell electron

Characteristic radiation an x-ray photon emitted from the atom when an outer-shell electron fills an inner-shell vacancy

Chauffer's fracture an intra-articular fracture of the distal radius primarily involving the styloid of the radius caused by axial compression

Chemically stable describes an atom that has exactly eight electrons in the outermost shell

Chondro sarcoma a malignant tumor of cartilaginous origin; it has a higher incidence in males than in females

Chronic diseases diseases that have a slow onset and may last for an extended length of time

Circuit breaker a device used to quickly shut down an electrical circuit in case of overload

Clay shoveler's fracture a fracture of the lower cervical spine caused by hyperflexion

Code of ethics a document that indicates the duties, ideals, values, and goals of a radiologic technologist

Collimation the process of restricting and confining a beam of radiation to a given area

Collimator shutters an adjustable x-ray beam restrictor that alters the quality and quantity of the x-ray beam

Common law a system of applied law that usually develops in the absence of codified written laws or laws enacted through legislation (pertinent statutes)

Communication a process by which information is exchanged between individuals through a common system of symbols, signs, or behavior

Compound a substance composed of like molecules

Compression one of the factors that influence density and contrast of the x-ray image; has the effect of reducing tissue thickness

Computed radiography (CR) digital radiography that records radiographic images on photostimulable phosphor plates instead of film/screen image receptors

Computed tomography a medical imaging procedure that provides clinical information in the detection and differentiation of disease

Conductor a material that carries electricity easily

Cone a simple beam-limitation device consisting of a circular metal tube with a flared end

Confidentiality a patient's legal and ethical right to privacy

Congenital existing at birth and acquired during development in the uterus

Constitutional law the highest order of law; the branch of public law of a nation or state

Consumer-Assurance of radiological excellence (RadCARE) Bill a bill passed in the U.S. Senate that directs the U.S. Secretary of Health and Human Services to establish minimum educational and credentialing standards for personnel who plan and deliver radiation therapy and perform all types of diagnostic imaging procedures except medical ultrasound

Consumer-Patient Radiation Health and Safety Act (Public Law 97-35) a law enacted in response to growing concern and awareness about potential long-term effects from radiation exposure

Contact gonadal shielding a shielding procedure wherein flat or shaped gonadal shields are placed directly on the patient

Continuing education formal educational programs, which are usually short-term and specific, designed to promote knowledge, skills, and professional attitudes

Contrast radiographic contrast is defined as the visible differences between any two areas of radiographic density

Contrast agents substances used in many x-ray examinations to increase or decrease the tissue density

Contusion any mechanical injury (usually caused by a blow) resulting in hemorrhage beneath unbroken skin

Coronal one of the three primary body planes, also referred to as the frontal plane

Coulomb per kilogram the S.I. unit of exposure dose for x-rays or gamma rays; formerly known Roentgen.

Crest the uppermost point, the position of maximum positive value, of a progressive wave

Cultural diversity the cultural differences that exist between people, such as language, dress and traditions, and the way societies organize themselves

Current the flow of electrons in an electrical circuit

Cystic Fibrosis a disease resulting from a defective autosomal recessive gene that affects the endocrine glands and involves the respiratory system and many other organs

Decubitus body position lying down with a horizontal x-ray beam

Defamation the act of bringing harm to another person's reputation through libel (written word) or slander (spoken word)

Degenerative disease diseases generally associated with the aging process, which may, in some cases, develop following traumatic head injuries

Density overall blackness of the radiographic image; controlled by mA

Developer solution used for converting the exposed silver halide crystals into metallic silver

Diagnosis the determination of the nature of a disease, injury, or congenital defect

Diagnostic imaging the use of radiographic, sonographic, and other technologies to create a graphic depiction of the body part(s) in question

Diagnostic mammography mammography that provides additional information about patients who have signs and/or symptoms of breast disease

Digital imaging the creation of computerized image files and transferring them to computers located elsewhere in a network or across the internet

Digital imaging and communications in medicine (DICOM) system that transfers images and other medical information between computers

Digital imaging processing a complex technology that involves the use of a computer to prepare digital images. Digital imaging also refers to film-less imaging

Digital imaging production a methodology that includes data acquisition; image processing; image display, storage, and archiving; and image communication

Digital radiography (DR) technique in which x-ray absorption is quantified by assignment of a number to the amount of x-rays reaching the detector; the information is manipulated by a computer to produce an optimal image

Digital tomosynthesis digital tomography that involves x-ray tube movement and multiple low-dose exposures, which blurs out the tissue above and below the plane of interest

Digital-to-analog Converter (DAC) a process in which the digital image is converted into an analog signal that can be displayed on a monitor

Direct effect effect that occurs when x-ray photons directly interact with a "target" or master (critical) DNA molecule

Direct-capture method the process of recording a radiographic image without a separate image reader of cassette

Disinfection the destruction of microorganisms by using chemical methods

Dislocation the displacement of a bone such that the bones on opposite sides of a joint do not line up

Distance or source-to-image distance (SID); has a significant influence on density

Distortion variation from normal shape; a misshapen radiographic image

Dose fractionation and protraction two methods of radiation delivery. A protracted dose of radiation is delivered continuously at a lower dose rate. A fractionated dose is delivered at the same dose rate but divided into equal fractional quantities of radiation. Dose fractionation is used in radiation therapy since it allows time for tissue repair and recovery between the radiation treatments.

Dose-response relationship a point or level of radiation exposure (dose) at which a response or reaction first occurs

Dual energy x-ray absorptiometry a bone density test that measures bone density in grams/centimeter squared. A DEXA machine uses an x-ray source to obtain the measurement.

Dysplasia abnormal tissue development that often results from prolonged chronic irritation or inflammation

Dyspnea difficult or labored breathing

 E

Early somatic effects physiological effects that appear in the individual within days or weeks after

a significant external exposure to radiation; symptoms may include nausea, loss of hair, sore throat, hemorrhage, and diarrhea

Edema the accumulation of abnormal amounts of fluid in the intercellular tissue spaces or body cavities

Effective dose limiting system a prescribed set of dose limits that are based on calculations of the various risks of cancer and genetic effects to tissues and organs exposed to radiation

Effective focal spot the size of the focal spot that is perceived on the film

Electrification the process of imparting a charge to objects

Electrodynamics the movement of electrical charge

Electromagnetic radiation radiation consisting of an electrical component and a magnetic component; described in terms of energy, wavelength, and frequency

Electron a negatively charged fundamental particle found in atomic orbitals

Element a chemically distinguishable substance consisting of only one kind of atom

Embolization an interventional imaging procedure that employs the use of a catheter to restrict blood flow by creating an embolus in a vessel

Embolus a foreign substance, such as a cholesterol plaque, fat, or air bubble circulating in the blood

Empathy the ability to understand another's situation, such as fear, pain, anger, without actually having the emotion

Energy the ability to do work; usually divided into kinetic energy, the energy of motion, and potential energy, the energy of position; measured in joules

Environmental radiation see background radiation

Epistaxis bleeding or hemorrhage from the nose

Ergonomics the science of fitting the job to the worker

Ethics the philosophical study of human behavior or conduct

Etiology the study of the causes of disease and their mode of operation

Ewing's tumor a highly malignant, metastatic, small round cell tumor of bone, usually in the diaphyses of long bones, ribs, and flat bones of children and adolescents

Exposure factors factors that control production of the visible radiographic image

Exposure index number sensitivity range of exposure of computed radiographic image receptors, relative to the manufactures imaging plate exposure data. Determines overexposure or underexposure of the image as set by the radiographer.

False imprisonment the conscious restraint of the freedom of another without proper authorization, privilege, or consent of that individual

Filament the heated wire in the cathode of an x-ray tube where electrons are produced

Filament circuit the electric circuit to produce the heating current to the filament wire of an x-ray tube

Film badge a personnel radiation monitor that measures radiation exposure by the use of film

Film base a polyester that provides a rigid yet flexible support for the emulsion

Film contrast the ability of the film emulsion to react to radiation and to record a particular range of densities

Film emulsion the most important layer of the film which contains the crystals that will hold the latent image formation

Film fog "undesirable" density (film darkening); obscures image details

Film markers methods used to both medically and legally mark a film. Left and right side of the body must be marked on the film, as well as name, sex, age, facility name, and other critical database generally included

Film resolution ability of the crystals within the film emulsion to efficiently record information

Filtration (x-ray tube) the use of a filter to attenuate x-rays

Fixed kilovoltage technique an exposure or technique chart that uses an optimum kilovoltage to penetrate a given part of the body

Fixer an acidic solution which removes the unexposed and undeveloped silver halide crystals from the emulsion and hardens the soft gelatin

Fluoresce a type of luminescence or "lighting up" that occurs when certain phosphors (calcium tungstate) absorb radiation

Fluoroscopy an imaging modality that uses an x-ray source to obtain real-time images of internal structures of a patient through the use of a fluoroscope

Focal spot the region of the x-ray tube target where the electron beam is focused

Focusing cup the metal cup surrounding the filament in an x-ray tube that focuses the electron beam in the x-ray tube

Fomite an object that has been contaminated with a pathogen and serves to spread disease

Full-wave rectification a type of rectification that utilizes both halves of the AC voltage pulse

Fungi any of the eukaryotic spore-producing and typically filamentous organisms that lack chlorophyll, such as yeasts and molds

Fusion imaging also referred to as hybrid imaging, which combines modalities as PET/CT and SPECT/CT. Advantages include better diagnostic accuracy, treatment planning and response evaluation, and enhanced guided biopsy methods

Gamekeeper's thumb a deformity of the thumb that results from an abduction injury in which the ulnar collateral ligament is torn from the base of the proximal phalanx

Gamma radiation high-energy electromagnetic radiation resulting from radioactive decay of nucleus

Genetic effects effects that may not be apparent in the exposed individual but which may be passed on to future generations through genetically damaged chromosomes

Geometric factors factors connected with the geometry of image formation

Geometric properties properties of a quality diagnostic radiograph, namely, recorded detail and absence of distortion and magnification. Degree of blurring and size of the image affect accuracy

Germs microscopic organisms that are harmful and are capable of causing diseases

Giant cell tumor a bone tumor, ranging from benign to frankly malignant, composed of cellular spindle cell stroma containing multinucleated giant cells resembling osteoclasts

Gonadal shielding protection of the patients' gonads from direct primary exposure by placing shielding material between the x-ray beam and the patients' gonads

Gray (Gy) the S.I. unit of radiation absorbed dose; also expressed as joules per kilogram

Greenstick-type fracture a type of fracture which the cortex breaks on one side without separation or breaking of the opposing cortex

Grid a radiographic accessory constructed with lead strips to reduce the amount of scattered radiation from a given exposure reaching the image receptor (IR)

Gross negligence the intentional failure to perform a manifest duty in reckless disregard of the consequences as affecting the life or property of another

Ground glass sign an increased opacity of the lung parenchyema that is not dense enough to obscure underlying pulmonary vessels

Growth plate injuries injuries caused by a fall or blow to the limb or from overuse; includes shin splints, Achilles' tendon, and stress fractures

Half-wave rectification a type of rectification that utilizes only one half of the AC voltage pulse

Hangman's fracture a bilateral pedicle fracture involving the arch of the second cervical vertebral body; it is associated with hanging type injuries and often results from motor vehicle accidents

Health Insurance Portability and Accountability Act (HIPAA) a law written and implemented to provide health insurance reform and administrative simplification

Heat units (HU) a measure of the heat accumulated in the anode of an x-ray tube due to self-absorption in the anode

Heel effect diminished x-ray intensity at the anode end of an x-ray tube due to self-absorption in the anode

Hemoptysis expectoration of blood from some part of the respiratory tract

Hemorrhage the rupture of a blood vessel, either an artery or a vein

Hereditary the transmission of genetic characteristics from parent to offspring

Heredofamilial refers to any disease that occurs in families due to an inherited defect or process

Hertz the S.I. unit of frequency; expressed as 1/s

Hierarchy of human needs needs that must be met for physiological and psychological survival and growth. Physiological needs are related to survival (food, water, air, shelter), whereas psychological needs relate to requirements for love, belonging, and self-esteem.

High kVp technique a technique designed to utilize high kilovoltage for penetration, usually 100 kVp and greater

High-voltage cables two large cables used to connect the radiographic tube to the high-voltage generator

High-voltage transformer the transformer in an x-ray machine circuit that steps up the voltage prior to use in the x-ray tube

Hospital information system (HIS) a electronic database used in a hospital to store, generate, and retrieve patient information. Also used to manage administrative and financial aspects of a hospital

Host a reservoir in which microorganisms live and grow, such as human beings, animals, soil, water, and food

Hydrocephalus the condition of dilation or widening of the ventricles that is associated with increased intracranial pressure

Hyperechoic term used in ultrasound that refers to the increased brightness of an object relative to other things in the image

Hyperplasia the excessive proliferation of normal cells in the normal tissue arrangement of an organ

Hypersthenic a body type that is large and stocky and represents about 5% of the population

Hypertension a condition of high blood pressure created and exacerbated by a variety of conditions including disease, emotional stress, and environmental stress

Hypertrophy a general increase in bulk or size of a part or organ, which is not related to tumor formation

Hypoechoic term used in ultrasound that refers to the decreased brightness of an object relative to other things in the image

Hyposthenic a body type that is slender or thin and represents about 35% of the population

Hypotension a condition of low blood pressure that is not necessarily indicative of an illness unless accompanied by other symptoms

Iatrogenic a class of diseases that is caused by the medical treatment itself

Idiopathic a disease for which the underlying cause is unknown

Image evaluation the assessment of the image in terms of photographic effect for photographic factors, geometric factors, and accurate radiographic position

Image production using a set of criteria or a checklist in preparation of image production in order to avoid errors

Image quality a characteristic of an image that measures the perceived image degradation (typically, compared to an ideal or perfect image)

Implied consent an exception to the rule of informed consent, implied consent refers to a situation in which a person is unconscious or when a life-threatening emergency exists and no one is available to provide legal permission

Incandescence the emission of visible light by a body when heated to a high temperature

Indirect effect effect that occurs when a photon strikes a noncritical molecule, usually water, and the noncritical molecule then transfers the ionization energy to the critical DNA molecule

Inert devoid of active chemical properties, as the inert gases

Inertia the tendency of a moving body to remain in motion or a stationary body to remain at rest

Infarction the localized death of tissue resulting from a sudden insufficiency of arterial or venous blood supply

Infection an inflammatory process in response to a disease-causing organism

Infection control the prevention of the spread of infectious conditions and diseases

Inflammation a local response to cellular injury that is marked by capillary dilatation, leukocytic infiltration, redness, heat, pain, swelling, and often loss of function

Informed consent an individual's right to disclosure of all information related to a medical procedure or treatment to assure the person's full understanding for voluntary consent to accept medical care

Inherent filtration attenuation of the primary x-ray beam as a result of its passage out of the x-ray tube through the insulating medium and tube window

Insulator a material that resists the flow of electricity

Intensifying screens screens composed of fluorescent phosphors that intensify the action of radiation

Interventional imaging procedure used to intervene with the course of certain disease conditions without subjecting the patient to the risks of surgery or other invasive procedures

Inverse square law the intensity of radiation is inversely proportional to the square of the distance

Ion an electrically charged particle

Ionization the imparting of charge to an atom by the removal or addition of an electron

Ionizing radiation radiation that causes production of charged particles (ions)

Ischemia the disruption of the blood supply to an organ or part of an organ depriving cells and tissues of oxygen and nutrients

Isotope a nuclear arrangement with differing neutron numbers and the same atomic numbers

Joint Review Committee on Education in Radiologic Technology (JRCERT) the profession's largest programmatic accrediting agency; reviews a program's admission policy, curriculum, academic practices, and faculty qualifications

Joule the S.I. base unit of energy

Justice the balancing and fair distribution of medical care, facilities, and resources for society

Kerley's A lines relatively long septations that radiate from the right and left pulmonary hilum

Kerley's B lines small septations in the lung that contain lymphatics and venules that are visible on chest radiographs only when they are abnormally thickened

Kilovolt peak meter the device that measures the energy of an x-ray beam

Kilovolt peak meter the device that measures the energy of an x-ray beam

Kilovoltage a factor sometimes that needs to be adjusted for various thickness ranges of anatomical structure

Kilovoltage peak (kVp) one of the exposure factors

Kinetic energy the energy of motion

Kyphosis an abnormal or exaggerated thoracic "humpback" curvature with increased convexity

Large focal spot the larger filament in the focusing cup of the cathode assembly of the x-ray tube

Late somatic effects physiological effects that appear in the individual after months to years of significant external exposure to radiation; effects include cancer (leukemia), birth defects, cataracts

Latent image an invisible image produced in a film emulsion by x-rays or visible light that can be converted into a visible image by development

Law of Bergonié and Tribondeau the relation of radiation sensitivity to mitotic state and differentiation

Law of conservation the physical principle that energy can neither be created nor destroyed

Leakage radiation any x-ray photons that escape from the housing except at the window or port

Left anterior oblique a positioning terminology, refers to the body position in which the body is rotated with the left anterior portion closest to the film

Left posterior oblique a positioning terminology, refers to the body position in which the body is rotated with the left posterior portion closest to the film

Licensing used in referring to state laws

Light absorption deals with the absorption characteristics of x-ray film to light, especially in the darkroom

Limited radiographer an individual other than a radiologic technologist who performs diagnostic x-ray procedures on selected anatomical sites

Limited x-ray machine operator standards A set of norms instituted by the ASRT basic elements to be incorporated in credentialing programs of states that allow persons to perform limited x-ray procedures

Line focus principle the effect whereby the apparent focal spot is smaller than the actual focal spot of an x-ray tube

Line voltage compensation a technique that uses a component in the primary circuit to the autotransformer to increase or decrease the line voltage if there is a drop or surge in the line voltage

Linear energy transfer (LET) the loss of energy to matter by radiation; measured in keV

Lordosis a term meaning "bent backward" and describing the normal anterior concavity of the lumbar and cervical spine

Lucent areas (within the lung fields) areas where there is increased penetration by the x-ray beam within the lungs

Magnetic resonance imaging procedure used in medical imaging to visualize the structure and function of the body

Magnetism the ability of certain materials to attract iron and other metals

Magnification enlargement of the size of the actual anatomical part

Malignant the quality of being invasive and destructive; usually attributed to tumors and other abnormal growths

Mallet fingers abnormality is visible where the fingertip is curled downward and the patient cannot straighten the finger out

Mammography quality standard act act that requires the technical aspects of mammography to meet minimum standards, and which also requires those performing and interpreting mammograms have mammography training and demonstrate clinical competency

Manifest image the change on an x-ray film that becomes visible when the latent image undergoes appropriate chemical processing

Mass the amount or quantity of matter

Matrix the basic formation of a two-dimensional image that consists of columns (M) and rows (N)

Maximum Permissible Dose (MPD) the maximum amount of radiation allowed under radiation safety standards; defined for the whole body, body parts, and calendar periods. MPD has been replaced by effective-absorbed dose-equivalent limits

Meiosis also called reduction division, creates two identical cells produced each containing only one-half (23) of the usual forty-six chromosomes

Mental capacity ability to function or reason based on age, condition, illness, memory, judgment, or other status

Metabolic diseases diseases that interfere with the normal physiologic function of the body; examples are osteoporosis and cystic fibrosis

Metastasis the characteristic of malignant growths of spreading to distant locations

Meter the S.I. base unit of length

Microorganisms extremely small organisms: bacteria, fungi, protozoa, rickettsiae, and viruses

Milliammeter (mA) an instrument used to measure x-ray tube current

Milliamperage the unit of x-ray tube current

Milliamperage seconds (mAs) the product of x-ray tube current and exposure time; a measure of x-ray quantity

Mitosis division of cells resulting in two cells

Mixture a combination or two or more substances

Molecular imaging procedure that enables the visualization of the cellular function and the follow-up of the molecular process of living organisms

Molecule chemical combination of atoms into substances

Molybdenum a desirable filament material because of its high melting point

Momentum the product of mass and velocity

Monteggia fracture a fracture that occurs at the proximal third of the ulna with anterior dislocation of the radial head

Motion a major factor in reducing image clarity and increasing distortion

Myeloma a tumor composed of cells of the type normally found in the bone marrow

NCRP Report No. 116 report that states that for educational and training purposes, radiation workers less than 18 years old be limited to an annual dose limit of 1 mSv (0.1 rem)

NCRP Report No. 54 a report on Medical Exposure of Pregnant and Potentially Pregnant Women that discusses the risks associated with fetal exposure

Necrosis the pathologic death of one or more cells, or of a portion of tissue or organ, resulting from irreversible damage

Negligence the omission to do something that a reasonable person (guided by those considerations which ordinarily regulate human affairs) would do, or the doing of something that a reasonable and prudent person would not do

Neoplastic diseases diseases characterized by new, abnormal growths in the body

Neutron an uncharged fundamental particle found in the nucleus of an atom

Night-Stick fracture a fracture that occurs at the mid-shaft of the ulna, resulting usually from a direct blow to the forearm

No Manual Lift policy A policy prohibiting staff from manually lifting or transporting patients

Non-ionizing radiation radiation that does not cause the production of charged particles (ions)

Nonmaleficence in the health professions, to prevent harm or to cause no harm to another person

Nonpathogenicorganisms microscopic organisms that are not harmful

Nonstochastic effects somatic effects that are directly related to the dose of ionizing radiation received

Nosocomial infections opportunistic infections; a group of pathogenic microorganisms that are common in medical settings

Nuclear medicine referred to as "emission imaging," where photons are emitted from inside the patient and subsequently detected by a gamma camera imaging system

Nuclear Regulatory Commission (NRC) a U.S. government agency responsible for regulating the nuclear energy industry

Nucleus (1) the center of an atom containing neutrons and protons; (2) the portion of a cell containing the DNA

Object-to-image receptor distance (OFD) the practice/rule of placing the object (anatomy) as close to the image receptor (the cassette) as possible

Oblique position a positioning terminology, refers to the body position (erect or lying down)

Occlusion See *infarction*

Occult not visible (or) hidden

Occupancy factor (T) Used to modify the shielding requirement for a particular barrier by taking into account the fraction of the workweek that the space beyond the barrier is occupied

Occupational exposure Radiation required by radiation workers in the course of performing their professional responsibilities

Octet rule the rule that the number of electrons in the outermost shell of an atom can never exceed eight electrons

Ohm the S.I. unit of electrical resistance

Optical imaging an imaging technique that involves inference from the deflection of light emitted from a laser or infrared source to anatomic or chemical properties of material

Osgood-Schlatter disease a condition caused by repetitive stress on part of the growth area of the upper tibia and is characterized by inflammation of the patellar tendon and surrounding soft tissue

Osteoarthritis the most common type of arthritis; a degenerative joint disease that affects the cartilage that covers the ends of bones that meet to form a joint

Osteochondroma a benign tumor composed of bone and cartilage

Osteoma a benign, slow-growing tumor composed of well-differentiated, densely sclerotic, compact bone, occurring particularly in the skull and facial bones

Osteomalacia a condition characterized by increasing softness of bones so that they become flexible and brittle, caused by lack of calcium in tissues

Osteopenia a condition of low bone mass

Osteophytes small deposits of bone

Osteoporosis an age-related disorder related to the decrease in bone mass and atrophy of skeletal tissues with increased susceptibility to fractures

Osteosarcoma a tumor that arises from bone-forming cells and affects chiefly the ends of long bones; its greatest incidence is in the age group of 10 to 25 years

Paget's disease a skeletal disease of the elderly characterized by thickening and softening of bones and the bowing of long bones

Particulate radiation ionizing radiation consisting of physical particles such as electrons or neutrons

Pathogenesis the origin and development of a disease

Pathogenic organisms microscopic organisms that are harmful and are capable of causing diseases

Pathology a branch of the medical sciences that attempts to discover the nature of disease and its causes, processes, development, and consequences

Patient advocate a person who speaks on behalf of a patient in order to protect their rights and help them obtain needed information and services

Percutaneous vertebroplasty A treatment that involves injecting a special liquid cement into fractured vertebral sections

Periodic table of elements a tabular arrangement of the elements according to their atomic numbers so that elements with similar properties are in the same column

Pertussis an acute infectious inflammation of the larynx, trachea, and bronchi caused by *Bordetella pertussis*; characterized by recurrent bouts of spasmodic coughing

Philosophy learning related to a search for truth and a general understanding of values and reality

Photoelectron an electron released or ejected from a substance by photoelectric effect

Photographic properties (factors) properties of a quality diagnostic radiograph, namely, density and contrast

Photon the massless particle that conveys electromagnetic force, x-rays, and light

Photostimulable phosphor (PSP) a material used to capture radiographic images in computed radiography systems

Phototimer an exposure-timing device that uses a light-sensitive photomultiplier tube placed behind a fluorescent screen

Physics a branch of science that deals with matter and energy and their relation to each other

Picture archiving and communication systems (PACS) a systematic network for sending, receiving, and storing all digital images within the medical imaging department

Pixel picture element and is the smallest piece of a two-dimensional, rectangular image array of square pixels that make up the matrix

Pneumonia an inflammation of lung tissue mostly due to infection by bacteria or viruses

Pocket ionization chamber a small, pocket-sized ionization chamber used for monitoring radiation exposure of personnel

Port a window segment constructed at the point where the primary x-ray beam exits the glass envelope of the x-ray tube

Positive beam limitation (PBL) system a collimation device that automatically limits an x-ray beam according to the size of the image receptor

Positron emission tomography a nuclear medicine imaging technique that produces a 3-dimensional image or map of functional processes in the body

Posterior a positioning terminology, refers to the body position facing the radiographic tube

Potential difference the difference in electrical potential between two points on an electrical conductor

Potential energy the energy of position

Pott's fracture a fracture of the lower part of the fibula, with serious injury of the lower tibial articulation (Dorland's Medical Dictionary

Prehypertension a condition of blood pressures between 120–130 millimeters of mercury systolic or 80–89 diastolic

Primary and secondary circuits the primary circuit is the part of an x-ray machine circuit on the input side of the high-voltage transformer; the secondary circuit is the part of an x-ray machine circuit on the output side of the high-voltage transformer

Primary Protective Structural Shielding a protective barrier that is located perpendicular to the line of travel of the primary x-ray beam

Primary radiation the light source used to produce x-rays

Professional ethics in the health-related professions, standards of conduct that relate to duties and obligations of health care practitioners

Prognosis a forecast of the probable course and/or outcome of a disease

Prone a positioning terminology, refers to the body position lying face downward

Proton a positively charged fundamental particle found in the nucleus of an atom

Protozoa microscopic one-celled organisms that may be pathogenic

Pulse rhythmic dilation of an artery produced by the flow of blood into the vessel by the contraction of the heart

Quanta separate packets of energy constituting the electromagnetic radiation

Quantum see quanta (singular of quanta)

Radiation electromagnetic waves or particular matter emitted as a result of electronic or atomic transitions

Radiation absorbed dose is 100 ergs of energy absorbed by 1 gram of absorbing material

Radiation biology a branch of the biological sciences, which involves the study of the effects of ionizing radiation on living tissue

Radiation equivalent man (REM) The unit of the quantity, absorbed dose equivalent of any type of ionizing radiation that produces the same biologic effect as one rad of radiation

Radiation oncology commonly referred to as radiation therapy, which involves the use of ionizing radiation for the treatment of malignancy and some benign diseases

Radiographic film the recording medium which plays a critical role in production of diagnostic radiographs

Radiographic position a specific body part position, such as supine or prone; refers to the patient's physical position

Radiographic projection the path of the central ray

Radiographic tube the most important component of a radiographic unit, which creates the electrons used to produce the x-rays

Radiographic view the body part seen by the x-ray film or other recording medium, such as a fluoroscopic screen

Radiography the making of film records (radiographs) of internal structures of the body by passing x-rays or gamma rays through the body to act on specially sensitized film

Radiologic technologist an individual graduated from a nationally accredited education program in the radiologic sciences; registered with the ARRT or an equivalent national organization or holds a full-state license

Radiology information system (RIS) a computerized database used by radiology departments to store, manipulate, and distribute patient radiological data and imagery

Radiolucent any material that permits the penetration and passage of x-rays or other forms of radiation

Radiolysis an event in which a water molecule is ionized resulting in free ions capable of recombining with other free radicals to form new molecules

Radiosensitivity the measure of the response of a biological organism to radiation

Rapport a relationship marked by harmony, accord, or affinity

Recorded detail sharpness of the structural lines as recorded in the radiographic image

Rectifier an electrical device that allows the flow of electricity in one direction only

Recumbent a positioning terminology, refers to the body position lying down

Registration a procedure required to maintain an active status of the certification

Relative biological effectiveness (RBE) a measure of the biological effects of different types of radiations; the ratio of the effect of a standard radiation to a test radiation

Rem Roentgen equivalent man; the obsolete unit of dose equivalent

Remnant radiation also exit radiation or image-forming radiation, refers to radiation being responsible for the film darkening resulting in the latent image

Repeat examination a patient examination that is repeated due to inadequate patient preparation

Res ipsa loquitur "the thing speaks for itself," a situation where the injured person in no way contributed to her/his injury

Respiration the exchange of oxygen and carbon dioxide in the lungs

Rhenium a desirable filament material because of its high melting point

Rickets a condition in which osteomalacia occurs before the growth plate closes

Rickettsiae microscopic life forms found in tissues of fleas, lice, ticks, and other insects

Right anterior oblique a positioning terminology, refers to the body rotated with the right anterior portion closest to the film

Right posterior oblique a positioning terminology, refers to the body rotated with the right posterior portion closest to the film

Roentgen (R) the S.I. unit of exposure dose for x-rays or gamma rays; now known as Coulomb per kilogram

Rotor the moving part of a motor

Sagittal one of the three primary body planes; divides the body into right and left portions

Scatter radiation the secondary radiation produced as a result of interactions of the primary radiation beam with atoms

Scoliosis an abnormal or exaggerated lateral curvature of the vertebral spine

Screen film film used with intensifying screens that emit light during the x-ray exposure, thereby allowing a reduction in the x-ray exposure

Screen film contrast determined by the combination of screen-film phosphor type light sensitivities

Screening mammography procedure used for the detection of breast cancer and breast diseases

Secondary Protective Structural Shielding a protective barrier runs parallel to the primary beam and protects diagnostic radiology personnel from secondary (leakage and scattered) radiation

Sensitivity speck tiny particles of atomic silver and silver sulfide, these sensitized specks will react to the developer chemicals during film processing

Sensitometry study of how radiographic film responds to radiation exposure photographically and to processing conditions chemically

Sepsis bacterial infection of the blood

Shadow gonadal shielding a shielding procedure wherein the shields are suspended from the beam-limiting system

Sievert (Sv) the S.I. unit of dose equivalent; also expressed as one joule per kilogram;

Signs and symptoms key indicators of disease or injury

Silver halide crystals active ingredient of the radiographic film emulsion

Silver recovery a chemical or electrolytic process used to remove silver from radiographic fixer solution

Small focal spot the smaller filament in the focusing cup of the cathode assembly of the x-ray tube

Somatic effects effect of radiation on the human body other than the gonads; responsible for cancer and cataracts

Source-to-image receptor distance (SID) a factor that influences recorded detail; greater (increased) the SID, smaller the geometric blur, which leads to improved recorded detail

Speed the screen's ability to produce density with a given exposure to x-rays; there are three major speed categories of calcium-tungstate screens: medium speed, high speed, and fine detail (slow) speed

Sprain any trauma to a joint and its associated ligaments with resulting in pain, rapid swelling, limited function, and localized warmth over the area

Stator the stationary part of a motor

Statues laws; principles and rules that are enacted by legislative bodies, such as the Congress of the United States or state legislative bodies

Stenting procedure used to introduce a stent (a device or mold of a suitable material, used to hold a skin graft in place

Sthenic a body type that is the average or normal body shape and represents about 50% of the population; means strong and physically fit

Stochastic effects effects that occur in a random way and the severity of the effects are not dose dependent

Stress fracture fractures occuring most in the lower extremity resulting from the bending of the bone almost to the point of breakage due to repetitive trauma; the fracture is generally hairline crack

Subject contrast contrast resulting from the amount of radiation transmitted by a particular body part as a result of the differential absorption characteristics of the tissues and structures of the part

Subluxation a partial or incomplete dislocation

Substance a material that has definite and constant composition

Supine a positioning terminology, refers to the body lying on the back

Surface landmarks exterior landmarks that may be palpated to locate specific vertebral bodies

Surgical Asepsis procedures and techniques used to destroy microorganisms before they enter the body

Sympathy acknowledgment of another person's grief, hurt, or loss

Symptomatic patient a patient exhibiting signs of disease or illness

Synchronous timer an exposure-timing device that is controlled and driven by an electrical synchronous motor

System Internationale d'Unites (SI) The International System of Units which gives the internationally agreed metric and nonmetric units for weights and measures

Tachycardia increased heart rate

Tachypnea increased respiration rate

Target theory the theory which states that there are one or two critical targets for radiation damage in a cell

Teardrop fracture an avulsion fracture of one of the short bones, such as a vertebra, causing a tear-shaped disruption of bone tissue

Teleradiology procedure in which images may be electronically transmitted over distances to other health care facilities

Ten-day rule a guideline that states that pelvic or abdominal x-ray examinations of women of child-bearing age be done only in the first ten days following the onset of menstruation

Tendinitis the condition of inflammation of a tendon

Thermionic emission the production of electrons by the heating of the x-ray tube filament

Thermoluminescent dosimeter a personnel radiation monitoring device, which, when heated, produces light proportional to the radiation exposure

Thrombolysis Dissolution or destruction of a thrombus

Thrombus a clot of blood formed and lodged within a blood vessel

Time one of the exposure factors; the period when something occurs; measured in seconds or milliseconds

Torts Negligence, which may be unintentional, and gross negligence, which is intentional, are both referred to legally as torts

Transmission-based precautions a set of safeguards designed for patients documented or suspected to be infected with highly transmissible or epidemiologically important pathogens for which additional precautions beyond standard precautions are needed to interrupt transmission in hospital

Transverse one of the three primary body planes; horizontal or axial plane that is at right angles to the vertical axis of the body

Traumatic injuries injuries that result from impacts to the body

Triage medical screening of patients to determine their relative priority for treatment

Trigger finger a condition where a finger intermittently becomes locked in a bent position

Tube heat capacity the maximum heat capacity of an x-ray tube

Ultrasound an imaging technique that uses sound waves that are well above the frequency audible to humans or animals for diagnostic or therapeutic purposes

Universal precautions a set of procedural directives and guidelines published by the Centers for Disease Control and Prevention (CDC) to prevent parenteral, mucous membrane, and nonintact skin exposures of health care workers to bloodborne pathogens

Valence the number of electrons in the outermost shell of an atom; also called chemical combining characteristic

Vaporize an element turning into its vapor state

Variable kilovoltage technique an exposure or technique chart that is rarely, if ever, used today with modern equipment and is mentioned only for information and background

Vector an infected insect or animal that passes disease through a bite, e.g., ticks, fleas, lice

Velocity the rate of motion of an object; measured in meters per second

Viruses the smallest known organisms, which cannot survive outside a living organisms as it requires host cells for replication

Vital signs measures that let us know how a patient is doing on very basic levels of functioning—body temperature, pulse rate, blood pressure, and respiration rate

Volt the S.I. unit of potential difference

Voxel volume of pixels

Whiplash a term encompassing soft tissue neck injuries from a variety of causes

Wilhelm Conrad Röentgen discovered X rays in 1895

Window an opening provided in the x-ray tube housing to permit unrestricted exit for the useful x-ray photons from the glass envelope (see also Port)

Work the expenditure of energy

Workload (W) the radiation output weighted time during the week that the x-ray unit is actually delivering radiation

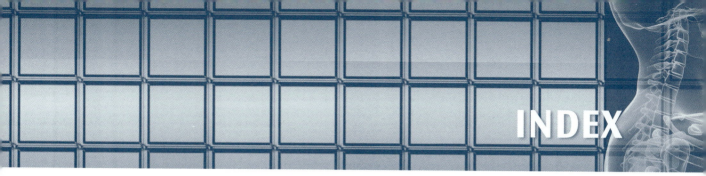

INDEX

Page numbers followed by "*f*" denote figure; those followed by "*t*" denote tables

A

Abdomen
    anatomy of, 356–357
    anterior-posterior projection of, 358*f*, 422, 422*f*
    computed tomography of, 429
    radiographs of, 208
    trauma of, 357
    x-ray examination of, 357–359, 358*f*
Absorbed dose, 459–460, 469
Absorbed dose equivalent, 470, 492*t*
Absorption, 459–460
Abuse
    child. *See* Child abuse
    diagnostic imaging of, 361–363
    fractures and, 363
    physical, 363
    reasonable suspicion or belief of, 362
    reporting of, 362
Accidents, 93–94
Acetic acid, 394
Acromegaly, 360
Acromioclavicular joint dislocation, 340
Active matrix array, 280
Actual focal spot, 170
Acute diseases, 290
Acute radiation syndrome, 475, 480–482
Acute respiratory distress syndrome, 311
ADA. *See* Americans with Disabilities Act
Added filtration, 499–500

Additive pathology, 292–295
Administrative regulations, 54
Adolescents, 216–217
Advocacy for patients, 32, 34
Aerial image, 247, 247*f*
Air bronchograms, 307, 312
Airborne pathogens, 83
Airborne transmission, 84*t*
Air-gap technique, 500
Air-space disease, 312, 318
ALARA, 294, 494, 510
Alpha 1-antitrypsin, 313
Alpha particles, 143, 144*t*
Alternating current, 162, 190
Aluminum, 262–263
Alzheimer's disease, 222–223
Ambulatory patients, 98
American College of Radiology, 293–294, 324, 325*f*, 509
American Registry of Radiologic Technologists
    certifications offered by, 4–5, 5*f*, 12–13, 17*t*, 449
    continuing education requirements, 18
    ethics standards of, 13, 15
    history of, 4, 12
    limited scope of practice, 15, 16*f*, 17*t*
    mission of, 4
    primary pathways of, 6*f*
    radiographic positions and projections, 213